FIRST AID FOR THE® ABSITE

Jennifer LaFemina, MD
Resident in Surgery
Department of Surgery
Massachusetts General Hospital
Boston, Massachusetts

R. Todd Lancaster, MD
Resident in Surgery
Department of Surgery
Massachusetts General Hospital
Boston, Massachusetts

Series Editor

Tao Le, MD
Assistant Clinical Professor
Chief, Section of Allergy and Clinical Immunology
Department of Medicine
University of Louisville
Louisville, Kentucky

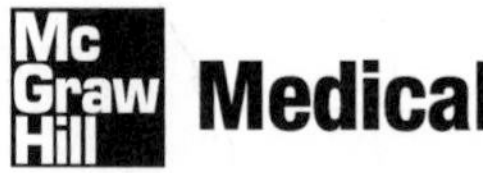

New York / Chicago / San Francisco / Lisbon / London / Madrid / Mexico City
Milan / New Delhi / San Juan / Seoul / Singapore / Sydney / Toronto

The McGraw-Hill Companies

First Aid for the® ABSITE

1 2 3 4 5 6 7 8 9 0 QPD/QPD 0 9 8

ISBN 978-0-07-154547-1
MHID 0-07-154547-6

NOTICE

Medicine is an ever-changing science. As new research and clinical experience broaden our knowledge, changes in treatment and drug therapy are required. The authors and the publisher of this work have checked with sources believed to be reliable in their efforts to provide information that is complete and generally in accord with the standards accepted at the time of publication. However, in view of the possibility of human error or changes in medical sciences, neither the authors nor the publisher nor any other party who has been involved in the preparation or publication of this work warrants that the information contained herein is in every respect accurate or complete, and they disclaim all responsibility for any errors or omissions or for the results obtained from use of the information contained in this work. Readers are encouraged to confirm the information contained herein with other sources. For example and in particular, readers are advised to check the product information sheet included in the package of each drug they plan to administer to be certain that the information contained in this work is accurate and that changes have not been made in the recommended dose or in the contraindications for administration. This recommendation is of particular importance in connection with new or infrequently used drugs.

This book was set in Electra LH by International Typesetting and Composition.
The editor was Catherine A. Johnson.
The production supervisor was Sherri Souffrance.
Project management was provided by Aparna Shukla, International Typesetting and Composition.
Quebecor World Dubuque was printer and binder.

This book is printed on acid-free paper.

Library of Congress Cataloging-in-Publication Data

LaFemina, Jennifer.
First aid for the ABSITE / Jennifer LaFemina, Robert Todd Lancaster.
p. ; cm.
Includes index.
ISBN-13: 978-0-07-154547-1 (pbk.)
ISBN-10: 0-07-154547-6 (pbk.)
1. Surgery—Examinations, questions, etc. I. Lancaster, Robert Todd. II. Title.
[DNLM: 1. Surgical Procedures, Operative—Examination Questions. 2. Surgical Procedures, Operative—Handbooks. 3. Clinical Medicine—Examination Questions. 4. Clinical Medicine—Handbooks. 5. Specialty Boards. WO 18.2 L162f 2009]
RD37.2.L34 2009
617.0076—dc22 2008008599

DEDICATION

To our contributors, for your time, dedication, and contribution of knowledge and insight into this project. Without you, this project would not have been possible.

To our mentors, for your guidance, wisdom, and knowledge. Your daily display of mastery of this craft drives us to excel.

To our families, loved ones, and friends, for your patience and support. Because, above all, you are the inspiration for everything we do.

CONTENTS

Color insert appears after page 112

AUTHORS

Janivette Alsina, MD, PhD
Resident in Surgery
Massachusetts General Hospital
Pancreas

Emily R. Christison-Lagay, MD
Resident in Surgery
Massachusetts General Hospital
Pediatric Surgery

Danielle Gottlieb, MS, MD, MPH
Resident in Surgery
Massachusetts General Hospital
Cardiac

Alex Bernard Haynes, MD, MPH
Resident in Surgery
Massachusetts General Hospital
Esophagus

Kaitlyn J. Kelly, MD
Resident in Surgery
St. Vincent's Hospital
Stomach

Jennifer LaFemina, MD
Resident in Surgery
Massachusetts General Hospital
Small Intestine/Surgical Principles

R. Todd Lancaster, MD
Resident in Surgery
Massachusetts General Hospital
Surgical Principles

Ugwuji N. Maduekwe, MD
Resident in Surgery
Massachusetts General Hospital
Breast

Miguel A. Medina III, MD
Resident in Surgery
Massachusetts General Hospital
Plastic and Reconstructive Surgery

Mark M. Melendez, MD, MBA
Resident in Surgery
Stony Brook University Medical Center
Skin and Soft Tissue/Surgical Subspecialties

Nicolas Melo, MD, MS
Resident in Surgery
Massachusetts General Hospital
Hernias/Colorectal

Andrew J. Meltzer, MD
Resident in Surgery
Massachusetts General Hospital
Perioperative Care/Vascular

Ellen C. Meltzer, MD
Fellow in Internal Medicine
Boston University Medical Center
Perioperative Care

Timothy M. Millington, MD
Resident in Surgery
Massachusetts General Hospital
Thoracic/Transplantation

Elizabeth A. Sailhamer, MD, MMSc
Resident in Surgery
Massachusetts General Hospital
Trauma, Burns, and Critical Care

Gregory R. Veillette, MD
Resident in Surgery
Massachusetts General Hospital
Endocrine

Yanghee Woo, MD
Resident in Surgery
New York-Presbyterian Hospital, Columbia University Medical Center
Liver, Biliary System, and Spleen

SENIOR REVIEWERS

Hasan B. Alam, MD
Associate Professor of Surgery
Harvard Medical School
Division of Trauma, Emergency Surgery, and Surgical Critical Care
Massachusetts General Hospital
Trauma, Burns, and Critical Care

William Gerald Austen Jr, MD
Assistant Professor of Surgery
Harvard Medical School
Chief, Division of Plastic and Reconstructive Surgery
Massachusetts General Hospital
Plastic and Reconstructive Surgery

James H. Balcom IV, MD
Department of Surgery
Divisions of General and Vascular Surgery
North Shore Medical Center
Vascular

Frederick Y. Chen, MD, PhD
Assistant Professor of Surgery
Harvard Medical School
Division of Cardiac Surgery
Brigham and Women's Hospital
Cardiac

Alexander B. Dagum MD, FRCSC, FACS
Associate Professor of Clinical Surgery and Orthopaedics
Chief, Division of Plastic and Reconstructive Surgery
Stony Brook University Medical Center
Surgical Subspecialties

Marc A. deMoya, MD
Instructor of Surgery
Harvard Medical School
Division of Trauma, Emergency Surgery, and Surgical Critical Care
Massachusetts General Hospital
Perioperative Care

Dean M. Donahue, MD
Assistant Professor of Surgery
Harvard Medical School
Division of Thoracic Surgery
Massachusetts General Hospital
Thoracic

Shawn P. Fagan, MD
Assistant in Surgery
Harvard Medical School
Division of Burns
Massachusetts General Hospital
Surgical Principles

Charles M. Ferguson, MD
Associate Professor of Surgery
Harvard Medical School
Division of General Surgery
Massachusetts General Hospital
Hernias

Cristina R. Ferrone, MD
Instructor in Surgery
Harvard Medical School
Division of General Surgery
Massachusetts General Hospital
Pancreas

Richard A. Hodin, MD
Professor of Surgery
Harvard Medical School
Division of General Surgery
Massachusetts General Hospital
Small Intestine

Dicken S. C. Ko, MD, FRCSC
Assistant Professor of Surgery
Harvard Medical School
Surgical Director, Renal Transplant Program
Massachusetts General Hospital
Transplantation

Michael Lanuti, MD
Assistant Professor of Surgery
Harvard Medical School
Division of Thoracic Surgery
Massachusetts General Hospital
Esophagus

Daniel P. Ryan, MD
Associate Professor of Surgery
Harvard Medical School
Division of Pediatric Surgery
Massachusetts General Hospital
Pediatric Surgery

Marc J. Shapiro, MS, MD, FACS, FCCM
Professor of Surgery and Anesthesiology
Chief, General Surgery, Trauma, Critical Care, and Burns
Stony Brook University Medical Center
Skin and Soft Tissue

Paul C. Shellito, MD
Assistant Professor of Surgery
Harvard Medical School
Associate Visiting Surgeon
Department of Surgery
Massachusetts General Hospital
Colorectal

Michelle C. Specht, MD
Instructor of Surgery
Harvard Medical School
Division of Surgical Oncology
Massachusetts General Hospital
Breast

Antonia E. Stephen, MD
Instructor in Surgery
Harvard Medical School
Division of Surgical Oncology
Massachusetts General Hospital
Endocrine

Vivian E. Strong, MD
Assistant Professor of Surgery
Weill Medical College of Cornell University
Department of Surgery
Memorial Sloan-Kettering Cancer Center
Stomach

Warren D. Widmann, MD
Associate Clinical Professor of Surgery
Columbia University Medical Center
Department of Surgery
New York-Presbyterian Hospital
Liver, Biliary System, and Spleen

PREFACE

The American Board of Surgery In-Training Examination (ABSITE) is administered each January to every general surgery resident in the United States. This exam is an opportunity for residents to demonstrate their mastery of various basic science and clinical management problems. It also serves as a standardized instrument by which department chairpersons and residency directors can evaluate the progress of their trainees and the efficacy of their educational curricula.

As nearly any general surgery resident can attest, the ABSITE also represents a source of great stress. While it is true that this examination is not intended to be the sole assessment of any resident's progress, great import is often placed on the test results for a variety of reasons. First, ABSITE results are known to be an accurate indicator of an individual's ability to pass the Qualifying Exam of the American Board of Surgery. Additionally, because many residents plan to seek fellowship training after completion of their formal general surgery training, they recognize that many fellowship directors use ABSITE scores as a device for comparison of residents from different programs. Accordingly, it is only logical that everyone sitting for this exam hopes to score within the highest percentile. Finally, the other certainty to which all general surgery residents can attest is that the rigors of a surgical residency afford little time for preparation for such an important examination.

With this first edition of *First Aid for the ABSITE* we hope to provide surgical residents with the most useful, high-yield, and up-to-date review of surgical material for their ABSITE preparation. From the outset, every editing and content decision for this book was made with the singular purpose of helping the reader achieve a higher score and excel on the ABSITE.

This new addition to the *First Aid* series represents a dedicated effort by a number of residents and faculty members in order to create a book that includes

- A concise, all-in-one review book of highly tested basic science and clinical science components of surgery.
- A comprehensive preparation book for both the Junior and Senior ABSITE examinations.
- Hundreds of high-yield key facts, mnemonics, figures, diagrams, and tables to highlight high-yield, highly tested information.
- Sample questions to reinforce highly tested material, in some cases beyond what is presented in the chapters.

We hope that you find *First Aid for the ABSITE* a necessary and invaluable adjunct to your ABSITE preparation and surgical curriculum. We invite you to share your thoughts and ideas about the book and to contribute suggestions for the next edition of *First Aid for the ABSITE*. Good luck on the ABSITE.

Boston	Jennifer LaFemina
Boston	R. Todd Lancaster
Louisville	Tao Le

ACKNOWLEDGMENTS

First Aid for the ABSITE represents a collaborative effort among residents and surgical faculty. We would like to acknowledge the dedication and contributions of these people in the creation of this book.

To reinforce the resident-to-resident nature of this book, we would like to thank a number of surgical residents who reviewed the content to ensure its accuracy and high-yield nature.

- Robert E. Boykin, MD (Harvard Combined Orthopaedic Program)
- Ross F. Goldberg, MD (St. Vincent's Hospital)
- Daniel J. Krochmal, MD (Mayo Clinic at Scottsdale)
- Alvin Kwok, MD (Brigham and Women's Hospital)
- Amy R. Riley, MD (Detroit Medical Center)
- Stacy K. Ugras, MD (New York-Presbyterian Hospital)

For constant support, guidance, and commitment to excellence, we thank our publisher, McGraw-Hill, and our senior editor, Catherine A. Johnson. For helping organize and coordinate the project, we thank Midge Haramis and, for her enthusiasm and encouragement, we thank Selina Bush.

Boston	Jennifer LaFemina
Boston	R. Todd Lancaster
Louisville	Tao Le

HOW TO CONTRIBUTE

To continue to produce future high-yield editions of *First Aid for the ABSITE*, we invite you to submit comments, suggestions, or corrections to material in this book, as well as

- Recommendations for additional high-yield and highly tested facts on both the Junior and Senior ABSITE examinations.
- New key facts, mnemonics, diagrams, or illustrations.
- Comments about low-yield facts that should be removed from future editions of this book.

For each submission that is incorporated into the next edition, you will receive a personal acknowledgment in the next edition.

The preferred way to submit recommendations, suggestions, and new ideas is via electronic mail. Please include your name, address, institutional affiliation, phone number, and email address. Send your submissions to

firstaidabsite@gmail.com

NOTE TO CONTRIBUTORS

All entries become property of the authors and are subject to review and editing by the authors. In the event that similar or duplicate entries are submitted, only the first entry received will be used. With recommendations about high-yield facts, please provide appropriate references.

CHAPTER 1

Guide to the ABSITE

R. Todd Lancaster, MD
Jennifer LaFemina, MD

▶ INTRODUCTION TO THE ABSITE

The American Board of Surgery In-Training Examination (ABSITE) is an exam created and administered by the American Board of Surgery (ABS) to assess surgical residents' knowledge about the fundamentals of surgically-relevant basic science and clinical problems. The exam may be used by surgical residency programs as an evaluation tool to assess resident performance and understanding of general surgical principles.

▶ ABSITE—THE BASICS

What Is the Format of the ABSITE?

The ABSITE is divided into 225 multiple choice questions, incorporating five clinical content categories:

- Body as a whole
- Gastrointestinal
- Cardiovascular and respiratory
- Genitourinary, head and neck, skin, musculoskeletal, nervous system
- Endocrine, hematologic and lymphatic systems, breast

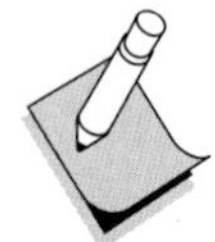

The ABSITE is divided into Junior and Senior exams. Both versions have 225 multiple choice questions.

As of 2007, the ABSITE is administered in two forms: a Junior and a Senior exam. The percentage of questions representing each of the categories is dependent on the version of the exam.

What Is the Difference Between the Junior and Senior ABSITE Examinations?

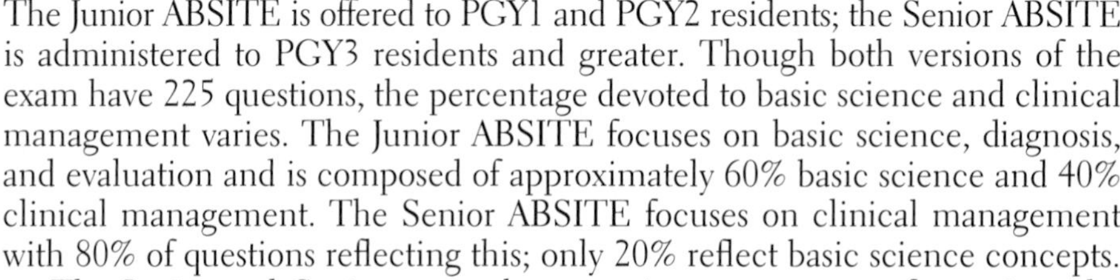

The Junior ABSITE is offered to PGY1 and PGY2 residents; the Senior ABSITE is administered to PGY3 residents and greater. Though both versions of the exam have 225 questions, the percentage devoted to basic science and clinical management varies. The Junior ABSITE focuses on basic science, diagnosis, and evaluation and is composed of approximately 60% basic science and 40% clinical management. The Senior ABSITE focuses on clinical management with 80% of questions reflecting this; only 20% reflect basic science concepts.

The majority of Junior ABSITE questions cover basic science. The majority of Senior ABSITE questions focus on clinical management.

The Junior and Senior exams have varying percentages of questions devoted to the five clinical content categories: the Junior ABSITE has a significant number of questions related to the "body as a whole" category and the Senior exam has a more equal distribution of the five clinical content categories.

Do I Need to Register for the Examination?

If you are taking the exam at your home institution, there is no additional registration required.

When and Where Is the ABSITE conducted?

The ABSITE is administered every January.

The ABSITE is conducted annually at the end of January. Exams are administered by each residency program. If you are away from your home institution at the time of the exam (ie, doing research at an outside institution), you may be able to coordinate with your residency program to complete the test at another institution.

How Is the ABSITE Scored?

Examination scores are available to program directors at the end of March. The scores are distributed to the program directors, and you may receive your Report of Performance from your program director.

Your Report of Performance summarizes the percent of questions answered correctly in both clinical management and basic science. It also summarizes the percentage of questions answered correctly in each of the five clinical content categories. You will also receive a percentile score, which reflects your performance compared to residents of your same PGY level.

Your Report of Performance includes key words—divided into the five clinical content categories and into basic and clinical management—describing the tested content that you answered incorrectly.

The ABSITE is graded by the percentage of questions you answered correctly. Your performance is also compared to residents in your same PGY level.

Is the ABSITE Required by the ABS for Certification?

No. The ABS does not require the ABSITE to obtain board certification in surgery.

What Is the Importance of the ABSITE?

The ABSITE fulfills a number of functions.

- Expands the basic science and clinical general surgery knowledge base of surgical residents.
- Allows residency programs to evaluate and assess resident performance and knowledge of general surgical concepts.
- Predicts a resident's ability to pass the Qualifying Examination of the ABS.

There is a high correlation between ABSITE performance and Qualifying Exam performance (ABS report to AAST, 2007; www.aast.org).

How to Best Utilize *First Aid for the ABSITE*?

First Aid for the ABSITE is designed to maximize your success on both the Junior and Senior ABSITE exams. This book presents high-yield, highly tested, up-to-date facts in an attempt to highlight pertinent points and increase your score. As both exams have basic science and clinical management sections, *we recommend reviewing the entire book to maximize success*. Residents taking the Junior ABSITE should pay particular attention to the basic science components; residents taking the Senior ABSITE should focus on the clinical management sections.

CHAPTER 2

Surgical Principles

R. Todd Lancaster, MD
Jennifer LaFemina, MD
Reviewed by Shawn P. Fagan, MD

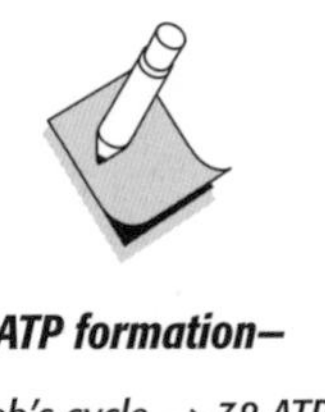

ATP formation–

Kreb's cycle → 38 ATP

Anaerobic cycle → 2 ATP

Cell and Molecular Biology

Cell Structures

Cell structures and functions are summarized in Table 2-1.

Nucleic Acid to Protein

DNA is a double-stranded double helix with purine (ie, adenine, guanine) and pyrimidine (ie, cytosine, thymine) nitrogen-containing bases. After the addition of sugar moieties and phosphates, adenosine forms hydrogen bonds with thymidine while guanosine pairs with cytidine. RNA is similar except that it is single-stranded, has a ribose rather than 2'-deoxyribose sugar moiety, and has uracil in place of thymine.

During transcription, RNA polymerase creates a complementary **messenger RNA** (mRNA) from DNA. Posttranscriptional modification (eg, splicing,

TABLE 2-1. Cellular Structures and Functions

Cellular Structures	Structures and Functions
Cell membrane	Lipid bilayer with embedded proteins (60% protein, 40% lipid) involved in transport (eg, pumps, channels, carriers), enzyme reactions, cell adhesion, signaling.
Nucleus	**Largest organelle.** Nuclear membrane limits macromolecule transport. Nuclear pores allow for transport to cytoplasm. Houses nuclear genome and regulates gene expression.
Mitochondria	Site of ATP production via **oxidative phosphorylation**. Has independent, circular, double-stranded DNA.
Cytoskeleton	Involved in structural support, cell division, cytokinesis, intracellular trafficking. Includes microfilaments (smallest, made of **actin**, involved in cytokinesis and cell shape), intermediate filaments (stronger and longer than microfilaments, provide mechanical support), microtubules (largest, made of **tubulin**, involved in MTOC, intracellular trafficking).
Centrosome	Anchors microtubules during mitotic spindle formation to allow cell division and cell cycle progression.
Golgi apparatus	Involved in protein processing and transport.
Endoplasmic reticulum (ER)	Rough ER harbors ribosomes and is involved in protein synthesis and folding. Smooth ER lacks ribosomes and is involved in detoxification and steroid synthesis.
Ribosome	Composed of ribosomal RNA and protein, found on the rough ER or in the cytoplasm. Involved in **translation** of mRNA into protein.
Telomere	$(TTAGGG)_n$ repeat located on chromosome ends to protect against degradation and end-to-end fusion. Plays a role in **senescence** and neoplasia.
Lysosome	Contains an acidic environment with digestive enzymes to degrade viruses, bacteria, nonfunctional organelles.

5′-capping, 3′-polyadenylation) creates mature mRNA, which is translated at the ribosome into a polypeptide. Posttranslational modification then changes the structure, chemical nature, or functional groups of the original protein.

Nitrogen bases are converted to nucleosides and nucleotides by the addition of sugar moieties and phosphates. Purines are named with "-osine" (adenosine, guanosine) and pyrimidines are named with "-idine" (cytidine, thymidine).

Cell Cycle

Divided into four phases: M, G_1, S, and G_2. M phase involves mitosis. G_1 follows M phase and involves cell growth and protein synthesis. The cell's DNA content doubles during synthesis (S) phase. G_2 involves cell growth and preparation (eg, microtubule creation) for mitosis. Complexes of cyclins and cyclin-dependent kinases drive cell cycle progression via phosphorylations. Inhibitors of cell cycle progression are abundant (see Figure 2-1). Two main regulators include **p53** and **pRB**.

> Pyrimidine nucleotide bases—**PYR**amids **CUT**: **PYR**imidines → **C**ytosine, **U**racil, **T**hymine

Mitosis and Meiosis

Mitosis results in two identical sister cells. During meiosis a diploid cell divides into four haploid germ cells, allowing for sexual reproduction (see Table 2-2).

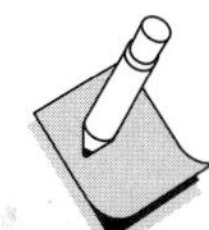

Posttranslational modification of preproinsulin (ie, folding, removal of the C-peptide, and creation of disulfide bonds) results in the active insulin molecule.

↑ Proinsulin, ↑ C-peptide, ↑ Insulin → Insulinoma.

↑ Insulin, ↔/↓ C-peptide → Factitious hyperinsulinemia (eg, injection).

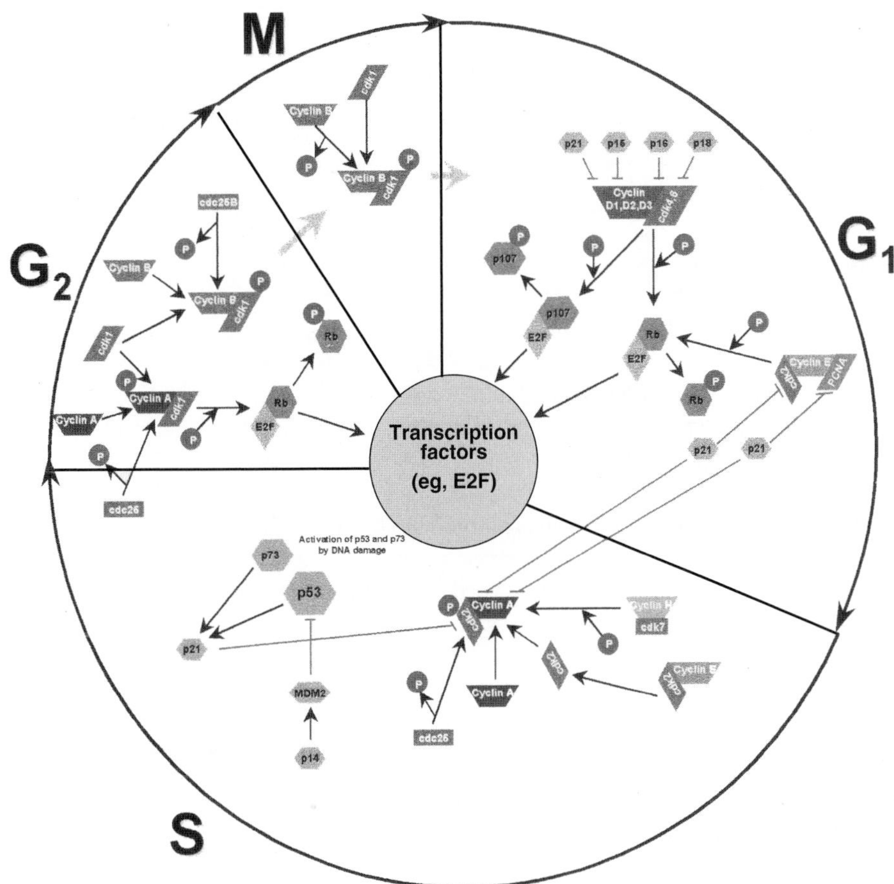

FIGURE 2-1. Cell cycle.

(Reproduced, with permission, from Lichtman MA, et al. *Williams Hematology*, 7th ed. New York: McGraw-Hill, 2006:160.)

G_1, S, and G_2 make up interphase.

TABLE 2-2. Phases of Mitosis and Meiosis

Phase	Description
Mitosis	
Prophase	Chromatin condenses to form chromosomes, identical centrosomes migrate to opposite poles, spindle begins to form, nuclear membrane disintegrates.
Metaphase	Chromosomes are maximally condensed and aligned at equator.
Anaphase	Sister chromatids separate to opposite poles.
Telophase	Chromosomes are released from spindle and decondense. Nuclear membrane begins to re-form to form new nucleus.
Cytokinesis	Division of cell cytoplasm to create new identical daughter cell.
Meiosis I & II	
Prophase I	Chromatin condenses to form chromosomes, spindle begins to form, nuclear membrane disintegrates. **Coupling of homologous chromosomes** creates four stranded tetrad. **Recombination** may occur.
Metaphase I	Tetrads align at equator and attach to spindle.
Anaphase I	Pairs of homologous chromatids separate to opposite poles.
Telophase I	Homologous pairs are released from spindle. Nuclear membrane begins to reconstitute to make new nucleus.
Cytokinesis I	Division of cytoplasm results in two cells, each with one copy of the chromosome.
Prophase II	Similar to prophase I, except tetrad does not form.
Metaphase II	Chromosomes align at equator and attach to spindle.
Anaphase II	Chromatids separate to opposite poles.
Telophase II	Chromatids are released from spindle. Nuclear membrane begins to re-form to make new nucleus.
Cytokinesis II	Division of cytoplasm results in four cells, each with 1/2 of the daughter cell's genetic material.

Apoptosis

Programmed cell death through biochemical events → characteristic morphologic changes: Cell shrinkage, chromatin condensation, karyorrhexis, blebbing of plasma membrane, and formation of vesicular apoptotic bodies. Critical in suppression of tumor formation, normal development, and removal of damaged cells. Involves multiple signals, including **tumor necrosis factor (TNF)** and **caspase**.

Proto-oncogenes and Tumor Suppressor Genes

Proto-oncogenes and tumor suppressor genes (TSGs) are **normal** genes that have the potential to cause malignancy when mutated. Oncogenes arise

TABLE 2-3. Commonly Mutated Proto-oncogenes

PROTO-ONCOGENE	CHROMOSOME	TUMOR TYPE OR SYNDROME
K-ras	12p	Soft-tissue sarcomas, pancreatic cancer (90%), biliary cancers
RET	10q	Multiple endocrine neoplasia-2 (MEN-2), medullary thyroid cancer
c-myc	8q	Breast, colon, cervical, small cell lung carcinomas
HER2/neu	17q	Breast (30%), ovarian, lung, gastric, oral cancers

HER2 = human epidermal growth factor receptor-2

through **gain of function** mutations of proto-oncogenes that code for growth factors, growth factor receptors, signal transduction molecules, or nuclear transcription factors (see Table 2-3). Mutations in **one of two copies of the proto-oncogene** results in persistent autostimulation and uncontrolled cell proliferation.

TSGs in the native state function as negative regulators of the cell cycle, but **loss-of-function** mutations lead to uncontrolled cell proliferation (see Table 2-4). Unlike proto-oncogenes, TSGs require **mutations in both copies** of the gene to result in deregulation.

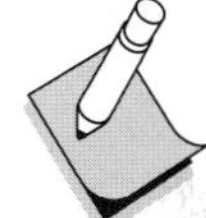

High-yield cancer markers–

Carbohydrate antigen 19-9 (CA-19-9): Pancreatic cancer
Carcinoembryonic antigen (CEA): Colorectal cancer
Cancer antigen 125 (CA-125): Ovarian cancer
Prostate-specific antigen (PSA): Prostate cancer
α-Fetoprotein (AFP): Hepatocellular cancer (only + in 60% of tumors < 2 cm)
Human choriogonadotropin (hCG): Nonseminomatous testicular cancer
Tyrosinase: Melanoma
HER2/neu: Breast cancer

TABLE 2-4. Commonly Mutated Tumor Suppressor Genes

TSG	CHROMOSOME	TUMOR TYPE/SYNDROME
RB1	13q	Retinoblastoma, osteosarcoma
P53	17p	Sarcoma, breast cancer, **Li-Fraumeni** syndrome
BRCA1	17q	Familial breast cancer, **ovarian** cancer.
BRCA2	13q	Familial breast (**male**/female), pancreatic, prostate cancers
STK11	19p	Peutz–Jeghers syndrome
MENIN	11q	Multiple endocrine neoplasia-1 (MEN-1); not MEN-2
CDKN2	9p	Familial atypical multiple mole melanoma syndrome, pancreatic cancer
PTEN	10q	Cowden's syndrome (hamartomas)
WT1	11p	Wilms' tumor
VHL	3p	von Hippel-Lindau (renal cell carcinoma, pheochromocytoma, retinal angioma)
APC	5q	Familial adenomatous polyposis

SURGICAL PRINCIPLES

Immune System

Humoral and Cellular Immunity

The immune system is divided into 1° and 2° lymphoid tissues. B and T lymphocytes are **produced in the 1° lymphoid tissues** (eg, bone marrow, thymus). Lymphocytes interact with antigen presenting cells to **initiate an immune response** in the 2° lymphoid tissues.

B cells produce antibodies and are the cornerstone of **humoral immunity**. When B cells recognize a nonself antigen via the IgM receptor, they differentiate into **plasma cells**, which secrete antibodies.

- IgM: First antibody produced.
- IgG, IgM: Activate complement cascade.
- IgG: Crosses the placenta.
- IgA: Crosses mucosal barriers and present in secretions.
- IgE: Binds to mast cell involved in hypersensitivity reactions.

> Acute Phase Reactants—
> **A**cute **P**hase **H**elps **F**ight **C**omplicated **D**isease:
> α-1 **A**ntitrypsin
> **P**realbumin
> **H**aptoglobin/**H**eat shock protein
> **F**ibronectin/**F**erritin
> **C**-reactive protein
> **D**-dimer

T cells mediate **cellular immunity**. These cells mature in the thymus, where tolerance to self is assured. **MHC I are on all nucleated cells** and activate CD8 cells; **MHC II are on monocytes and B cells** and activate CD4 cells. The three T cell classes are

- **Helper T cells**: Carry CD4 on surface. Synthesize growth factors, which lead to proliferation of all T cells.
- **Cytotoxic T cells**: CD8 on surface. Kill target cells via osmotic lysis or induction of apoptosis.
- **Suppressor T cells**: CD8 on surface. Modulate antibody formation and cellular immunity.

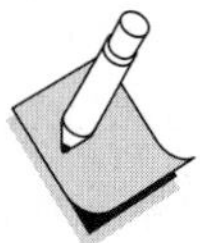

Acute phase reactants ↑ with inflammation. Albumin ↓ with inflammation.

Complement System

Collection of proteins that provides **innate** (nonspecific) immune defense. Activated via the "classical" pathway (eg, opsonin [IgG, IgM] binding) or the "alternative" pathway (eg, bacteremia, endotoxin, activating surfaces [bypass pump circuitry]). The pathways converge as C3 is cleaved; resultant C3b attaches to the antigen surface. The **membrane attack complex** (C5-C9) is then recruited to disrupt membrane integrity, leading to lysis. In the normal host, this system is regulated by another protein, **C1 inhibitor**.

NK cells (non-T, non-B lymphocytes) are another component of the **innate** immune system. NK cells lack antigen specific receptors and are important for early immune defense (ie, before a specific immune response is mounted) and, with cytotoxic T cells, tumor cell response.

*Platelet COX is **irreversibly** inhibited by aspirin and **reversibly** inhibited by NSAIDs. COX-2 inhibitors do not inhibit platelet COX. Other antiplatelet agents (eg, clopidogrel) do not affect the COX pathway but function by blocking platelets' ADP receptors.*

Hypersensitivity Reactions

Classified according to the immunologic mechanism involved (see Table 2-5).

Inflammation

Inflammatory responses are critical to host defense and tissue repair. **Acute inflammation** is marked by accumulation of leukocytes, local ↓ in BP, and ↑ in vascular permeability. **Chronic inflammation** is persistent and is marked by fibroblast proliferation and capillary growth.

Leukocyte chemotaxis is signaled by bacterial peptides, complement byproducts (C5a), platelet activating factor, and various cytokines. Two critical cytokines are **TNF-α** and **IL-1α**. Primary functions include initiation of the

TABLE 2-5. Hypersensitivity Reactions

Type	Mediator	Description	Examples
Type I	IgE-mediated	Cross-linking of IgE receptors on mast cells → activation, degranulation → vasodilation, secretory stimulation, vascular permeability, inflammation.	Atopy (allergic rhinitis, hay fever), anaphylaxis
Type II	Antibody-mediated	IgG or IgM binds to antigen on a cell surface, activating the complement cascade.	Immune-mediated hemolysis (Rh factor)
Type III	Immune complex–mediated	Rather than binding to a cell-surface antigen, IgG and IgM form circulating immune complexes. Complexes may deposit in tissues or vascular endothelium → immune response (eg, complement, PMNs, phagocytosis).	Serum sickness or Arthus reaction (localized cutaneous inflammation)
Type IV (Delayed)	Cell-mediated	Activated T cells accumulate in an antigen rich environment. Usually occurs 24–48 hrs after exposure.	Contact dermatitis, hypersensitivity pneumonitis

Low affinity adhesion (rolling)–
L-selectin: Continually expressed by Leukocytes
E-selectin: Expressed by Endothelial cells in response to TNF-α or IL-1
P-selectin: Expressed by Platelets and endothelial cells in response to histamine or thrombin

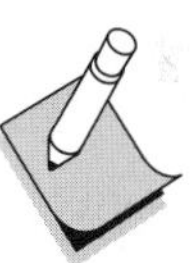

High affinity adhesion (transmigration)–
Ig superfamily: Expressed by endothelium. Involved in cell recognition, binding, firm adhesion, diapedesis
Integrins: Expressed by PMNs. Involved in firm cell-ECM adhesion, cell-ECM signal transduction, cell migration

acute phase response (eg, fever, shock, acute phase reactants), activation of endothelial cells (eg, leukocyte recruitment and adherence), and activation of fibroblasts (eg, collagen synthesis).

Prostaglandin and leukotrienes are chemoattractants and inflammatory mediators derived from the cell membrane stores of the lipid, **arachidonic acid**.

- **Cyclooxygenase** (COX) activation → prostaglandin → vasodilation, vasoconstriction, ↑ vascular permeability, platelet aggregation.
- **Lipoxygenase** activation → leukotriene synthesis → chemotaxis, degranulation, ↑ vascular permeability.

Cell adhesion molecules (CAM) are integral to leukocyte recruitment and activation (see Table 2-6).

A day in the life of CAMs–
Leukocyte rolling on vessel wall → Selectin.
Leukocyte stops rolling and adheres to endothelial wall → Integrin.
Leukocyte migrates into subendothelial space via diapedesis → PECAM1.

Hematologic System

Coagulation

Vascular injury involves a breach in a vessel's endothelial layer. Primary hemostasis involves **endothelium-initiated** vascular constriction and formation of **platelet plug** by collagen and von Willebrand factor (vWF). Platelets then release arachidonic acid, which is converted to **thromboxane A2** (TXA_2) by COX. TXA_2 stimulates further vasoconstriction and platelet aggregation. **Platelets also release ADP, Ca^{2+}, serotonin, and α-granules**, which change the membrane to form a surface for Ca^{2+} and other clotting factors, which then combine and form enzymatically active complexes.

The **coagulation cascade** involves intrinsic and extrinsic pathways (see Figure 2-2). The pathways converge as Factor X is activated to Factor Xa.

TABLE 2-6. Cell Adhesion Molecules

TYPES	DESCRIPTION
Cadherins	**Ca^{2+}-dependent** transmembrane proteins involved in cell adhesion via cytoskeletal interactions. Epithelial **E-cadherin** binds **β-catenin**.
Selectins	**Ca^{2+}-dependent** proteins with carbohydrate-binding domains that resemble **lectin** and allow for leukocyte "**rolling**" (necessary first step of inflammation). Includes **L**-selectin (on **l**eukocytes; acts as a "homing device"), **E**-selectin (on **e**ndothelial cells; involved in immediate inflammatory response/leukocyte recruitment), **P**-selectin (on **p**latelets and endothelial cells; similar function as E-selectin).
Integrins	Often activated after selectins. Involved in **firm cellular adherence** to extracellular matrix (ECM), cell-ECM signal transmission (growth, death, differentiation, division), cell migration.
Ig superfamily	**Ca^{2+}-independent** proteins with Ig-like domain that binds specific ligands. Involved in cell recognition, binding, firm adhesion, diapedesis. Includes ICAMs, VCAMs, PECAM1, NCAM.

SURGICAL PRINCIPLES

> Thromboxanes and prostacyclins **TAP** the **PIE:**
> **T**hromboxane causes vasoconstriction and platelet **A**ggregation; derived from **P**latelets.
> **P**rostacyclin causes vasodilation and **I**nhibits platelet aggregation; derived from **E**ndothelial cells.

Factors Xa and Va require the addition of Ca^{2+} and form a highly active enzymatic complex (prothrombinase) that converts prothrombin to thrombin. Thrombin then cleaves fibrinogen into fibrin monomers and activates Factor XIII to XIIIa. As fibrin monomers polymerize, additional cross-links are created by XIIIa to form a stable clot.

INTRINSIC pathway → All necessary components for clot formation are intrinsic to the circulating plasma. EXTRINSIC pathway → Requires endothelial disruption and exposed tissue factor (thromboplastin) for activation.

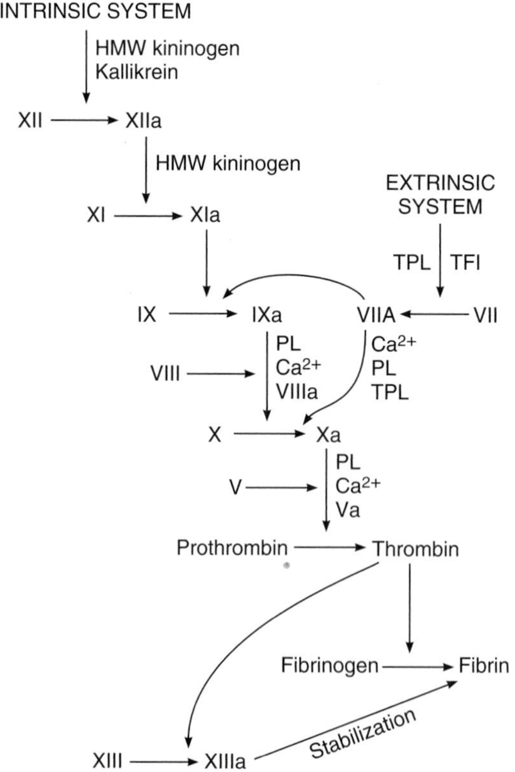

FIGURE 2-2. Coagulation cascade.

(Reproduced, with permission, from Ganong WF. *Review of Medical Physiology*, 22nd ed. New York: McGraw-Hill, 2005:542.)

The **extrinsic** pathway is of paramount importance for surgical procedures. Most factors are **liver-derived serine proteases**. However, Factor XIII is released by platelets, and Factor VIII is made by endothelial cells. Factor XII is activated by cardiopulmonary bypass. Factor VII has the shortest half-life ($t_{1/2}$ = 2-6 hours).

Extrinsic pathway—**WEPT**:
Extrinsic pathway → **PT**

Heparin and low molecular weight heparin (LMWH) augment the antithrombotic activity of ATIII.

ANTICOAGULATION AND FIBRINOLYSIS

Anticoagulation and fibrinolysis balance the coagulation cascade. Anticoagulation system inhibits coagulation via:

- **Antithrombin III** (ATIII): Circulating serine protease inhibitor produced by the **liver**. Binds and inhibits activity of Factors II (thrombin), IX, X, XI, and XII to prevent thrombosis. Augmented by heparin.
- **Protein C**: Circulating protein activated by the thrombin-thrombomodulin complex on the (intact) endothelial surface. With protein S, it cleaves Factors Va and VIIIa to halt the coagulation cascade.
- **Protein S:** Cofactor for activity of protein C.

Activated protein C (APC; recombinant) and its uses are discussed in Chapter 18.

The fibrinolysis-thrombolytic pathway initiates as circulating plasminogen is cleaved by either thrombin or medications (eg, tPA) to form active plasmin. Plasmin then cleaves organized fibrin clots and inactivates thrombin. Inhibitors of the fibrinolysis pathway include **ε-aminocaproic acid** and **aprotinin**.

BLEEDING DISORDERS

Due to disruption in platelet number or function or an inability to form a fibrin clot (see Table 2-7).

__Fondaparinux__ is a synthetic molecule that specifically inhibits Factor Xa. Unlike heparin, does not require monitoring.

- **Disseminated intravascular coagulation (DIC):** Widespread stimulation of thrombosis that ultimately results in hemorrhage. Thrombin stimulates platelet aggregation → extensive thrombosis. Also activates plasminogen

TABLE 2-7. Bleeding Disorders and Associated Lab Values

DISORDER	RELEVANT LABORATORY FINDINGS
DIC	↓ Fibrinogen, ↑ fibrin split products, ↓ platelets, ↑ PT, ↑ PTT, fragmented red blood cells on peripheral smear.
vWD	Nl platelet number and morphology, ↑ BT (+/– aspirin challenge), ↑ PTT, ↓ ristocetin activity (types I and IIb).
Hemophilia A and B	↓ PTT, ↓ factor levels on specific factor assays (VIII or IX), **mixing tests** result in nl **PTT.**
Glanzmann Thrombasthenia	Nl platelet number and morphology, ↑ BT, **no aggregation** in response to ADP, collagen, or thrombin.
Bernard–Soulier	↓ Platelets, large platelets on peripheral smear, ↑ BT, **no aggregation** in ristocetin assay.
ITP	↓ Platelets, nl PT/PTT/BT, nl bone marrow, may see enlarged (immature) platelets on peripheral smear.
TTP	↓ Platelets, ↓ RBC, ↑↑ **LDH**, fragmented RBC on peripheral smear, (–) Coombs test.
Uremia	↑ BUN/Creatinine, nl platelet count.

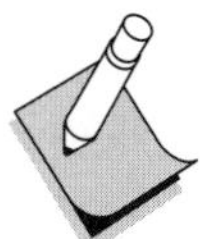

*ε-**Aminocaproic acid** blocks activation of plasminogen to plasmin. **Aprotinin** is a serine protease that also inhibits plasmin and has anti-inflammatory effects. Consider after cardiac bypass surgery for postoperative bleeding or for tPA overdose.*

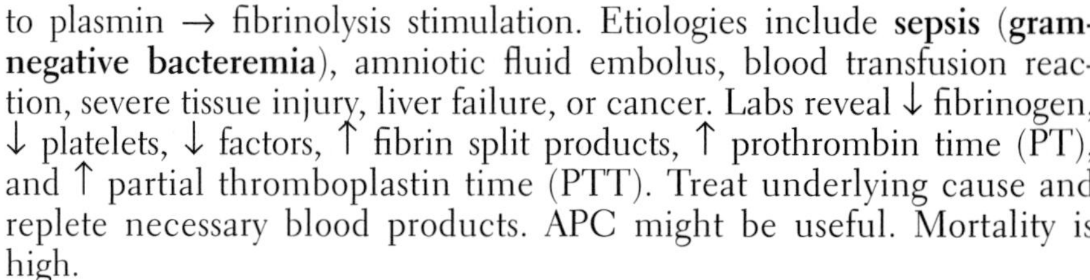

to plasmin → fibrinolysis stimulation. Etiologies include **sepsis** (**gram-negative bacteremia**), amniotic fluid embolus, blood transfusion reaction, severe tissue injury, liver failure, or cancer. Labs reveal ↓ fibrinogen, ↓ platelets, ↓ factors, ↑ fibrin split products, ↑ prothrombin time (PT), and ↑ partial thromboplastin time (PTT). Treat underlying cause and replete necessary blood products. APC might be useful. Mortality is high.

- **von Willebrand disease's (vWD): Most common congenital bleeding disorder**, usually inherited in autosomal dominant fashion. Involves a deficiency or functional defect of vWF. vWF is endothelial-derived and normally binds platelets (via **glycoprotein Ib**) to collagen to cause platelet adherence at bleeding site. Suspect vWD in patients with frequent nosebleeds, extensive bruising, or significant blood loss during menstrual period, childbirth, or surgical procedures. Labs might reveal ↑ **bleeding time** (BT), ↓ **Factor VIII,** ↑ PTT, and ↓ **ristocetin cofactor activity**.
  - Type I: Most common form (80%). **Quantitative** ↓ in vWF levels. Treat with **DDAVP**.
  - Type IIa: **Qualitative** vWF deficiency with abnormally small vWF multimers (large multimers are required for platelet adhesion).
  - Type IIb: **Qualitative** vWF deficiency due to rapid clearance of the large multimers. **Avoid DDAVP**. Treat with **cryoprecipitate**.
  - Type III: Exceedingly rare and most severe form with near absence of vWF. **Autosomal recessive**. Treat with cryoprecipitate.
- **Hemophilia**: Hemophilia A (Factor VIII deficiency; **most common form**) and hemophilia B (Factor IX deficiency; Christmas disease) are usually due to low levels of specified protein. Primarily affects men (**X-linked recessive**). Signs include spontaneous **hemarthroses**. Labs reveal ↑ PTT and normal BT. Preoperative management includes repletion of deficient factors: administer **Factor VIII to normal level** and **Factor IX to 50% of normal** prior to major procedures.
- **Inherited platelet disorders**: **Glanzmann thrombasthenia** is an autosomal recessive disorder marked by the absence of glycoprotein IIb-IIIa receptors (fibrinogen receptor), preventing platelet-fibrinogen adhesion. Labs reveal ↑ BT. **Bernard–Soulier syndrome** is an autosomal recessive abnormality of the glycoprotein Ib (vWF receptor)-Factor V-Factor IX complex, resulting in abnormal platelet adhesion. Treatment for both includes platelet transfusion.
- **Acquired platelet disorders**:
  - Idiopathic thrombocytopenic purpura (ITP): Caused by IgG, which binds to platelet surface and results in platelet sequestration and destruction. Signs can include petechiae and bleeding gums. Rule out initiating causes (eg, HIV, hepatitis C virus [HCV], drug reaction, systemic lupus erythematosus). Initial treatment includes steroids and IVIG. Platelet transfusions are reserved for severe cases after other therapies have failed. Most patients ultimately require **splenectomy**.
  - Thrombotic thrombocytopenic purpura (TTP): Caused by an inability to degrade large vWF multimers → platelet aggregation → microangiopathic hemolysis. May be idiopathic or induced by a specific cause (eg, medications [quinine], cancer, HIV). Signs include the pentad of **thrombocytopenia, anemia, altered mental status, renal failure, and fever**. First line treatment is large volume plasmapheresis.
  - Uremia: Results in platelet dysfunction and possibly severe bleeding. Treat with dialysis or DDAVP, if needed.
  - Antiplatelet therapy: Treatment with glycoprotein IIB-IIIa inhibitors or ADP receptor blockers ↑ BT. Drug effects persist 5-10 days.

vWF binds Factor VIII and prevents its degradation. Severe vWD can cause a coagulation disorder that is similar to hemophilia A.

Hypercoagulable Disorders

Hypercoagulable diseases include

- **Factor V Leiden: Most common inherited hypercoagulable disorder.** Caused by autosomal dominant genetic mutation resulting in Factor Va **resistance to APC inactivation**. Associated with **spontaneous arterial or venous thrombosis** and **pregnancy loss**. Confirm by identifying Factor V mutation. Treat with warfarin if other hypercoagulability risk factors are present.
- **ATIII deficiency:** Associated with more severe thrombosis than Factor V Leiden. If mutation affects heparin binding site (rather than active site), there is no ↑ risk for spontaneous clot, but there is an attenuated response to heparin. Treat with fresh frozen plasma (FFP, which contains ATIII), followed by heparin and warfarin.
- **Protein C or protein S deficiency:** Usually autosomal dominant. Deficiency of either vitamin K-dependent protein results in inability to inactivate Factors Va or VIIIa. Diagnose with protein activity assays, which use snake venom to activate proteins C and S. Treat with heparin, followed by warfarin.
- **Lupus anticoagulant:** Characterized by autoantibodies against phospholipid component of the PTT assay, yielding ↑ **PTT**. Associated with **thrombosis rather than bleeding**. **PTT will not correct after a plasma mixing test**. Confirm with ↑ **Russell viper venom time**. Can be associated with + RPR and anticardiolipin levels. If needed, treat with warfarin or heparin (difficult to monitor due to PTT anomaly).

Heparin-Induced Thrombocytopenia (HIT) Alternatives—Direct Thrombin Inhibitors:

Lepirudin: Cleared by kidney

Argatroban: Cleared by liver

Dose according to PTT levels as INR is not reliable.

Warfarin inhibits the synthesis of vitamin K–dependent proteins (Factors II, VII, IX, X, and proteins C and S) resulting in ↑ PT. FFP and vitamin K may reverse supratherapeutic levels.

A 64-year-old man presents to the emergency department with swelling and pain in his left leg. Questioning reveals that he underwent femoral angioplasty 14 days earlier. You are appropriately concerned about deep vein thrombosis (DVT) and start therapy with a direct thrombin inhibitor. Why? Your choice of anticoagulant is appropriate because the patient may have a unique presentation of HIT. Delayed-onset HIT can occur after heparin has been discontinued and even after minimal heparin exposure. Do not give heparin but send CBC (for platelet count) and HIT antibody test to confirm diagnosis.

Heparin-Induced Thrombocytopenia

Most common drug-induced thrombocytopenia. Symptoms usually develop 4-14 days after initiation of heparin **(risk is lower with LMWH).** Type I is associated with a transient, asymptomatic ↓ in platelets that is rarely < 100,000 platelets/μL; platelet count normalizes after heparin discontinuation. Type II is mediated by **IgG** antibodies against **platelet factor 4** (**PF4**) → platelet degranulation → arterial and possibly venous clots (**white clot**). Treatment includes **heparin** discontinuation and initiation of nonheparin anticoagulation (eg, direct thrombin inhibitors such as lepirudin or argatroban).

Methemoglobinemia

Oxidized iron (Fe^{3+}) cannot carry O_2. Symptoms include confusion, lethargy, and seizures. Signs include **resistant cyanosis** and anemia. Confirm with ↑ methemoglobin and cyanosis in the setting of normal PaO_2. Treat with **methylene blue**.

Blood group O is the universal donor. If crossmatched blood is not available in an emergent setting, consider using type O blood.

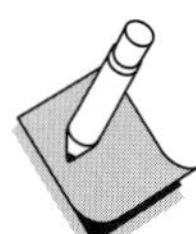

PRBC have ↓ 2,3-DPG and ↓ ATP

↓ 2,3-DPG → ↑ O_2-Hgb binding.

Transfusion-Associated Lung Injury (TRALI)**–Anti-HLA **antibodies in donor plasma** bind to **recipient leukocytes.

TRANSFUSION MEDICINE

There are four blood groups: O, A, B, and AB. Blood group **O is a universal donor**; group **AB is a universal recipient**. Blood products are summarized in Table 2-8.

Three categories of adverse reactions associated with blood product transfusions include

- **Infectious**: HCV (1/1.6 million), HIV (1/1.9 million), HBV (1/63,000), CMV (↓ risk if leukocyte-reduced).
- **Immune mediated**: Acute hemolysis (recipient has preformed antibodies; results from ABO mismatch), delayed hemolysis (amnestic response after previous transfusion), **febrile nonhemolytic reaction** (most common), anaphylaxis (common in IgA-deficient patients), transfusion-associated lung injury (**TRALI**). TRALI results from anti-HLA antibodies in donor plasma binding to recipient WBCs. Complex deposition occurs in the pulmonary vessels → ↑ permeability. CXR shows bilateral infiltrates. Treatment is supportive.
- **Non-immune mediated**: Fluid overload, hypothermia, hyperkalemia, hypocalcemia, iron toxicity.

TABLE 2-8. Blood Products

COMPONENT	SHELF LIFE	CONTENT	USES
Packed red blood cells (PRBC)	21-42 days	75% RBC, 25% plasma	Anemia, ↓ O_2 carrying capacity
Platelets (pooled)	5 days	$3\text{-}6 \times 10^{11}$ platelets	Inherited platelet disorders; severe ITP with failure of therapy
FFP	1 year if frozen; 24 hours if thawed	200 U of each coagulation factor; 400 mg of fibrinogen	Warfarin reversal, correction of coagulopathy
Cryoprecipitate	1 year if frozen	80 U **factor VIII**, 225 mg fibrinogen, variable amounts of **vWF**	Factor VIII deficiency, vWD (type II or III)
Recombinant factor VIII or IX	Must be reconstituted at time of use	Factor VIII > 3000 U/mg, Factor IX 270 U/mg	Hemophilia A or B
Factor VIIa	Must be reconstituted at time of use	30,000 U/mL	Refractory bleeding from GI bleed or trauma

(Adapted, with permission, from Kasper DL, et al. *Harrison's Principles of Internal Medicine,* 16th ed. New York: McGraw-Hill, 2005:664.)

A 59-year-old woman is status post liver transplant in the surgical ICU. Extensive intraoperative bleeding resulted in multiple transfusions of PRBC and FFP. On postoperative day 0, it is noted that she is requiring increasing ventilator support, and CXR shows bilateral patchy infiltrates. How do you proceed? This appears to be a case of TRALI. This disorder is managed similarly to acute respiratory distress syndrome (ARDS; low volume ventilation), but is expected to resolve within 48 hours.

Physiology of Aging and Pregnancy

Elderly patients account for half of surgical emergencies and three-fourths of perioperative deaths. Generally have more comorbid conditions and smaller physiologic reserve → ↑ risk of morbidity and mortality. Age is rarely a contraindication to surgery, but specific physiologic changes should be considered:

- Cardiovascular: Increased prevalence of coronary artery disease (CAD). As maximum HR ↓ with age, cardiac output is dependent on volume status. Calcification of conduction system may lead to ↑ incidence of arrhythmia. Early ambulation is vital to prevent deconditioning.
- Pulmonary: ↓ Alveoli surface area → ↑ risk of pneumonia or difficulty weaning from ventilator.
- Renal: ↓ Glomerular filtration rate predisposes to acute renal failure and drug toxicity.
- Central nervous system: ↓ Ability to maintain cerebral perfusion pressure during hypotension → ↑ risk of transient ischemia attack and cerebrovascular accident.
- Body composition/metabolism: ↑ Fat and ↓ muscle alter the volume of distribution for many drugs. Impaired ability to metabolize medications.
- Immune system: Increased susceptibility to infection.

Pregnancy **does not** ↓ risk of surgical illness, thus an approach to the pregnant patient should be considered. Special considerations for pregnant women include

- Avoid radiographic studies (when possible) during the first trimester.
- ↑ Blood volume and altered hepatic function will alter medication doses.
- **Appendicitis** should be managed with appendectomy in all trimesters.
- **Cholecystitis** should be managed nonoperatively until the second trimester.
- **Hiatal hernias** should be managed conservatively during pregnancy as many cases will resolve after delivery.
- Other **hernias** should be surgically repaired during pregnancy only if strangulated or incarcerated.
- **Breast cancer** should be **surgically** treated as soon as cancer is suspected.

Statistics and Epidemiology

Research Study Designs

Study designs include

- **Case series: Observational**, nonexperimental study that describes a group of patients with a similar intervention and outcome. Often used to describe unique presentations, conditions, or treatments. Cannot establish a cause-effect relationship. **Case report** is a subtype that focuses on the disease process in a small subset of patients.

- **Meta-analysis:** Study that combines results from different publications as a means of increasing power and making an overall conclusion about the effect of a treatment. Drawbacks include difference in quality and clinical definitions between studies as well as publication bias.
- **Case-control: Retrospective** comparison of **people who already have disease** (cases) with similar individuals without disease (controls) to determine possible risk factors. Advantages: quick, inexpensive, requires few subjects (good for rare diseases), and able to evaluate multiple risk factors simultaneously. Drawbacks: recall bias, selection bias, and inability to prove a cause-effect relationship.
- **Cohort (longitudinal) study: Prospective** comparison of **subjects with a similar exposure** within a specific time period in order to determine relationships between exposure and disease (not useful for rare conditions). Advantages: ability to estimate absolute risk of a disease due to exposure and unbiased data collection. Disadvantages: expensive, time-intensive, and only able to control for **known** confounders.
- **Cross-sectional study:** Similar to the cohort study except that analysis is conducted for a specific time point.
- **Randomized controlled trial:** Clinical trial in which subjects are randomly selected and exposed to treatment or control. May be open, blinded, or double-blinded. Major advantage is that both **known and unknown confounders are evenly distributed** between two groups.

A new endoscopic intervention has been shown to decrease the risk of postoperative DVT from 1/10 to 1/20. What is the number needed to treat? Divide 100 by the absolute risk reduction: 100 / (10% – 5%) = 100/5 = 20 patients must be treated for one to have a benefit.

EPIDEMIOLOGIC TERMS

Relevant ideas are summarized in Table 2-9.

TABLE 2-9. Epidemiologic Terms

EPIDEMIOLOGICAL TERMS	DEFINITION
Incidence	Number of **new** cases of a disease over a specific time period/number of people at risk.
Prevalence	Number of cases of disease/number of people in population. Greater in **chronic disease.**
Birth rate	Number of live births/1000 population (per year).
Maternal mortality rate	Number of maternal deaths due to childbearing/100,000 live births.
Infant mortality rate	Number of deaths children < 1 year of age/1000 live births.
Mortality rate	Number of deaths/1000 people.

STATISTICAL TERMS

Relevant ideas are summarized in Table 2-10.

TABLE 2-10. Statistical Terms

STATISTICAL TERM	DEFINITION
Sensitivity	True positive / (true positive + false negative). Probability that the test will be positive in the presence of disease.
Specificity	True negative / (true negative + false positive). Probability that the test will be negative in the absence of disease.
Positive predictive value (PPV)	True positive / (true positive + false positive). Probability of disease in the setting of positive test.
Negative predictive value (NPV)	True negative / (true negative + false negative). Probability of health in setting of negative test.
Accuracy	Relation of the calculated value to the actual value.
Precision	Reproducibility of value.
Relative risk (RR)	Risk of disease in exposed group / risk of disease in unexposed group. RR < 1 = less likely to occur in experimental group (compared to control). RR > 1 = more likely to occur in experimental group.
Absolute risk reduction (ARR)	(Events / subjects in control group) – (Events / subjects in experimental group).
Relative risk reduction	([Events / subjects in control group] – [Events / subjects in experimental group]) / (Events / subjects in control group).
Number needed to treat	1 / ARR.
Odds	The ratio of the probability of occurrence of an event to the probability of no occurrence (p / [1 – p]).
Odds ratio	Odds in exposed group / Odds in unexposed group.
Power	1-β. Probability that data will show a difference when a true difference exists. The larger the sample size, the greater the power.
Type I error (α error)	Rejecting a **true** null hypothesis (ie, reporting a significant finding when none truly exists; actual difference found is due to chance).
Type II error (β error)	Accepting a **false** null hypothesis (ie, not finding a difference when one does exist); usually due to limited power of a study.

	DISEASE PRESENT	DISEASE NOT PRESENT
Test Positive for Disease	A (true positive)	B (false positive)
Test Negative for Disease	C (false negative)	D (true negative)

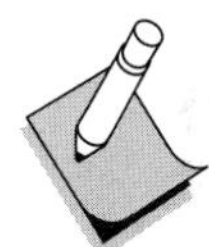

Sensitivity = A / (A + C)
Specificity = D / (B + D)
PPV = A / (A + B)
NPV = D / (C + D)
RR = (A / [A + B]) / (C / [C + D])
Accuracy = (A + D) / (A + B + C + D)

Sensitivity and specificity—**SP**in/**SN**out:
Specificity → ability to "rule **IN**"
Se**N**sitivity → ability to "rule **OUT**"

Statistical Tests

- **T-tests** assess the difference in **means** of a **continuous variable** between two groups and determine if the difference is statistically significant. Used for normally distributed data.
- **Analysis of variance** assesses the difference in the means of a **continuous variable** over three or more samples. Can be thought of as a t-test for > 2 groups.
- **Fisher's exact test** is a test for proportions of **discrete variables** when the number of groups is small (eg, 2 × 2 table).
- **Chi-square** is a test for proportions of **discrete variables** when the number of groups is larger (eg, 5 × 5 table). Sometimes referred to as a contingency table.
- ***P*-value < 0.05 is generally accepted to be statistically significant** and implies a < 5% probability of results being due to chance alone.

▶ SAMPLE QUESTIONS

A cohort of 50 men and 50 women is followed for one year; 10 women develop uterine cancer. What is the incidence of uterine cancer?	The incidence is 20%. Incidence only refers to the population at risk. Men are not at risk.
Which of the following marker: disease associations is incorrectly matched? CA 19-9: Pancreatic cancer CA 125: Hepatocellular cancer hCG: Testicular cancer Tyrosinase: Melanoma	CA 125 is not associated with hepatocellular cancer. Rather, it is a marker for ovarian cancer. AFP is sometimes used as a marker for hepatocellular cancer (large tumors).
From which surgical diseases do pregnant women enjoy a decreased risk?	None. Special attention must be paid to uncommon symptoms in these patients (ie, RUQ pain with appendicitis).
Which CAMs are important for leukocyte recruitment?	Leukocyte rolling is mediated through low affinity molecules (selectins), while adhesion is through high affinity molecules (integrins, ICAM, PECAM).
In what setting is the Mann-Whitney U-test used?	Also called a Wilcoxon rank-sum test. Used in the setting of ordinal data or continuous data that is not normally distributed. Compares the distribution of two samples and determines similarity or difference.
A man with known ITP presents with petechiae and nosebleeds. Platelet count is 8000/µL. He has undergone steroid and IV Ig therapy, with no result. How do you proceed?	Consider platelet transfusion if bleeding leads to hemodynamic compromise, but transfused platelets will bind IgG as well. This patient needs to undergo splenectomy.
Describe the mutations associated with MEN-1 and MEN-2.	MEN-1: Mutation of TSG, *MENIN*. MEN-2: Mutation of proto-oncogene, *RET*.
Why does heparin primarily affect PTT over PT?	Heparin augments the activity of ATIII, further inhibiting the conversion of Factor XI → XIa and XII → XIIa in the intrinsic pathway. Intrinsic pathway is assessed via PTT.
A young female complains of frequent nosebleeds, bruising, and heavy menstruation. Labs show ↑ BT. What are the diagnosis and plan?	This is likely von Willebrand's disease. The first line of therapy is DDAVP. If this fails, she may have type II or III vWD. Treat these with cryoprecipitate.

After anesthesia induction, a man develops angioedema of the skin, airway, and intestines. What is the presumed cause? Management?	Hereditary angioedema is an autosomal dominant disease caused by ↓ production or function of **C1 inhibitor.** Treat with steroids, antihistamines, and epinephrine. Prophylaxis includes FFP.
Will transfusion of leukocyte-reduced PRBCs result in a lower incidence of TRALI?	No. TRALI is caused by **donor antibodies** reacting with **recipient leukocytes**. The complexes then aggregate in the alveoli, triggering the syndrome.

CHAPTER 3

Perioperative Care

Andrew J. Meltzer, MD
Ellen C. Meltzer, MD
Reviewed by Marc A. deMoya, MD

Preoperative identification of risk factors allows thoughtful planning of intra- and post-operative management in an effort to optimize outcomes.

In **all** patients, a comprehensive medical and surgical history should be obtained with specific attention paid to prior surgical complications and any underlying cardiac, pulmonary, endocrine, renal, or hematologic disorders. Preoperative evaluation should include **ECG and CXR for men > 40 years and women > 55 years**. Patients > 40 years should have basic laboratory evaluation (eg, electrolytes, complete blood count [CBC]).

Risk Assessment and Preoperative Planning

Cardiac

The prevalence of coronary artery disease necessitates preoperative cardiac risk assessment. Significant risk factors for heart-related complications include **age > 70 years, current or previous angina, history of myocardial infarction (MI), Q wave on ECG**, and **congestive heart failure** (CHF). Patients with none of these comorbidities are at a low risk for cardiac complications. Patients with ≥ 3 are at high risk, and all others are at a moderate risk.

Another risk assessment tool is the **Goldman index,** which uses clinical, ECG, and laboratory data to determine preoperative cardiac risk (for noncardiac surgery). Points are assigned to risk factors (see Table 3-1), and the total is predictive of postoperative outcome (see Table 3-2).

Patients in the **lowest risk** groups may proceed to elective surgery without further testing. Patients at **highest risk** likely require specialist consultation. Those at **moderate risk** require further testing to determine a clinical pathway. These further tests may consist of exercise ECG, dipyridamole thallium scan (if unable to exercise), echo, or dobutamine stress echo, all of which identify those who will benefit from risk modification.

High-risk patients and those with moderate risk and + follow-up tests should delay elective procedures and be evaluated by a cardiologist for medical optimization or coronary intervention. Risk modification may include **perioperative β-blockade** (to continue until discharge), noninvasive cardiac output monitoring, or postoperative ICU care.

A 75-year-old man is evaluated in the ER with the acute onset of lower abdominal pain. His medical history is significant only for diverticulosis and a MI 10 years ago. Exam reveals hemodynamic instability and a systolic murmur radiating to the carotid arteries. Upright CXR shows free air under the diaphragm, and a clinical diagnosis of perforated diverticulitis is made. Is a cardiology consult needed? According to the Goldman index, his risk score is 15 (age, aortic stenosis, emergency procedure, intraperitoneal procedure), and his expected risk of cardiac death is 2%. For elective surgery, evaluation by a cardiologist is appropriate. In this emergent setting, however, he should proceed directly to surgery with plans for postoperative ICU care.

Pulmonary

After cardiac occurrences, **pulmonary complications** represent the greatest source of morbidity and mortality. In the postoperative period, many indices

TABLE 3-1. Goldman Criteria for Perioperative Cardiac Risk

RISK FACTOR	POINTS	RISK FACTOR	POINTS
S2 Gallop or jugular venous distention (JVD)	11	MI in previous 6 months	10
> 5 PVCs/minute ever on ECG	7	Nonsinus rhythm on ECG	7
Age > 70 years	5	Emergency operation	4
Intrathoracic procedure	3	Intraperitoneal procedure	3
Significant aortic stenosis	3	Poor general health	3

of pulmonary function are diminished (eg, forced expiratory volume in 1 second [FEV_1], forced vital capacity [FVC], functional residual capacity [FRC]). Problems such as atelectasis, pneumonia, chronic obstructive pulmonary disease (COPD) exacerbations, and respiratory failure are more common in smokers, patients with chronic respiratory illness, obese or malnourished patients, and those of poor functional status. Preoperative pulmonary function tests (PFTs) should be performed on select patients. **Failure to improve PFTs with appropriate therapy is highly predictive of postoperative respiratory failure.** Pulmonary risk reduction is achieved through smoking cessation, pre- and postoperative chest physiotherapy, laparoscopic approach (when possible), and appropriate pain control (especially for thoracic and upper abdominal incisions). Additionally, obese patients (body mass index [BMI] > 40 kg/m^2) benefit from perioperative continuous positive airway pressure (CPAP) and intraoperative use of ↑ positive end-expiratory pressure (PEEP; 10 cm H_2O).

DIABETES MELLITUS

Type I diabetics are generally at risk for hyperglycemia and diabetic ketoacidosis (DKA) in the perioperative period due to the absence of insulin secretion. The perioperative care of **type II** diabetics is complicated by insulin resistance and impaired insulin secretion. Prior to surgery, it is generally appropriate to

PERIOPERATIVE CARE

TABLE 3-2. Morbidity and Mortality Associated with Goldman Score

POINT TOTAL	CLASS	MAJOR COMPLICATION (%)	CARDIAC DEATH (%)
0-5	I	0.7	0.2
6-12	II	5	2
13-25	III	11	2
≥ 26	IV	78	56

hold all oral antihyperglycemics and reduce insulin doses by half on the day of surgery. Preoperative evaluation should include assessment for cardiac, neurologic, renal, and peripheral vascular disease. Diabetic patients with **CHF, valvular disease, end-organ failure, or peripheral vascular disease (PVD)** are at ↑ risk for perioperative mortality. Poor perioperative glucose control can lead to ketosis, dehydration, acidosis, poor wound healing, and impaired immune function. All diabetics should receive glucose infusion and insulin replacement (IV or subcutaneous) to maintain normoglycemia until preoperative regimen is resumed.

ANEMIA

Preoperative anemia warrants a detailed history and exam as well as appropriate hematologic laboratory evaluation, including iron studies and a hemolysis panel. Correctable causes of anemia (eg, deficiencies of iron, folate, and vitamin B_{12}) should be treated; arrange for availability of crossmatched blood. **In adults > 50 years of age, anemia of an unknown source represents malignancy until proven otherwise.** CXR, colonoscopy, or CT scan should be performed as indicated.

DEEP VEIN THROMBOSIS

Hematologic disorders that predispose to perioperative bleeding or thrombosis are discussed in Chapter 2.

A **detailed personal and family history** is the most appropriate first test to screen for hypercoagulable diseases. Inquire about recurrent clots, spontaneous abortion, or recurrent exposure to heparin. Without appropriate prophylaxis, the incidence of **deep vein thrombosis** (DVT) approaches 25% for abdominal procedures and 50% for some orthopedic procedures. Prophylaxis should begin preoperatively with elastic stockings and pneumatic compression devices placed **prior** to induction of anesthesia. Major abdominal procedures and malignancy-related procedures also require chemical prophylaxis prior to incision. Current recommendations are summarized in Table 3-3.

TABLE 3-3. DVT Prophylaxis Recommendations

INDICATION	ACCEPTED PROPHYLAXIS METHODS
Low risk (minor surgery, age < 40 years, no risk factors)	Early ambulation
Moderate risk (minor surgery with risk factors; major surgery, age > 40 years, no risk factors)	Low-dose heparin (LDH), low-molecular weight-heparin (LMWH), elastic stockings (ES), *or* intermittent pneumatic compression (IPC).
High risk (minor surgery with risk factors, age > 60 years; major surgery, age > 40 years, additional risk factors)	Mechanical (ie, ES or IPC) *and* chemical (ie, LDH or LMWH) prophylaxis.
Very high risk (multiple risk factors present)	As above

Anesthetics and Pain Control

Just prior to elective surgery, patients should receive **amnestic** or **anxiolytic** medications, **H_2-receptor blockers** (to ↑ gastric pH and ↓ risk of aspiration pneumonitis), an α-adrenergic agonist (to ↓ salivation and gastric secretions), and a prophylactic antiemetic.

Intraoperative anesthesia consists of **amnesia**, **analgesia**, and **muscle relaxation** or **paralysis**. Anesthesia may be local, regional, or general. The anesthetic agents employed, method of delivery, and induction techniques are determined by patient- and procedure-specific factors.

General anesthesia is usually induced with IV medications (anxiolytic and paralytic). In emergent cases, or in patients with a high risk of aspiration, **rapid sequence intubation** is employed. This calls for administration (in order) of a **sedative-amnestic** (eg, thiopental, propofol), a depolarizing **paralytic** agent (eg, succinylcholine), and rapid endotracheal intubation. Opioid medications are sometimes added to this cocktail. **Inhalational induction** requires delivery of nitric oxide along with a volatile anesthetic (eg, halothane, isoflurane, sevoflurane, desflurane). Intubation can then be attempted without administration of paralytic. The advantage of this form of induction is that the patient continues to **breathe spontaneously** (should intubation be unsuccessful).

Succinylcholine is contraindicated in patients with malignant hyperthermia, skeletal myopathies, acute burns, trauma, and upper motor neuron injury.

> Amide anesthetics all have **2 "Is"** and esters have **1 "I"**–
> Amides: L**I**doca**I**ne, bup**I**vaca**I**ne, mep**I**vaca**I**ne, pr**I**loca**I**ne, rop**I**vaca**I**ne.
> Esters: Coca**I**ne, proca**I**ne, chloroproca**I**ne, tetraca**I**ne, benzoca**I**ne.

Regional anesthesia (eg, spinal, epidural, nerve block) provides local pain control while allowing the patient to remain conscious during the procedure. Additionally, it does not require induction of general anesthesia, thus avoiding possible hemodynamic lability associated with large boluses of anxiolytics or sedatives. Low doses of sedatives are given for patient comfort. An additional advantage is that postoperative pain control is generally excellent. Urinary catheterization should be maintained for duration of epidural use as bladder distension may otherwise occur. Potential complications include epidural headache (spinal only), failure of adequate anesthesia, epidural hematoma (especially with LMWH), and peripheral nerve damage (rare).

Local anesthesia involves intradermal injection of anesthetics, resulting in a **reversible block of neural conduction** by continuous closure of Na^+ channels. Local anesthetics are divided into **amides** (metabolized by the liver) and **esters** (metabolized by plasma cholinesterase). Due to the similar chemical structure within each group, a documented allergy to one drug implies that all agents from that family are unsafe for use. Toxic reactions (eg, **seizures**, **cardiac arrhythmias**) are the same for both classes and are related to membrane instability.

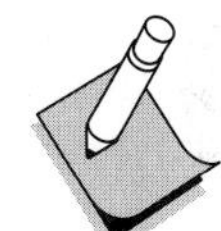

Maximum single dose of lidocaine in an adult = 4.5 mg/kg.
Maximum single dose of bupivacaine in an adult = 2 mg/kg.

Intraoperative pain control is attained with the use of both opioid and nonopioid agents. **Opioid agents** (eg, morphine, fentanyl) act via agonist activity at central **μ receptors** and suppress respiratory drive. **Nonopioid agents** (eg, ketamine, ketorolac) do not act at the μ receptor and do not suppress respiratory drive. Ketamine is a **dissociative anesthetic** (amnestic) but is associated with significant hallucinations and delirium, which would require concomitant use of a benzodiazepine. Other side effects of ketamine are tachycardia and HTN. Ketorolac (an nonsteroidal anti-inflammatory drug [**NSAID**]) is another nonopioid anesthetic frequently used intraoperatively. It carries a theoretical bleeding risk (ie, inhibits platelet aggregation) and may cause renal impairment.

Malignant Hyperthermia

Occurs in 1 in 50,000 patients. Caused by an inherited abnormality of the **ryanodine receptor**. This mutation (when **triggered by volatile anesthetics, succinylcholine, or amide local anesthetics**) leads to **high Ca^{2+} levels** in the sarcoplasmic reticulum of skeletal muscle. This leads to prolonged muscle contraction, hypermetabolism, rhabdomyolysis, hyperthermia, and acidosis. Early recognition, withdrawal of anesthetic, supportive treatment, and administration of **dantrolene** are the first-line therapy.

Intraoperative Monitoring

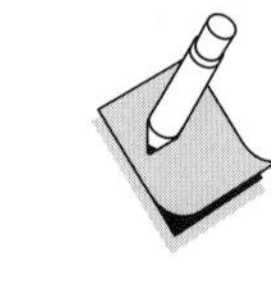

Advanced hemodynamic monitoring is discussed further in Chapter 15.

Intraoperative monitoring involves frequent or continuous assessment of the level of sedation, end tidal CO_2 (capnography), pulse oximetry, and hemodynamic parameters (eg, BP, HR). Urine output is frequently measured to assess volume status and end-organ perfusion.

▶ POSTOPERATIVE CARE

Fluids and Electrolytes

Total body water (TBW) comprises 45-60% of total body weight, depending on the patient's age and lean muscle mass. Intracellular fluid comprises two-thirds of the TBW; extracellular fluid (ECF) comprises the remaining one-third. The ECF is further divided into plasma (25%) and interstitial (75%) compartments. Because of active transport and electrolyte-specific channels, the various compartments maintain different electrolyte concentrations in the steady state (see Figure 3-1).

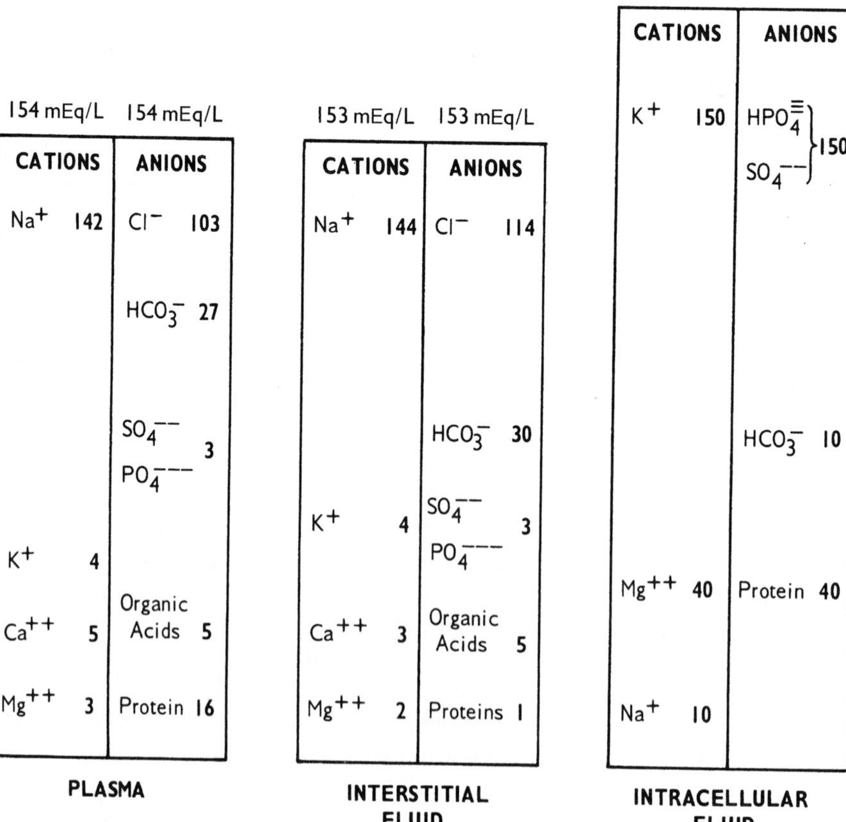

FIGURE 3-1. Electrolyte composition of body compartments.

(Reproduced, with permission, from Brunicardi FC, et al. *Schwartz's Principles of Surgery*, 8th ed. New York: McGraw-Hill, 2005:45.)

TABLE 3-4. **Electrolyte Composition of Gastrointestinal Fluids**

TYPE OF SECRETION	VOLUME (mL/24h)	NA (mEq/L)	K (mEq/L)	CL (mEq/L)	HCO_3^- (mEq/L)
Stomach	1000–2000	60–90	10–30	100–130	0
Small intestine	2000–3000	120–140	5–10	90–120	30–40
Colon		60	30	40	0
Pancreas	600–800	135–145	5–10	70–90	95–115
Bile	300–800	135–145	5–10	90–110	30–40

(Reproduced, with permission, from Brunicardi FC, et al. *Schwartz's Principles of Surgery,* 8th ed. New York: McGraw-Hill, 2005:46.)

Fluid maintenance and repletion are dictated by electrolyte and volume status with attention paid to expected electrolyte levels in fluid losses (see Table 3-4). Fluid resuscitation plan should account for the patient's cardiac and pulmonary status. It is expected that approximately one-third of administered crystalloid volume will remain in the extracellular space after osmotic equilibration.

After establishment of the euvolemic state, oral intake is often sufficient to match normal fluid losses. In patients who are NPO or who have limited oral intake, maintenance IV fluids should be provided to replace free H_2O and electrolyte losses. The volume requirement can be estimated based on the patient's dry body weight: 4 mL/kg/h for the first 10 kg of body weight; 2 mL/kg/h for the next 10 kg; and 1 mL/kg/h for each kg thereafter.

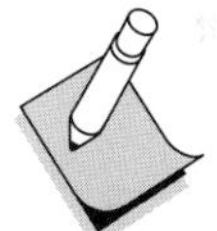

4/2/1 rule for hourly maintenance IV fluids–
4 mL/kg/h for first 10 kg
2 mL/kg/h for next 10 kg
1 mL/kg/h for each kg > 20 kg

Disorders of Electrolytes

Signs and symptoms of electrolyte abnormalities are summarized in Table 3-5.

DISORDERS OF SODIUM

Due to fluid shifts, pain- or anesthesia-related hormonal disturbances, and iatrogenic causes. Plasma Na^+ abnormalities are common postoperative complications.

Diabetes insipidus (central) should be considered in all postoperative patients with ↑ Na^+ levels, particularly those who have undergone intracranial or intrathoracic procedures. Hypernatremia can also be the result of a free H_2O deficit. Initial therapy is dictated by the calculated deficit. The calculated volume of free H_2O should be repleted slowly, such that plasma Na^+ does not fall > 1 mEq/L/h.

Hyponatremia may be seen postoperatively even in healthy patients and is often caused by excessive administration of hypotonic maintenance IV fluids. Less commonly, hyponatremia is caused by a **syndrome of inappropriate ADH secretion (SIADH)**. Lab results may mistakenly report a low Na^+ level in patients with markedly ↑ plasma levels of protein, glucose, or lipid. In cases of true hyponatremia, the fractional excretion of Na^+ (FENa) may help determine etiology: FENa > 1% (or urine Na^+ > 20 mEq/L) implies SIADH. As with hypernatremia, care must be taken to avoid rapid changes in Na^+ level.

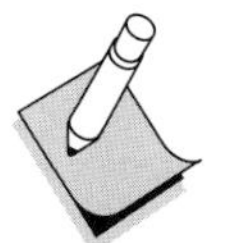

Key electrolyte formulas–
% TBW = 60% (males), 50% (females).
Free H_2O deficit (L) = (kg) × (% TBW) × ([Serum Na^+ / 140] – 1).
Na^+ deficit (mEq/L) = (125 – Serum Na^+) × (kg) × (% TBW).

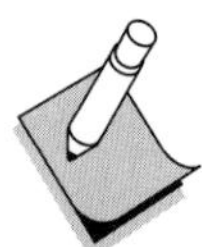

Effect of hyperglycemia on Na^+ level—

Corrected Na^+ = Measured Na^+ + ([Serum glucose − 100] / 100 × 1.6)

Formula for the fractional excretion of Na^+—

FENa(%) = $(Plasma_{Cr} \times Urine_{Na}) / (Plasma_{Na} \times Urine_{Cr})$

Pathology associated with correction of Na^+—

Rapid correction of hypernatremia → cerebral edema.

Rapid correction of hyponatremia → central pontine myelinolysis.

Correction of chronic hyponatremia should be kept < 10 mEq/L in any 24-hour period.

TABLE 3-5. Signs and Symptoms of Electrolyte Abnormalities

	HYPO-	HYPER-
Sodium	Related to cerebral swelling: nausea, headache, lethargy, confusion, obtundation → seizures, coma (Na^+ < 120 mEq/L).	Altered mental status, weakness, ↑ thirst, polyuria. Severity related to acuity of change.
Potassium	Fatigue, myalgia, muscle weakness, hypoventilation. ECG demonstrates T wave inversion → ST depression → widened QRS.	Weakness, flaccid paralysis, metabolic acidosis. ECG demonstrates peaked T wave → widened QRS → ventricular fibrillation (VF) or asystole.
Calcium	↑ Nerve/muscle excitation, cramps, tetany, laryngospasm, perioral paresthesias, **Chvostek's** and **Trousseau's** signs. ECG shows prolonged QT.	Constipation, nausea, vomiting, anorexia, nephrolithiasis, weakness, depression, lethargy.
Magnesium	Weakness, muscle cramps, central nervous system (CNS) irritability, tremors, nystagmus, +Babinski	Weakness, ↓ reflexes, obtundation, confusion, urinary retention
Phosphorus	Rhabdomyolysis, paresthesias, encephalopathy, respiratory failure	Symptoms of hypocalcemia, extraosseous tissue calcification

Treat with **free H_2O restriction**; hypertonic saline and **demeclocycline** may be given if SIADH is present.

DISORDERS OF POTASSIUM

Treatment of **hyperkalemia** includes removal (eg, sodium polystyrene, dialysis) or relocation (eg, intracellular shift with glucose and insulin or HCO_3^-) of K^+. Immediate steps are taken to prevent cardiac effects by giving **Ca^{2+}** (to **stabilize myocardial cellular membrane**). **Hypokalemia** can usually be managed with oral or IV repletion.

DISORDERS OF CALCIUM

Symptomatic **hypercalcemia** is treated with volume resuscitation and concomitant diuresis. Severe or malignancy-related hypercalcemia is treated with bisphosphonates. Correction of **hypocalcemia** requires oral or IV supplementation after correcting any abnormalities of Mg^{2+}.

DISORDERS OF MAGNESIUM

Hypermagnesemia requires dialysis in rare, symptomatic cases that are unresponsive to withdrawal of exogenous supplementation. **Hypomagnesemia** is treated with IV repletion.

DISORDERS OF PHOSPHORUS

Hyperphosphatemia is treated with phosphate binders and dialysis (in the setting of renal failure). **Hypophosphatemia** can be treated with oral or IV supplementation.

After pancreaticoduodenectomy, a 62-year-old woman develops a pancreatic fistula. She is noted to be moderately confused and dehydrated. Laboratories are remarkable for pH = 7.30, Pco_2 = 32 mm Hg, Po_2 = 98 mm Hg, HCO_3^- = 18 mEq/L, Cl^- = 118 mEq/L, and Na^+ = 140 mEq/L. Describe the patient's acid-base imbalance. She is suffering from non–anion gap metabolic acidosis, likely caused by GI losses through the pancreatic fistula. Pancreatic exocrine secretions are rich in HCO_3^-.

Formula for anion gap–

Anion Gap =

$Na^+ - (HCO_3^- + Cl^-)$

Normal < 11 mEq/L

Anion gap metabolic acidosis is caused by **MUDPILES:**
Methanol
Uremia
DKA
Paraldehyde
Iron/**I**NH
Lactic acid
Ethanol/**E**thylene glycol
Salicylates

Acid-Base Imbalances

Acid-base disorders can be either respiratory or metabolic and have varying levels of compensation. Table 3-6 describes etiologies and treatments for common disorders in the perioperative period.

TABLE 3-6. Perioperative Acid-Base Disorders

DISORDER		CLUES	POSSIBLE CAUSES	TREATMENT
Metabolic acidosis	Anion gap	↓ pH ↓ HCO_3^-	Shock, renal failure, ketoacidosis	Volume resuscitation, hemodynamic support
	Non–anion gap	↓ pH ↓ HCO_3^- ↑ Cl^-	Gastrointestinal (GI) losses (diarrhea, fistula), acetazolamide administration, renal tubular acidosis (RTA).	Treat underlying cause, stop offending drugs, administer HCO_3^- (for RTA).
Metabolic alkalosis	NaCl responsive	↑ pH ↑ HCO_3^- ↓ U_{Cl} "dry"	Diuretic therapy (contraction), nasogastric tube (NGT) suction, pyloric obstruction.	Volume expansion, acetazolamide (in setting of CHF), stop diuretics.
	NaCl nonresponsive	↑ pH ↑ HCO_3^- ↔ U_{Cl}	Severe hypokalemia, hyperaldosteronism, citrate (blood) or acetate (total parenteral nutrition [TPN]) load in setting of ↓ glomerular filtration rate (GFR).	K^+ repletion, adjust TPN (if necessary), treat underlying cause.
Respiratory acidosis		↓ pH HCO_3^- ↑ pCO_2	CNS depression, atelectasis, mucous plug, effusion, ↑ pain, abdominal distension.	↑ Ventilation (deep breaths, CPAP, BiPAP, intubate), pain control, naloxone (if needed).
Respiratory alkalosis		↑ pH ↓ pCO_2	Hyperventilation (pain, anxiety, pulmonary embolism [PE]), Gram-negative sepsis.	Treat underlying cause; rebreathing of CO_2.

Non-anion gap metabolic acidosis is caused by **USED CAR:**
Ureterostomy
Small bowel or pancreatic fistula
Extra Cl^-
Diarrhea
Carbonic anhydrase inhibitors
Adrenal insufficiency
RTA

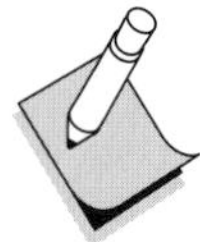

Specific mechanisms for nutrient absorption are discussed in Chapter 9.

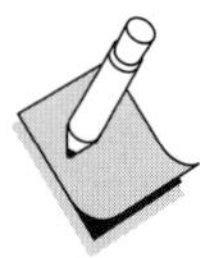

ATP energy production–
Aerobic respiration yields 36-38 ATP/glucose molecule. Anaerobic respiration yields 2 ATP/glucose molecule.

Nitrogen balance formula–
Nitrogen balance = [Consumed protein (g) / 6.25] – [Urine urea nitrogen (g) + 4 g]

Surgical Metabolism and Nutrition

Malnutrition is disproportionately prevalent in surgical patients due to ↑ caloric needs. Failure to meet energy requirements has important consequences with respect to wound healing, immune function, respiratory status, and gut function.

CELLULAR METABOLISM

Aerobic cellular respiration is the final common pathway for energy synthesis. Amino acids, fatty acids, and glucose can each provide substrate for the electron transport chain in the mitochondria, which results in formation of adenosine triphosphate (ATP).

Carbohydrates are the 1° energy source (40% of caloric intake), yielding **4 kcal/g**. Nearly all enterally consumed carbohydrate is broken down by brush border enzymes to glucose and then absorbed. As plasma glucose ↑, pancreatic β-cells release insulin, which stimulates protein synthesis and limits proteolysis and lipolysis. In the absence of circulating glucose (starvation state), glucagon is released and allows for breakdown of protein, lipid, and glycogen, leading to ↑ plasma glucose. As glycogen is depleted, **gluconeogenesis** ensues in the liver and kidneys.

Enterally consumed **protein** also yields **4 kcal/g**. Daily protein requirements are estimated at 0.8 g/kg. This estimate ↑ as protein loss ↑ (eg, diarrhea, burn exudate, fistula, nephrotic syndrome). In the nonstarvation state, there is a + nitrogen balance. A **nitrogen balance is indicative of starvation** as protein breakdown then exceeds protein synthesis. In this state, most amino acids are converted to pyruvate or oxaloacetate, which are used for gluconeogenesis. As the amino group is removed from these protein substrates, the **urea cycle** is the pathway for nitrogen elimination via the urine. This deaminated amino acid backbone is now used for gluconeogenesis or the tricarboxylic acid (TCA) cycle.

Dietary **lipid** provides 40% of caloric intake, providing **9 kcal/g. Triglycerides (TG)** are the storage form of lipid; in the starvation state, TGs are hydrolyzed (**lipolysis**) to fatty acids and then to fatty acyl-CoA, which can either be oxidized in the TCA cycle or used to form **ketone bodies**. Though this ketogenesis occurs in the liver, the liver itself cannot use ketone bodies as an energy source for its metabolic pathways.

Nitrogen balance is calculated by subtracting nitrogen output from nitrogen intake. Output consists of urinary nitrogen (urea component is measured; 3 g/d nonurea nitrogen estimated) and fecal nitrogen (estimated at 1 g/d). Nitrogen intake is calculated from protein intake (6.25 g protein = 1 g nitrogen).

Gluconeogenesis provides an exhaustible source of glucose in the starvation state. The substrates for gluconeogenesis are proteolysis-derived amino acids (except leucine and lysine) and the glycerol carbon backbone generated by lipolysis. The **Cori cycle** is an additional pathway for producing glucose in the starvation state. These reactions use lactate (byproduct of anaerobic respiration) as a substrate. Lactate is transported to the liver; at a net cost of 4 ATP, it is used to create glucose (with pyruvate as an intermediate). The glucose is then transported back to peripheral tissues for use.

SURGICAL NUTRITION

Nutritional assessment includes physical exam or laboratory evaluation. Must evaluate relative weight for height, body fat, temporal bulk, extremity strength, and presence of ascites. Laboratory values indicate nutritional status over various time periods based upon their half-life ($t_{1/2}$). Frequently used metrics (with $t_{1/2}$) include **albumin** (18 days), **transferrin** (7-10 days), and **prealbumin** (2 days).

Metabolic requirements vary with physiologic stress. Basal energy expenditure (BEE) estimates the body's caloric needs in the unstressed, steady state and is approximately **25 kcal/kg/d**. This value is ↑ in certain clinical conditions. The **respiratory quotient** (RQ) is sometimes used to more accurately estimate metabolic needs. The RQ is **1.0 for glucose** oxidation, **0.8 for protein** oxidation, and **0.7 for fat** oxidation.

If not contraindicated, it is always preferable to feed patients enterally. **Enteral feeding** (eg, orally consumed diet or feeding via a NGT, gastrostomy, or jejunostomy) preserves mucosal barrier function and is associated with ↓ mortality, infection, and hospital stay. **Contraindications** to enteral nutrition are usually temporary and relative (eg, bowel rest in the setting of small bowel obstruction [SBO]). Consideration should be given for feeding tube placement at the time of initial surgery if long-term therapy may be required. Various nutritional supplements are available (see Table 3-7).

When the gut cannot be utilized for nutrition, **parenteral nutrition** (central or peripheral) is indicated. Clinical settings may include the preoperative care of a malnourished patient or the postoperative care of a patient with protracted (> 7 days) inability to tolerate enteral feeds. Preoperative nutritional support should only be used if therapy can be provided for a **minimum of 7 days** before a procedure. Preoperative therapy shorter than this has not been shown to be effective and will expose patients to risk. Approximately 15% of exposed patients experience **complications of TPN,** including catheter-related infection, sepsis, complications associated with gaining and maintaining venous access, electrolyte disorders, acid-base abnormalities, refeeding syndrome, hepatic steatosis, and biliary stasis.

Physiologic stress requires you to **E**at **T**o **S**tay **B**ig and **T**all:
Elective surgery = 1.2 × increase in BEE
Trauma = 1.3 × ↑ in BEE
Sepsis = 1.5 × ↑ in BEE
Burns = 2.0 × ↑ in BEE
Temperature = 1.1 × ↑ in BEE for each degree over 37.5°C

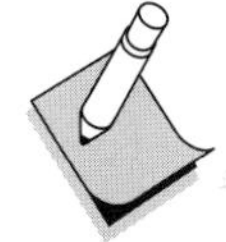

Respiratory quotient formula–

Respiratory quotient = CO_2 produced (L/min) / O_2 consumed (L/min)

TABLE 3-7. Nutritional Supplements

Additive	Effect	Caution
Arginine	↑ Growth hormone and insulin release → ↑ protein synthesis and wound healing.	Not used in septic patients (↑ nitric oxide production → vasodilation, ↓ inotrope).
Omega-3 fatty acids	Incorporated in cell membranes → cyclooxygenase pathway shunts to ↓ inflammatory cytokines.	Risk of ↑ lipid in diet.
Glutamine	Vital for nitrogen transport in rapidly dividing cells; maintains GI mucosa.	Enteral delivery is inefficient (metabolized by liver). Consider parenteral dosing.
Trace metals (zinc, selenium, copper)	Cofactors for antioxidant enzymes. Deficiency → damage from O_2 free radicals.	Poor evidence to support use.
Antioxidants (vitamins A, C, E, β carotene)	As antioxidant enzyme pathways are saturated, these are used as second-line scavengers of reactive O_2 species.	Poor evidence to support use.

Postoperative Complications

Mental Status Changes

May be due to many factors including electrolyte abnormalities, retained anesthetic, adrenal insufficiency, narcotic or benzodiazepine overdose, dementia, delirium, sepsis, steroid psychosis, and cerebrovascular accident (CVA). Initial evaluation should include neurologic exam and routine laboratory evaluation. Carotid bruits, recent hypotension, or asymmetric motor and sensory deficits should prompt noncontrast head CT to rule out CVA.

Atrial Fibrillation

Most common postoperative arrhythmia, which coincides primarily with interstitial fluid mobilization. Resultant **atrial stretch** causes myocardial membrane instability and the development of arrhythmogenic focus. Evaluation should include CXR, chemistries, cardiac enzymes, and thyroid function tests. Electrolytes (eg, K^+, Mg^{2+}) must be aggressively corrected. Initial treatment is aimed at **HR control and BP maintenance**. Carotid massage is rarely sufficient to treat atrial fibrillation (AF). First-line medications act by slowing atrioventricular conduction. β-blockers and Ca^{2+}-channel blockers are effective, though each has potential limitations (eg, β-blockade → hypotension, Ca^{2+}-channel blockade → CHF exacerbation). **Cardioversion** is required in the setting of hemodynamic instability. AF persisting > 48 hours may require long-term anticoagulation if the risk-benefit profile allows.

A 55-year-old man is one day s/p left thoracotomy for left upper lobectomy. His temperature is 102°F. Evaluation of the wound shows no cellulitis, urinalysis lacks white blood cells (WBC), and serum WBC is normal. Pulmonary auscultation reveals fine rales at the left lung base with diminished breath sounds. CXR shows an elevated left hemidiaphragm. What is the treatment? The patient's fever is likely caused by atelectasis, which is in turn likely due to suboptimal pain control. Encourage deep breathing, ambulation, and consider placement of epidural for pain control.

Pulmonary Complications

Incidence is 7% following major noncardiac surgery. **Atelectasis**, a segmental collapse of the airway, is often caused by poor inspiratory effort in the setting of poorly controlled postoperative pain. It may manifest as early postoperative fever with an abnormal CXR. Primary treatment is prevention (eg, incentive spirometry, chest physical therapy, ambulation, sitting position). Preventive measures, when employed, ↓ pneumonia risk. **Pneumonia** is a common nosocomial infection affecting up to 15% of ventilated patients. Diagnose with history and exam (eg, fever, rales, hypoxemia), laboratory studies (eg, leukocytosis, + blood or sputum cultures), and CXR (eg, lobar or multilobar infiltrates). Prompt intervention is warranted to minimize morbidity and mortality: after collection of sputum sample, initiate broad spectrum antibiotics for suspected pneumonia. Narrow coverage when culture and sensitivity data allows.

Acute Renal Failure

Common postoperative complication with an incidence of 0.6% (10× ↑ after cardiac surgery). Etiology varies by type of renal failure.

TABLE 3-8. Laboratory Findings in ARF

TYPE	FENA	URINE OSMOLARITY	URINE NA$^+$
Prerenal	< 1	> 500	< 20
Intrinsic	> 1	< 350	> 40

(Adapted, with permission, from Brunicardi FC, et al. *Schwartz's Principles of Surgery,* 8th ed. New York: McGraw-Hill, 2005:349.)

- **Prerenal:** Hypotension, CHF
- **Intrinsic:** Acute tubular necrosis, nephrotoxic drugs
- **Postrenal:** Obstruction

Determine type of acute renal failure (ARF) with urinary Na^+ excretion, FENa, and urine osmolarity (see Table 3-8). Treatment is directed at the type of ARF. Prerenal failure is treated by maintenance of renal perfusion. Postrenal failure is treated with urinary system drainage. Treatment of intrinsic failure depends on nephrotoxic source. **Sodium bicarbonate** infusion may prevent contrast-related nephropathy.

> A 77-year-old man is 2 days s/p exploratory laparotomy for perforated diverticulitis. He remains febrile and has markedly diminished urine output. Despite aggressive fluid resuscitation and vasopressor support, his mean arterial pressure is < 55 mmHg. What are your next steps? Order an adrenocorticotropin hormone (ACTH)-stimulation test. His cortisol level increases by 7 μg/dL. Based on this failed stimulation test, administer hydrocortisone 100 mg IV every 8 hours for his adrenal insufficiency.

ADRENAL INSUFFICIENCY

One of the differential diagnoses for a **hypotensive patient with a history of chronic steroid therapy**. Patients undergoing moderate or major surgery with documented or presumed hypothalamic-pituitary-adrenal axis suppression should receive stress dose steroids. Always rule out other common causes of hypotension (eg, hypovolemia, anemia, sepsis). See Chapter 12 for additional details.

> Indications for IVC filter placement—**P**lace **T**he **F**ilter, **C**lot **R**emains **B**enign:
> **P**rophylaxis for patient after trauma or with marginal pulmonary reserve.
> **T**hrombus free-floating in IVC or iliofemoral vein.
> **F**ailure of appropriate anticoagulation therapy.
> **C**ontraindication to anticoagulation.
> **R**ecurrent thromboembolism despite anticoagulation.
> **B**leeding complication while receiving anticoagulation therapy.

HEMATOLOGIC COMPLICATIONS

The surgical state, as well as underlying conditions, predispose patients to venous thromboembolism. Orthopedic, obstetric, and trauma patients are at an unusually high risk for DVT and PE. Patients with DVTs may present with calf pain or asymmetric leg swelling. Those with PEs may demonstrate ↑ central venous pressure, tachycardia, tachypnea, and the **classic $S_1Q_3T_3$ sign on ECG** (S wave in lead 1 suggesting right bundle branch block, Q and T wave inversions in lead 3). Confirm DVT with duplex ultrasound of the lower extremities; confirm PE with pulmonary CT angiography (CTA) or ventilation/perfusion (V/Q) scan. Management of postoperative DVT and PE generally consists of anticoagulation, though **inferior vena cava (IVC) filter** placement may be required if anticoagulation fails or if the risk of bleeding outweighs the benefits of treatment.

Anticoagulant medications are discussed in Chapter 2.

Infections of Surgical Patients

Wound Contamination Classification

Surgical wounds are classified as clean, clean-contaminated, contaminated, and dirty. Each is associated with a risk of surgical infection.

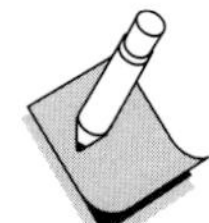

Surgical wound infection risk–

Clean: 1-5%

Clean-contaminated: 8-11%

Contaminated: 15-16%

Dirty: 28-40%

Clean

Atraumatic and uninfected wounds without entry into the GI, genitourinary (GU), or respiratory tracts. **1-5% risk of infection.**

Clean-Contaminated

Wounds associated with entry into the GI, GU, or respiratory tracts without significant spillage. **8-11% risk of infection.**

Contaminated

Traumatic wounds with gross contamination by GI tract or access into infected bile, urine, bone, or tissue. **15-16% risk of infection.**

Dirty

Wounds resulting from abscess drainage or debridement of infected soft tissue. **28-40% risk of infection.**

Surgical Site Infections

Infections of any surgically manipulated tissues. Generally categorized as **superficial** (eg, cellulitis), **deep** (eg, abscess at level of fascia), or **organ space** (eg, anastomotic leak, intra-abdominal abscess). Risk of **surgical site infections** is determined by procedure- and patient-specific factors. Most important risk factors are **wound class, patient immune status, obesity, diabetes mellitus (DM), and malnutrition.**

Clostridium Difficile Colitis

Nosocomial infectious colitis caused by antibiotic-induced imbalance in normal and pathologic colon flora. **Spread as a spore**, which is not killed with alcohol-based hand rubs. Commonly follows **recent antibiotic use**. Can present as abdominal pain, fever, leukocytosis, and watery or bloody diarrhea. Confirm diagnosis with *C. difficile* toxin in stool sample or with colonoscopy (**pseudomembranous colitis**). Initial treatment includes withdrawal of inciting antibiotics and initiation of vancomycin (oral or enema) or metronidazole (IV or oral) therapy. Recurrent cases may treated by repopulating the colon with normal flora (**probiotics**). Surgical intervention is warranted for perforation, toxic dilation, or sepsis.

Abscesses

Infected tissue isolated by the body to defend against widespread bacterial infection. First-line therapy is **drainage;** postdrainage antibiotics may be given if infection is complicated or if patient is immunosuppressed. Intra-abdominal abscesses are usually diagnosed by CT and can be percutaneously drained. Drainage catheters should remain in place until fluid no longer drains and cavity is collapsed. **Surgical drainage** is required if the collection is in a hazardous location, abscesses are multiple, or if there is reason to believe that peritoneal contamination is continuing (ie, anastomotic leak).

Line- and Catheter-Related Infections

Incidence ↑ with prolonged use and nonsterile insertion or manipulation. All tubes, lines, and drains should be removed as soon as clinically feasible. Central venous lines (CVL) can lead to infection in the blood or at the insertion site. Urinary drainage catheters lead to urinary tract infections (UTIs). **Any infection of this type should prompt catheter or line removal**. Diagnosis of UTI is confirmed by culture with 10^4 or 10^5 colony-forming units in symptomatic and asymptomatic patients, respectively. **Cystitis** should be treated with antibiotics for 1-3 days, while **pyelonephritis** requires treatment for 7-14 days. **Line-related bacteremia** is suspected when blood cultures from the line and the periphery isolate the same organism. **Routine CVL changes do not necessarily lead to fewer complications** (↓ risk of infection, but ↑ risk of insertion-related complications). If line-related bacteremia is suspected, empiric antibiotic therapy should be started and narrowed as soon as culture data permits.

Gram-Negative Bacteremia

Generally arises from **GI** or **GU system** source; less commonly associated with wounds, lines, or ulcers. Patients will often have a **rapid onset of fevers, chills,** and **rigors**. Lab tests may show leukocytosis (with left shift) or leukopenia, thrombocytopenia, and possibly, disseminated intravascular coagulation (DIC). If suspected, collect **blood cultures** and start empiric antibiotic treatment based on unit- and institution-specific resistance patterns. Narrow antibiotic regimen as cultures allow and continue antibiotics for 14 days, **even in the absence of + blood cultures** (due to risk of false negative result). Newer therapies based on the pathophysiology of gram-negative sepsis include **recombinant activated protein C (APC)**. APC is proven to ↑ survival for severely ill patients (APACHE II ≥ 25) but carries a high risk of bleeding complications. Additionally, if the source of infection is identified, this should be treated or removed.

Since gram-positive and gram-negative sepsis cannot be clinically differentiated, empiric treatment should cover both types of organisms.

A 48-year-old woman with known alcohol dependence is admitted to the ICU after being found unresponsive in her home. Her temperature is 104°F, and CXR shows patchy infiltrates in the dependent segments. What are your next steps? Recognizing possible aspiration pneumonia, you immediately start empiric antibiotics. Because of her alcohol dependence, you are concerned about anaerobic pathogens, so antibiotic coverage includes levofloxacin and metronidazole. Perform bedside bronchoscopy to obtain sputum cultures.

Aspiration Pneumonia

Aspiration of food, blood, gastric contents, or oropharyngeal secretions may occur during the induction of anesthesia or in patients who are unable to protect their airway (eg, recurrent nerve palsy, recent anesthetic application for bronchoscopy, narcotic overdose). **Posterior upper lobes and superior lower lobes are often involved.** May lead to airway obstruction, inflammation, pneumonia, bronchospasm, respiratory distress, or any combination. **Pneumonia**

PERIOPERATIVE CARE

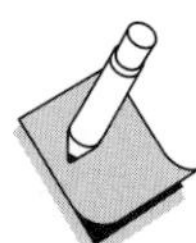

Aspiration of gastric contents with pH < 2.5 will cause immediate pneumonitis. Aspiration of anaerobic bacteria (eg, in alcoholics, patients with poor dentition) may result in pulmonary abscess.

refers to aspiration of oropharyngeal flora with subsequent bacterial infection. **Pneumonitis** refers to aspiration of sterile gastric contents, resulting in inflammation. Often, however, the inflammation and airway edema associated with pneumonitis leads to obstructed pulmonary segments and eventually pneumonia. In either scenario, **bronchoscopy with pulmonary toilet** are indicated. Pneumonia should be treated with two antibiotics (levofloxacin or ceftriaxone with either metronidazole or imipenem). Anaerobic coverage is particularly indicated in those with **poor dentition** or **alcohol dependence**. Suspected pneumonitis should be observed for 24 hours; if no improvement is noted, initiate treatment for aspiration pneumonia.

VENTILATOR-ASSOCIATED PNEUMONIA

Responsible for about **15% of hospital-acquired infections**, **ventilator-associated pneumonia** (VAP) begins after patient is mechanically ventilated ≥ 48 hours. **Early VAP** presents after 3-4 days of ventilation; **late VAP** presents after > 4 days of ventilation. Typically associated with fever, leukocytosis, purulent respiratory secretions, and a new or progressive pulmonary infiltrate on CXR. Diagnosis is confirmed with bronchoscopic cultures. Because of significant morbidity and mortality (30% mortality; ↑ with late VAP), broad spectrum antibiotic coverage should be selected for likely organisms.

- Early VAP: *Streptococcus pneumoniae, Haemophilus influenzae, Staphylococcus aureus*
- Late VAP: Typically antibiotic-resistant nosocomial organisms (eg, *Pseudomonas aeruginosa, Acinetobacter, Enterobacter*, methicillin-resistant *Staphylococcus aureus* [MRSA]).

BITES

Bites are most commonly from a dog or human ("fight bite"). All bites carry a high risk of infection, but dog bites also have a high risk of damage to deeper structures (**crush component**). Direct antibiotic therapy toward expected oral flora of the source: human bites are associated with *Streptococcus, Staphylococcus, Eikenella,* and *Haemophilus* species; dog and cat bites are associated with *Pasturella, Staphylococcus, Streptococcus, Eikenella, Actinomyces,* and *Fusobacterium*. For **human and dog bites**, initial antibiotic should be ampicillin-sulbactam, amoxicillin-clavulanic acid, or (if allergic) clindamycin plus a fluoroquinolone for 10 days. For **cat bites**, cefuroxime is preferred as ***Pasteurella multocida*** is the most common organism. If not delayed in presentation, most wounds can be closed after irrigation. It is **usually not appropriate to close puncture wounds or bites on the hand**. Tetanus booster should be given if not up to date. Tetanus toxoid plus tetanus immune globulin should be given if < 3 doses of toxoid have been given or if status is uncertain. Immobilization and elevation are also necessary.

NECROTIZING INFECTIONS

Includes soft tissue infections that progress rapidly and leave devitalized tissue behind. Risk factors are related to immunosuppression. **Necrotizing fasciitis** (including **Fournier's gangrene**) involves the fascia and the layer of tissue just superficial to this. Usually follows some degree of trauma to the skin and soft tissue (eg, surgery, bite, laceration, shaving). Exam will demonstrate an **exquisitely tender**, edematous (though not necessarily cellulitic) region, possibly with serous drainage. Underlying soft tissue lacks intact fascial planes. Infection is described by anatomic location and causative organism. Infection is most commonly polymicrobial (gram positive and gram negative; **type I**) in origin. **Type II** is more rapidly progressive and involves a single pathogen (**eg, Group A *Streptococcus pyogenes***). First-line therapy includes **early, aggressive debridement of all infected tissue**. Subcutaneous fluid and fascial biopsies should be collected for Gram stain and culture. Additional therapy consists of hemodynamic support, hydration, and IV antibiotics. Antimicrobial therapy is directed by culture results, but initial treatment includes **gentamicin, clindamycin, and penicillin** and should be tapered according to culture results.

Gas gangrene may present in the postoperative period. In contrast to necrotizing fasciitis, gas gangrene spreads to **all tissue layers** including skin and muscle. **Crepitance** is noted on exam as a result of the gas forming nature of the principle pathogens (***Clostridium*** species). Similar to necrotizing fasciitis, the wound is exquisitely painful, but gas gangrene differs in that the drainage is classically watery and brown ("**dishwater-like**"). Mainstays of therapy are excision and antibiotics (penicillin or metronidazole and chloramphenicol if penicillin-allergic). **Hyperbaric O_2** therapy may also be of value.

Cultures allow narrowing antibiotic spectrum for necrotizing infections–

Type I (polymicrobial) → gentamicin, clindamycin.

Type II (Group A S. pyogenes*) → penicillin, clindamycin.*

Gas gangrene → penicillin

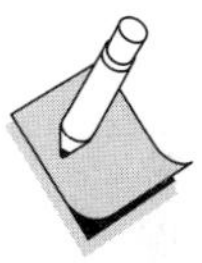

Risk factors for necrotizing infections–

Diabetes

Malnutrition

Obesity

Alcoholism

Lymphoma/leukemia

Vascular insufficiency

Steroid use

Cirrhosis

Human immunodeficiency virus (HIV)

POSTSPLENECTOMY SEPSIS

Occurs in < 1% of all patients after splenectomy. Infection is most frequently (80%) caused by **S. *pneumoniae***, although any encapsulated bacteria or parasite may precipitate sepsis. Because of their immature immune system, **children < 5 years of age are at greatest risk for sepsis**; daily prophylaxis with penicillin may be considered in this population. Encapsulated organisms often cause a **flulike prodrome**, which can quickly escalate to sepsis, shock, DIC, and organ failure. Initial treatment is with ceftriaxone (or vancomycin plus levofloxacin if penicillin-allergic).

BLOODBORNE VIRAL INFECTIONS

Transmission via transfusion is exceedingly rare (~1/3,000,000 units). Risk of HIV transmission after needlestick is low (0.3%), yet universal precautions are necessary. If **HIV exposure** is suspected, prophylactic therapy should be started within 4 hours. Risk of **hepatitis C virus (HCV)** infection after percutaneous exposure is greater (2%-3%). HCV prophylaxis is not available at this time.

Basic Pharmacology

DRUG PHARMACOKINETICS

Bioavailability is the effective portion of an administered medication that reaches the systemic circulation. **Volume of distribution** (V_d) is the theoretic volume over which a given dose of drug must be evenly distributed to yield a given plasma concentration. **Elimination** is the removal of pharmacologically active medication from the plasma either by metabolism to inactive product or by excretion.

Half-life ($t_{1/2}$) is the amount of time required for plasma level of a drug to fall by 50%. Half-life is determined by elimination as well as V_d. As lipid soluble drugs are eliminated from the plasma in the steady state, plasma concentration is quickly repleted (from fat stores) due to the concentration gradient (fat > plasma). Steady state plasma levels are achieved after the fourth or fifth $t_{1/2}$ regardless of administration regimen (infusion versus bolus).

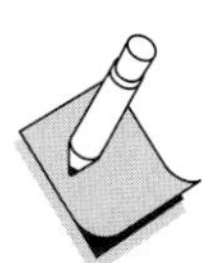

Splenectomy patients should receive pneumococcal, meningococcal, and H. influenzae *immunizations 2 weeks before surgery or after recuperation. Annual influenza vaccination should also be given.*

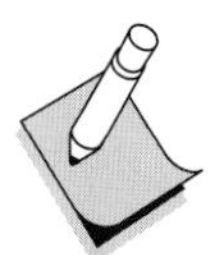

Volume of distribution–

V_d =

Dose administered / Plasma level of drug

Lipid-soluble drugs and those that poorly bind plasma protein will concentrate in the adipose tissue → ↓ plasma drug concentration → ↑ V_d.

Elimination can be of zero- or first-order kinetics. **Zero-order elimination** implies that a given amount of drug is eliminated per unit time. This occurs when the enzymatic pathway for elimination and metabolism becomes fully saturated, and higher plasma concentration does not result in ↑ elimination. **First-order elimination** implies that a constant fraction of the circulating drug is eliminated per unit of time.

Nonpolar molecules are minimally excreted by the body because of brisk reabsorption. Most **drug metabolism** involves transformation of fat-soluble (hydrophobic) substances into polar (hydrophilic) substances. These chemical changes usually result in hydrophilic, inactive molecules, though some metabolites are biologically functional (or toxic). Metabolism most commonly occurs in the **liver** but also occurs in the **kidney, lung, bowel wall,** and **in the circulation**.

Hepatic metabolism is primarily via the **cytochrome P-450** family of enzymes. This iron-dependent enzyme cascade is responsible for **conjugation** (ie, alkylation, hydroxylation, oxidation, methylation, deamination), **hydrolysis**, and **oxidation-reduction** of numerous pharmacologically active substances.

- **Common P-450 inducers**: Phenytoin, rifampin, nafcillin, carbamazepine, and phenobarbital.
- **Common P-450 inhibitors**: Diltiazem, verapamil, erythromycin, clarithromycin, fluconazole, itraconazole, ketoconazole, metoclopramide, allopurinol, and grapefruit juice.

Ethanol and aspirin are important drugs with zero-order elimination.

ANTIMICROBIAL MEDICATIONS

Antimicrobial medications are summarized in Table 3-9.

ANTIBIOTIC RESISTANCE

Seventy percent of hospital-acquired infections are caused by **antimicrobial-resistant bacteria**. Three basic mechanisms lead to resistance:

- Medication **cannot reach cellular target**: For example, bacterial wall porins (ie, protein channel through which antibiotics enter) are altered or absent, or drugs are actively expelled via an efflux pump. Can affect any antibiotic with an intracellular target (ie, those that act at the ribosome).
- Medication is **inactivated**: For example, bacteria may produce an enzyme or active site inhibitor, which prevents drug activity. Affects aminoglycosides and β-lactams.
- Medication's **cellular target is altered**: For example, bacterial site (surface or intracellular) may be physically changed or protected. Affects penicillins, quinolones, and macrolides.

Two important resistant bacteria are **MRSA** and **vancomycin-resistant** ***Enterococcus*** **(VRE)**.

- MRSA: Results from staphylococcal acquisition of genetic material that codes for a new penicillin-binding protein, which has a low affinity for penicillins. Now found to be community-acquired; in such cases, affects a younger, healthier population. Pathologic infections are treated with **vancomycin**. Carriers are treated with topical daptomycin or rifampin.
- VRE: Results from a single amino acid substitution (alanine → serine) on the enterococcus cell wall precursor (vancomycin-binding site). The gene for this resistance is carried on a **transposon**, rendering transmission to other bacteria possible. Treatment is with **linezolid**.

TABLE 3-9. **Properties of Selected Antimicrobials**

Antibiotic/Class	Activity	Mechanism	Excretion
Penicillins	-cidal	Bind penicillin-binding protein. Inhibit cell wall synthesis.	Renal
Cephalosporins	-cidal	Bind penicillin-binding protein. Inhibit cell wall synthesis.	Renal
Macrolides (eg, erythromycin)	-static	Act at ribosome (50s) to inhibit protein synthesis.	Hepatic
Lincosamides (eg, clindamycin)	-static	Act at ribosome (50s) to inhibit protein synthesis.	Hepatic
Carbapenems	-cidal	Bind penicillin-binding protein. Inhibit cell wall synthesis.	Renal
Quinolones	-cidal	Inhibit topoisomerase II and IV. Disrupt nucleic acid metabolism.	Renal, except moxifloxacin
Tetracyclines	-static	Acts at ribosome (30s) to inhibit protein synthesis.	Biliary accumulation; renal excretion
Glycopeptides (eg, vancomycin)	-cidal	Inhibit cell wall synthesis.	Renal
Aminoglycosides (eg, gentamicin)	Both	Acts at ribosome (30s) to inhibit protein synthesis. Disrupt cell wall synthesis.	Renal
Linezolid	-static	Act at ribosome (50s) to inhibit protein synthesis.	Metabolized in liver; excreted in urine
Chloramphenicol	-static	Acts at ribosome (50s) to inhibit protein synthesis.	Hepatic
Nucleic acid analogues (eg, acyclovir)		Selectively inhibits DNA polymerase.	Renal

▶ SAMPLE QUESTIONS

A 50-year-old male undergoes an exploratory laparotomy with colectomy. Six hours postoperatively, he has a temperature of 103.5°F with wound tenderness, erythema, and serous drainage. What organisms might be responsible?	*Clostridium perfringens*, β-hemolytic *Streptococcus*.
A 75-year-old woman has a prolonged hospital course following a bowel perforation. She reports "things don't taste right." Exam reveals a perioral rash. What is her likely nutrient deficiency?	Zinc.
During starvation, what supplies energy for the brain?	Ketones (from fatty acids).
A 25-year-old male sustains an injury. He has a documented allergy to lidocaine. What are options for local anesthesia?	Use an ester amide: benzocaine, cocaine, procaine, tetracaine, chloroprocaine.
A 20-year-old female with type I DM has a blood glucose of 500 mg/dL. Her Na^+ is 132 mEq/L. What is her corrected Na^+?	$132 + [(500 - 100) / 100] \times 1.6 =$ 138 mEq/L.
A 30-year-old male presents with an 80% total body surface area (TBSA) burn and a crush injury to the lower extremity. What muscle relaxant should be avoided?	Succinylcholine (depolarizing muscle relaxant that acts in noncompetitive manner). Contraindicated in burns, crush injuries, and paraplegia because of risk of hyperkalemic complications.
A 60-year-old male s/p liver transplant is found to have a $K^+ = 6.5$ mEq/L after an episode of nonsustained ventricular tachycardia. What is the next step in management?	Administer Ca^{2+} gluconate, perform stat repeat ECG, and repeat electrolytes. Correct K^+ with insulin (with glucose). Other options include β_2-agonist and sodium polystyrene. Discontinue offending agents (eg, tacrolimus).
Describe the benefits of epidural analgesia.	Pain relief, reduction of DVTs (total hip replacement, prostatectomy), reduction of pulmonary infections (thoracic, orthopaedic, abdominal operations), reduction of paralytic ileus (abdominal operations), enhanced vascular graft flow (major vascular operations).

What is the incidence of wound infection in a contaminated wound?	15-16%.
A 34-year-old female develops intraoperative tachycardia, tachypnea, HTN, arrhythmias, fever, ↑ $Pa\text{CO}_2$, and ↑ end tidal CO_2. What is your suspected diagnosis? Treatment?	Malignant hyperthermia. Administer dantrolene, perform cooling measures, correct hyperkalemia and acidosis.

CHAPTER 4

Esophagus

Alex Bernard Haynes, MD, MPH
Reviewed by Michael Lanuti, MD

Important congenital esophageal anomalies include–
Failure of separation of the dorsal foregut from the laryngeotracheal tree during development = tracheoesophageal fistula.
Failure of recanalization of tubular lumen = esophageal atresia, web, stenosis.
See Chapter 19 for more details.

Anatomic sites of esophageal narrowing–
ABCD:
Aortic arch
Bronchus (left main stem)
Cricopharyngeus
Diaphragm

Esophageal landmarks by endoscopic distances (from incisors)–
UES–15 cm
Thoracic inlet–18 cm
Aortic arch/Left mainstem bronchus–25 cm
LES/gastroesophageal junction (GEJ)–40 cm

▶ BASIC SCIENCE

Embryology

Esophageal development occurs primarily during the fourth week of gestation. The majority of the esophagus arises from the foregut, though the most proximal portion is derived from the pharyngeal apparatus.

Anatomy

MACROSCOPIC ANATOMY

Extends 18–25 cm from pharynx to stomach. Divided into cervical, thoracic, and abdominal regions.

- Cervical esophagus is ~5–6 cm and extends from the cricopharyngeus muscle (~C6) to thoracic inlet (~T1).
- Thoracic esophagus is ~15 cm and extends from the thoracic inlet (~T1) to esophageal hiatus of diaphragm (~T10).
- Abdominal esophagus is short (~5–6 cm) and may be absent in patients with a hiatal hernia or esophageal shortening from chronic inflammation.

The upper esophageal sphincter (UES) is created by the **cricopharyngeus** and innervated by the recurrent laryngeal nerve. The lower esophageal sphincter (LES) is **not an anatomic structure** but rather a functional zone. **Anatomic narrowing of the esophagus is present at the cricopharyngeus (narrowest region), left mainstem bronchus and aortic arch, and diaphragm.** These are the most common sites of foreign body impaction.

MICROSCOPIC ANATOMY

Esophageal wall is made of mucosa, submucosa, and muscularis and **lacks serosa.** Mucosa is composed of **nonkeratinizing, stratified squamous** epithelium except for the most distal few centimeters, which has columnar epithelium. Muscularis is divided into **outer longitudinal** and **inner circular** layers. Striated muscle is located in the upper one-third with smooth muscle in the remaining two-thirds.

BLOOD SUPPLY

Supplied by the inferior thyroid artery, descending thoracic aorta, bronchial arteries, left gastric artery, and inferior phrenic arteries. Extensive submucosal anastomotic plexus exists. Venous drainage is segmental to both systemic and portal systems.

INNERVATION

Vagus nerve provides parasympathetic innervation to the esophagus with **recurrent laryngeal branches** innervating the cricopharyngeus and cervical region. Sympathetic fibers arise from cervical and thoracic chain ganglia. The enteric nervous system, composed of the submucosal Meissner's plexus and myenteric Auerbach's plexus in the muscularis, coordinates swallowing.

Lymphatic Drainage

Submucosa contains rich, **nonsegmented** network of lymphatics with the upper two-thirds draining cephalad and lower one-third draining caudad.

Killian's triangle–
Site of cricopharyngeal weakness.
Most common location to find pseudodiverticula or iatrogenic perforation.

Physiology of Swallowing

The swallowing reflex is initiated by the central nervous system. Subsequent events include occlusion of the nasopharynx, elevation of the larynx with posterior displacement of the epiglottis to occlude the airway, relaxation of the cricopharyngeus, and pharyngeal relaxation as the bolus enters the esophagus. UES is tonically closed to limit air entry.

Primary peristalsis is an orderly wave, initiated by the bolus and the initiation of swallowing, propelling bolus to stomach. Secondary peristalsis occurs in the presence of esophageal distention. UES pressures are **50-70 mmHg at rest** and **12-14 mmHg with bolus**. LES is also referred to as the high-pressure zone, which prevents reflux of gastric contents into esophagus. Resting LES pressure is **10-20 mmHg**. LES relaxes with progression of peristalsis to permit entry of food to stomach.

A 35-year-old female presents with progressive heartburn and regurgitation of undigested food. She has a barium swallow that reveals a bird's beak tapering of the distal esophagus. What will her manometry studies show? Lack of peristalsis and failure of LES relaxation, consistent with achalasia.

*The esophagus **lacks serosa** and thus heals poorly after insult.*
*Esophageal submucosa is the **strongest layer** and of 1° importance for surgical repair.*

▶ CLINICAL SCIENCE

Achalasia

Demographics

Most common esophageal motility disorder. About 1–6 cases per 100,000 people diagnosed annually. Affects patients 25–60 years of age with equal distribution between genders. Characterized by **aperistalsis** and **failure of LES relaxation** during swallowing. **Not a 1° disorder**, as it is the result of neural degeneration.

Arterial supply to the esophagus–
Cervical esophagus supplied by inferior thyroid artery.
Thoracic esophagus supplied by aorta and bronchial arteries.
Abdominal esophagus supplied by left gastric and inferior phrenic arteries.

Signs/Symptoms

Patients most commonly present with **progressive dysphagia to solids and liquids**. May also present with heartburn, chest pain, and regurgitation of undigested food. Patients develop techniques to ameliorate dysphagia, often maintaining an upright position, keeping arms elevated over their heads, or consuming a liquid diet.

Diagnosis

Barium swallow reveals characteristic **bird's beak** tapering of distal esophagus with **dilation of proximal segment** (see Figure 4-1). Esophagoscopy is mandatory to rule out obstructing mass or stricture. Manometry reveals the characteristic **lack of peristalsis and failure of LES relaxation**. Resting LES pressures may be normal or high.

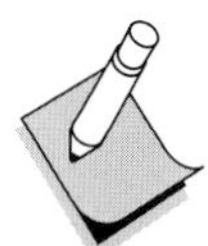

Esophageal sphincter pressures–

UES pressure (resting): 50–70 mmHg

UES pressure (bolus): 12–14 mmHg

LES pressure (resting): 10–20 mmHg

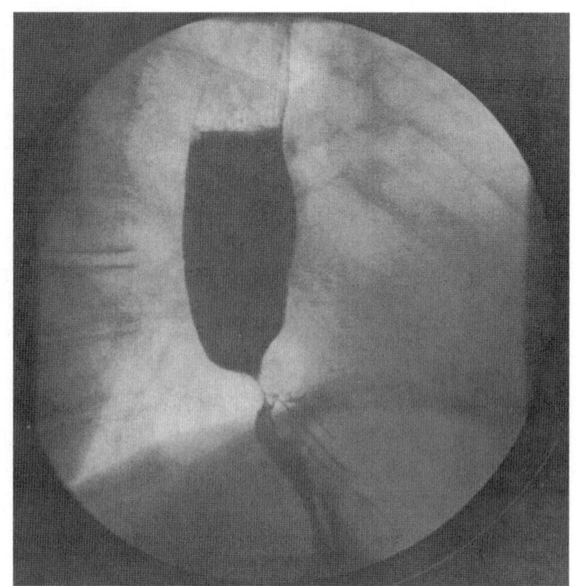

FIGURE 4-1. Esophageal achalasia. See also color insert.

(Reproduced, with permission, from Zinner MJ, Ashley SW. *Maingot's Abdominal Operations*, 11th ed. New York: McGraw-Hill, 2007.)

TREATMENT

Medical management with nitrates and Ca^{2+}-channel blockers are temporizing and associated with a number of side effects. Botulinum toxin injection into LES may provide temporary improvement but is not durable and makes future surgical intervention more difficult. Pneumatic dilation yields symptomatic improvement, but recurrence is high and risk of perforation is ~5%. **Heller myotomy is definitive therapy**; may be performed through chest or abdomen via open or videoendoscopic techniques. Myotomy must extend onto cardia and fully disrupt the LES. Reflux is common postoperatively, so concurrent fundoplication is often performed. In longstanding, severe achalasia, esophagus may be so dilated and nonfunctional (**sigmoid esophagus**) that esophagectomy is necessary.

Scleroderma

DEMOGRAPHICS

Rare disorder characterized by degeneration of smooth muscle, resulting in **LES failure** and **disordered peristalsis** of distal esophagus. Esophageal dysmotility affects ~80% of scleroderma patients, particularly women aged 40-50 years. Proximal **striated muscle is spared**.

SIGNS/SYMPTOMS

Associated with severe reflux (and esophagitis), dysphagia, and signs of scleroderma (eg, skin changes, sclerodactyly, calcinosis, Raynaud's, pulmonary HTN, renal impairment, telangiectasias).

DIAGNOSIS

Barium swallow reveals **dilated esophagus with distal narrowing.** Manometry reveals dysmotility or **aperistalsis of the distal esophagus** with ↑ **LES sphincter pressure.**

TREATMENT

Initial treatment with medical management includes H_2-blockers, proton pump inhibitors, and head of bed elevation. Surgical therapy is reserved for severe symptoms and loss of function and can include a fundoplication and gastroplasty (if a lengthening procedure is needed).

Diffuse Esophageal Spasm

Rare, 1° motility disorder characterized by **disordered, high-amplitude motility.** Predominant symptom is **substernal chest pain** that may radiate to the neck or upper extremities. **Dysphagia occurs with both solids and liquids.**

Diagnose with barium swallow, which demonstrates **corkscrew esophagus** and **segmentation** (see Figure 4-2). Manometry reveals **frequent, high-amplitude, simultaneous contractions** (≥ 20% of 10 simultaneous waveforms must demonstrate pathologic features) of esophageal body. LES is typically normal.

Medical therapy includes nitrates and Ca^{2+}-channel blockers. Botulinum toxin may relieve symptoms, but symptom recurrence is high. Pneumatic dilation is an alternative; risks are as for achalasia. Surgical therapy is indicated for intractable symptoms or the presence of esophageal diverticula. Long-segment myotomy provides relief of dysphagia in ~80% of cases but is not as successful in relief of chest pain.

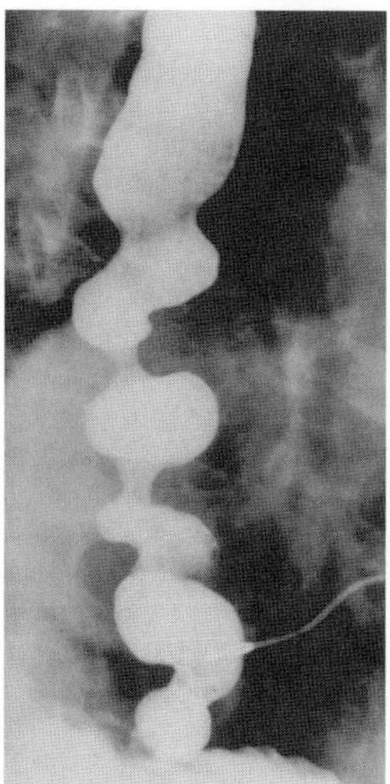

FIGURE 4-2. Diffuse esophageal spasm. See also color insert.

(Reproduced, with permission, from Brunicardi FC, et al. *Schwartz's Principles of Surgery*, 8th ed. New York: McGraw-Hill, 2005:88.)

Nutcracker Esophagus

Most common 1° esophageal motility disorder. Like diffuse esophageal spasm (DES), associated with substernal chest pain and dysphagia. Manometry demonstrates characteristic continuous, high-amplitude (> 2 standard deviations above normal) peristalsis. Treatment includes medical management to alleviate symptoms (see DES), but Heller myotomy may be used for refractory cases.

Esophageal Diverticula

Demographics

True diverticula (involving all layers of esophageal wall) or pseudodiverticula (involving mucosa only) are often found in association with other esophageal pathologies (eg, motility disorders, tumors). Increased incidence found with ↑ age.

Types

Differentiated by location.

- Pharyngoesophageal (Zenker's): **Pulsion diverticulum** usually found at Killian's triangle as a result of discoordination of UES relaxation and swallowing.
- Midesophageal: Either pulsion (because of motility disorders) or traction (because of extra-esophageal disease such as cancer or granulomatous infection).
- Epiphrenic: Most commonly caused by motility disorders, particularly achalasia. Commonly associated with gastroesophageal reflux disease (GERD) and occurs within 10 cm of the GEJ.

Signs/Symptoms

Often asymptomatic. May also present with regurgitation, halitosis, aspiration, chest pain, and dysphagia.

Diagnosis

Barium swallow demonstrates diverticulum. Manometry and pH studies reveal associated motility disorders and the presence of reflux. Esophagoscopy is necessary to rule out mechanical obstruction.

Treatment

If asymptomatic, no treatment is necessary. Perform **diverticulectomy with myotomy** to correct underlying motility disorder. Transoral stapled repairs may be option for Zenker's diverticula.

Esophageal Webs and Rings

May be congenital (incomplete recanalization) but are more commonly acquired. May involve all three layers (ie, mucosa, submucosa, muscularis) or only mucosa and submucosa. Patients are usually asymptomatic but can present with **dysphagia to solid food** or food impaction. May be associated with GERD (Schatzki's ring at the GEJ) or iron deficiency (webs of **Plummer-Vinson syndrome**). Barium swallow is diagnostic and should be followed by endoscopy to rule out malignancy. Therapy is indicated for symptomatic patients and includes gastric acid suppression, dietary modification, and esophageal dilation. Surgical therapy is rarely indicated.

The majority of paraesophageal hernias are type I (sliding hiatal).

Hiatal and Paraesophageal Hernias

DEMOGRAPHICS

More common in women. Incidence ↑ with ↑ age.

Cameron's ulcer–
Ulcer in a sliding hiatal hernia. Commonly found on the lesser curve. Associated with chronic blood loss but rarely with perforation.

TYPES

Paraesophageal hernias are caused by widening of the esophageal hiatus and subsequent herniation of intra-abdominal organs into the chest. Types II, III, and IV are paraesophageal hiatal hernias, while type I is a sliding hiatal hernia (see Table 4-1). In type II hernias, the GEJ remains intra-abdominal; in contrast, the GEJ herniates into the chest in types I, III, and IV.

SIGNS/SYMPTOMS

Often asymptomatic. May be related to GERD (especially type I). Chronic symptoms include dysphagia, early satiety, chest pain, and weight loss. **Cameron's ulcer** may cause bleeding and anemia. Incarceration and strangulation are rare but present with **Borchardt's triad** (ie, severe chest pain, painful retching without emesis, inability to pass a nasogastric tube [NGT]) and hemodynamic instability.

Borchardt's triad of an incarcerated paraesophageal hernia–
Severe chest pain
Painful retching without emesis
Inability to pass a NGT

DIAGNOSIS

Often found incidentally on upper endoscopy or CT. For paraesophageal hernias, auscultation may reveal bowel sounds in the chest. A CXR can demonstrate an air-fluid level in the chest and potentially, a coiled intrathoracic NGT. Barium swallow is diagnostic and useful for planning elective repair.

TABLE 4-1. Classification of Hiatal and Paraesophageal Hernias

TYPE	GEJ LOCATION	HERNIA CONTENTS	TYPE OF VOLVULUS
I (sliding hiatal)	Chest	GEJ +/- fundus	None
II (rolling paraesophageal)	Abdomen	Fundus	Organoaxial
III (mixed paraesophageal)	Chest	GEJ, fundus, body	Organoaxial or mesoaxial
IV (mixed paraesophageal)	Chest	GEJ, fundus, other abdominal organs	Organoaxial or mesoaxial

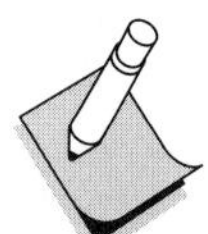

Regardless of approach and technique, all paraesophageal hernia repairs must involve hernia reduction, sac excision, and tension-free closure of the crural defect.

TREATMENT

Any patient with chest pain and a paraesophageal hernia must be treated as a surgical emergency (because of the potential risk of incarceration or strangulation). Elective repair is indicated for symptomatic patients with sliding hernias. Open or videoendoscopic techniques may be employed for transthoracic or transabdominal approaches. Transthoracic approach is preferred for chronic hernias. The classic teaching is that surgical repair is indicated for all asymptomatic paraesophageal hernias (due to possible risk of complications); current studies suggest this might not be necessary.

Mallory-Weiss Tears

Longitudinal tears in esophageal mucosa near the GEJ following **repeated retching** or other episodes of high intraluminal pressure. Commonly occur in **alcoholics**. Often associated with hiatal hernia and upper gastrointestinal bleed. Definitive diagnosis is by endoscopy. Episodes are usually self-limited and treated with supportive therapy. May occasionally necessitate endoscopic or angiographic therapy. Surgical intervention is rarely required and is reserved for bleeding that is unresponsive to other therapy.

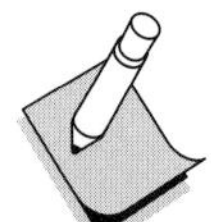

See Chapter 18 for a description of traumatic esophageal injuries.

Esophageal Perforations

DEMOGRAPHICS/RISK FACTORS

Most common cause of esophageal perforation is iatrogenic. Boerhaave's syndrome is the spontaneous rupture of the esophagus resulting from ↑ intra-abdominal pressure against a closed glottis, often during bouts of retching. Perforations may also be caused by malignancy or infection (eg, tuberculosis [TB]). More common in elderly and debilitated individuals; Most common location is in **distal thoracic esophagus**, with leak into the left chest.

SIGNS/SYMPTOMS

Most common presentation includes severe chest and back pain accompanied by dyspnea. Exam can reveal dullness to percussion of left chest, subcutaneous emphysema, tachycardia, hypotension, and severe sepsis with hemodynamic instability.

DIAGNOSIS

CXR may show **pneumomediastinum**, subcutaneous emphysema, left hydropneumothorax, or simple effusion. **Gastrograffin swallow** demonstrates leak. CT demonstrates extraluminal fluid and air in chest; oral contrast may help elucidate the location of the leak. Though esophagoscopy may worsen the perforation, it can localize the site of injury.

TREATMENT

Broad spectrum antibiotics, cessation of oral intake, and vigorous fluid resuscitation are essential. Drainage of pleural effusions and decompression of pneumothorax are mandatory. Most common operative therapy is irrigation and drainage of the pleural cavity with 1° repair of the perforation. If 1° repair is performed, reinforce with intercostal, pleural, or pericardial flap. In some perforations with delayed presentation or with associated esophageal pathology (eg, malignancy, severe stricture, end-stage achalasia), perform esophagectomy with immediate or delayed reconstruction. If delayed, esophageal diversion (eg, spit fistula) with placement of feeding jejunostomy is initially performed, followed by a second procedure to reestablish gastrointestinal continuity (eg, gastric pull-up, colonic interposition).

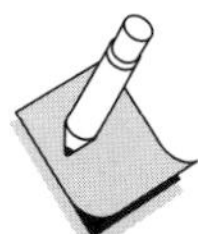

Stable patients without evidence of free pleural or peritoneal perforation or other underlying esophageal pathology may be treated conservatively.

Caustic Injuries

Alkali agents cause **liquefactive necrosis**; acids cause **coagulation necrosis.** Injuries most commonly occur in pediatric, mentally ill, and elderly populations. May be asymptomatic even with significant injury. Symptoms can include chest or abdominal pain and odynophagia. If full thickness injury occurs, signs and symptoms of perforation are present. Flexible esophagoscopy helps determine the extent of injury. **Always assess the airway and secure if necessary. Do not attempt to neutralize offending agent.** Asymptomatic patients can be observed. Patients with mild injury should be hospitalized and kept NPO for 1-2 days. Patients with full thickness injuries should be made NPO and started on total parenteral nutrition (TPN) and antibiotics. Plans should be made for esophageal resection with either delayed or immediate reconstruction. Any degree of injury may result in future strictures or squamous cell carcinoma (SCC). Alkali injuries have a worse prognosis.

> A 58-year-old man with a long history of GERD undergoes an endoscopy with biopsy. Pathology reveals mild dysplasia. What is the recommended followup? Endoscopic surveillance with biopsies at least every 2 years to monitor for development of dysplasia.

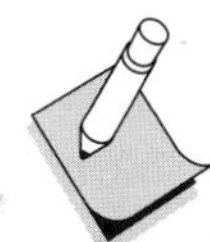

Endoscopic surveillance with biopsies every 2 years is mandatory in all patients with Barrett's to monitor for development of dysplasia.

Barrett's Esophagus

Premalignant condition characterized by **intestinal metaplasia** of the normal esophageal squamous mucosa. **Primary risk factor is GERD**; occurs in ~5-10% of patients with reflux. Symptoms are similar to those of GERD (see Chapter 5); signs of progressive disease can include worsening or persistent heartburn, dysphagia, unintentional weight loss, or hematemesis. Diagnose with endoscopy with random or directed biopsies. Correction of GERD by medical or surgical therapy prevents development of Barrett's or slows its progression, if it has already developed. Endoscopic surveillance with biopsies at least every 2 years is mandatory in all patients with Barrett's to monitor for development of dysplasia. **If severe dysplasia is present, perform esophagectomy, as severe dysplasia is associated with an ↑ risk of adenocarcinoma.**

20-50% of resected Barrett's specimens with severe dysplasia have adenocarcinoma on pathologic review.

Squamous Cell Carcinoma of the Esophagus

Previously the most common esophageal malignancy, though now adenocarcinoma is more common in the United States. Risk factors include tobacco or alcohol use, achalasia, alkali injury, and Plummer-Vinson syndrome. More common in elderly males. Signs and symptoms include **progressive dysphagia**, odynophagia, chest pain, dyspnea, weight loss, and fatigue. Barium swallow reveals narrowing. Esophagoscopy with biopsy is diagnostic. CT, positron emission tomography (PET), and endoscopic ultrasound can be used for staging. See Esophageal Adenocarcinoma section for details on staging and treatment.

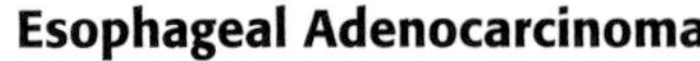

Esophageal Adenocarcinoma

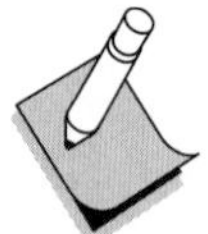

Benign lesions and motility disorders are associated with smooth narrowing of the esophagus. Malignant lesions demonstrate an irregular, apple core appearance.

DEMOGRAPHICS/RISK FACTORS

Most common esophageal malignancy in the United States. Primary risk factors are **GERD** and **Barrett's esophagus** (especially with severe dysplasia). Most common in middle aged males.

SIGNS/SYMPTOMS

Similar to SCC of the esophagus.

DIAGNOSIS

Barium swallow demonstrates characteristic malignant stricture. Esophagoscopy and biopsy confirm diagnosis. **CT, PET, and endoscopic ultrasound are used to stage disease.**

TREATMENT

Quick review of esophageal cancer therapy–
Stages I, IIA: Surgery (some T3N0 also receive neoadjuvant therapy)
Stages IIB, III: Chemoradiation (often neoadjuvant) plus surgery
Stage IV: Palliation (eg, esophageal stent)

Stage of disease determines treatment.

Surgical therapy involves resection of the tumor with negative margins, clearance of regional lymph nodes, and reconstruction with a tension-free, well-vascularized anastomosis. Various approaches to esophagectomy are summarized in Table 4-2.

The transhiatal approach avoids the morbidity of a thoracotomy but involves extensive blind dissection. Cervical anastomoses have lower morbidity if leaks occur. Concomitant jejunostomy tube placement allows early enteral nutrition. Minimally invasive approaches using laparoscopic and thoracoscopic techniques have been developed and are increasingly employed.

Esophagectomy-associated mortality at experienced centers is low (< 3%), and **most commonly is the result of pulmonary complications.** Postesophagectomy **pneumonia** results in the greatest morbidity. Anastomotic leaks are a major

TABLE 4-2. Surgical Approaches to Esophagectomy

APPROACH	INCISION(S)	ANASTOMOSIS LOCATION
Transhiatal	Laparotomy, neck	Neck
Ivor-Lewis	Laparotomy, right thoracotomy	Chest
Thoracoabdominal	Left thoracotomy	Chest
"Three hole"	Laparotomy, right thoracotomy, neck	Neck

source of morbidity (0-25%) with **worse outcomes if the leak occurs in the chest rather than the neck**. Small, contained leaks may be managed conservatively with antibiotics and NPO status. Larger leaks require drainage via interventional radiology or surgical debridement. If surgery is chosen, leaks without conduit necrosis may be managed by reinforced repair. Unstable patients or those with necrotic conduits should undergo resection of conduit and cervical esophagostomy with delayed reconstruction. Anastomotic stricture is common long-term complication (15-30%) and can be managed with endoscopic dilation(s).

Treatment of stage IIB or higher disease involves chemoradiation (commonly as neoadjuvant therapy). Some T3N0 (stage IIA) tumors also receive neoadjuvant therapy. Tumors that invade other organs may be resected en bloc if there is no evidence of distant spread. Primary chemoradiation is used for unresectable stage III tumors. Patients with metastatic disease or with tumors that erode into unresectable structures should be treated with palliative efforts: chemoradiation, intraluminal stenting, or ablation of tumor with laser or photodynamic therapy.

STAGING/OUTCOMES

Tumor, node status, metastasis (TNM) categories include

- T: T1 (invasion into lamina propria or submucosa), T2 (invasion into muscularis), T3 (invasion into adventitia), T4 (invasion into adjacent organs)
- N: N0 (- regional lymph nodes), N1 (+ regional lymph nodes)
- M: M0 (metastatic disease absent), M1 (metastatic disease present)

Staging includes

- Stage I: T1N0M0
- Stage IIA: T2-3N0M0
- Stage IIB: T1-2N1M0
- Stage III: T3N1M0 *or* T4, any N, M0
- Stage IV: Any T, any N, M1

Five-year survival varies from 80% for stage I, to 40% for stage II, and 10% for stage III disease. Five-year survival for patients undergoing esophagectomy is ~25%. There are no significant differences in survival between adenocarcinoma and SCC.

Majority of patients present with stage III disease.

▶ SAMPLE QUESTIONS

What layer is essential to esophageal anastomoses? Which layer is absent?	Submucosa is essential in repair. Esophagus lacks serosa.
A 50-year-old man develops an esophageal perforation. Where is the most common site of esophageal perforation during endoscopy? After repeated vomiting?	Endoscopy: Killian's triangle. Postemetic: Distal thoracic esophagus.
What are risk factors for SCC of the esophagus? Adenocarcinoma?	SCC: Tobacco use, alcohol, caustic injury, Plummer-Vinson syndrome. Adenocarcinoma: Chronic GERD, Barrett's esophagus, obesity.
What is the order of preference of conduit for esophageal reconstruction?	Stomach > colon > jejunum.
A 45-year-old man presents with progressive dysphagia to solids. What is the first diagnostic study?	Barium swallow.
What is the indication for esophagectomy in a patient with Barrett's esophagus?	Severe (high-grade) dysplasia on biopsy.
What is the main blood supply of the thoracic esophagus?	Branches from aorta and bronchial arteries.
What are manometric hallmarks of achalasia? DES?	Achalasia: Aperistalsis and failure of LES relaxation. DES: Disordered, high amplitude contractions.
What are long-term complications of caustic injury to the esophagus?	Stricture, SCC.
What determines resectability of esophageal malignancy?	Freedom from distant metastases or distant nodal involvement; ability to resect any adjacent, involved structures.
A 77-year-old female presents with severe chest pain, intractable retching, and inability to pass a NGT. What is her likely diagnosis? Treatment?	Incarcerated or strangulated paraesophageal hernia. Emergent surgical repair is necessary.
An 80-year-old man with dysphagia presents with aspiration pneumonia. For his esophageal study, what is the contrast agent of choice?	Nonionic (H_2O soluble) agent to minimize risk of pneumonitis.

A 30-year-old male has chest pain and dyspnea after upper endoscopy. What CXR findings suggest esophageal perforation?	Pneumomediastinum, subcutaneous emphysema, hydropneumothorax, pleural effusion.
What are the benefits of laparoscopic Heller myotomy with partial fundoplication compared to left thoracoscopic myotomy, for the treatment of achalasia?	↓ Length of stay and ↓ postopera tive reflux.
A 50-year-old man ingests a foreign body. Where are the most common locations where the foreign body may become impacted?	At the cricopharyngeus, at the level of the aortic arch or left mainstem bronchus, or at the diaphragmatic hiatus.
A 30-year-old male is incidentally found to have a Zenker's diverticulum. What is the appropriate treatment?	None if asymptomatic. If symptoms are present, surgical excision via neck or transoral stapling.
What is normal resting pressure of the LES? UES?	LES: 10-20 mm Hg. UES: 50-70 mm Hg.

CHAPTER 5

Stomach

Kaitlyn J. Kelly, MD
Reviewed by Vivian E. Strong, MD

▶ BASIC SCIENCE

Embryology

At the fifth gestational week, the embryonic stomach is suspended by ventral and dorsal mesenteries and develops as a dilated portion of the tubular embryonic foregut. By the seventh week, the stomach dilates further with the left side growing faster than the right to form the greater and lesser curvatures, respectively. This asymmetric growth causes rotation of the stomach into its normal anatomic position.

Anatomy

MACROSCOPIC ANATOMY

Divided into five segments: cardia, fundus, corpus, antrum, and pylorus.

- **Cardia:** Immediately distal to the gastroesophageal junction. Most proximal portion of the stomach.
- **Fundus:** Most superior portion of stomach; separated from esophagus by the cardial notch or **angle of His.** Highly distensible.
- **Corpus (body):** Extends from the fundus to pylorus. Largest portion of stomach.
- **Antrum:** Begins at the **angularis incisura** as a wider area that leads into a narrower pyloric canal and sphincter.
- **Pylorus:** Includes the pyloric sphincter, which controls release of gastric contents into duodenum.

MICROSCOPIC ANATOMY

Four layers include mucosa, submucosa, muscularis propria, and serosa.

- **Mucosa:** Composed of epithelium, lamina propria, and muscularis mucosa. Epithelium is composed of **simple columnar cells** with gastric pits that lead into deep glands. Each gastric segment has a characteristic glandular composition and structure (see Table 5-1). The lamina propria is a small connective tissue layer, which contains the vascular supply for the epithelium. The muscularis mucosa is a thin muscle layer that leads to formation of characteristic rugae or longitudinal folds.
- **Submucosa: Strongest layer of the gastric wall.** Composed of connective tissue and Meissner's plexus.
- **Muscularis propria (muscularis externa):** Composed of three smooth muscle sublayers including an **inner (oblique) layer unique to the stomach,** middle (circular) layer that thickens at the pylorus to form a sphincter, and an outer (longitudinal) layer that is continuous with the outer longitudinal muscle of esophagus. Auerbach's plexus is embedded in this layer.
- **Serosa:** Composed of visceral peritoneum.

Specialized cell types of the stomach include

- **Chief cells:** Forty-four percent of the gastric epithelium. Produce pepsinogen in response to food and acetylcholine. Pepsinogen is activated to pepsin at $pH < 5$. Pepsin cleaves peptide bonds breaking proteins into peptides and amino acids.
- **Parietal (oxyntic) cells:** Thirteen percent of gastric epithelium. Secrete HCl and intrinsic factor (IF). IF binds to vitamin B_{12}, facilitating its absorption at the terminal ileum.

TABLE 5-1. Gastric Glandular Distribution

ANATOMIC SEGMENT	GLANDULAR COMPOSITION	GLANDULAR STRUCTURE	1° CONTRIBUTION TO GASTRIC JUICE
Cardia	Surface epithelial cells,* mucous cells.	Cardiac glands: Nonbranching. Connected to short pits.	Mucous, HCO_3^-.
Fundus	Mucous cells, some parietal cells and chief cells.	Oxyntic glands: Tubular, some branching. Multiple glands empty into single pit.	Mucous, HCO_3^-, some HCl and IF.
Corpus	Mucous cells, parietal cells, chief cells, ECL cells, D cells.	Oxyntic glands (as in fundus).	HCl, IF, pepsinogen, mucous.
Antrum/ Pylorus	Mucous cells, G cells, some D cells.	Pyloric glands: Straight. Empty into deep pits.	Mucous, HCO_3^-, gastrin, somatostatin.

*Surface epithelial cells are distributed diffusely throughout gastric mucosa.

Quick review of gastric cells and their products–
Chief cells: Pepsinogen
Parietal cells: HCl, IF
Mucous neck cells: Mucous, HCO_3^-
G cells: Gastrin
D cells: Somatostatin
Enterochromaffin cells: Serotonin
Enterochromaffin-like cells: Histamine

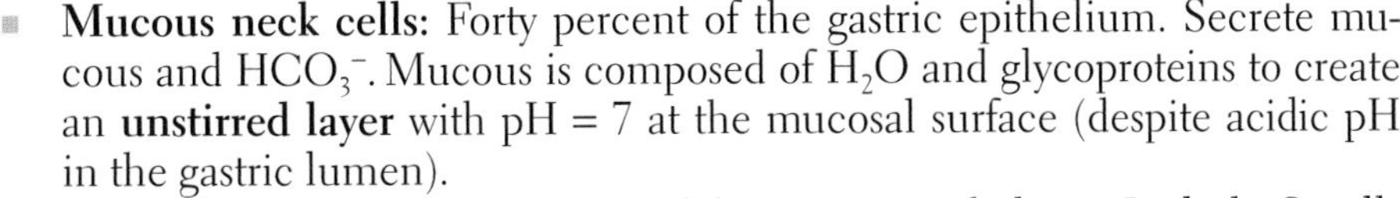

- **Mucous neck cells:** Forty percent of the gastric epithelium. Secrete mucous and HCO_3^-. Mucous is composed of H_2O and glycoproteins to create an **unstirred layer** with pH = 7 at the mucosal surface (despite acidic pH in the gastric lumen).
- **Endocrine cells:** Three percent of the gastric epithelium. Include G cells (secrete gastrin), D cells (secrete somatostatin), enterochromaffin cells (Kulchitsky cells; secrete serotonin), and enterochromaffin-like cells (ECL; secrete histamine).

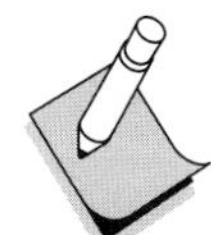

Left gastric vein is also called the coronary vein.

BLOOD SUPPLY

Arterial supply to the stomach is a highly anastomotic system. Specific vessels include

- **Left gastric artery:** Originates from the celiac axis. Supplies the proximal portion of the lesser curvature and gives off small branches to the diaphragm and distal esophagus.
- **Right gastric artery:** Originates from the common or proper hepatic artery. Supplies the distal portion of the lesser curvature.
- **Left gastroepiploic artery:** Originates from the splenic artery. Supplies the proximal portion of the greater curvature.
- **Right gastroepiploic artery:** Originates from the gastroduodenal artery (GDA). Supplies the distal greater curvature and pylorus.
- **Short gastric arteries:** Originate from the splenic artery. Contribute to the blood supply of the proximal stomach.

Venous system closely parallels the arterial supply and ultimately, all veins drain into the portal system. The right and left gastric veins drain into the portal vein directly, the right gastroepiploic vein drains into the splenic vein, and the left gastroepiploic vein drains into the superior mesenteric vein.

Clinical relevance of the left gastric vein–
Left gastric vein communicates with the portal system (via the portal vein) and the systemic venous system (via the esophageal plexus). Involved in the development of portal HTN-induced esophageal varices.

Relations of the left vagus live in **LA:**
Left vagus runs **A**nterior to stomach.
Laterjet nerve comes off **A**nteriorly.

INNERVATION

Vagus nerve supplies acetylcholine-mediated, parasympathetic innervation. Celiac plexus supplies sympathetic innervation. Enteric nervous system is composed of Auerbach's and Meissner's plexuses. Acetylcholine, serotonin, substance P, bombesin, cholecystokinin (CCK), nitric oxide, vasoactive intestinal peptide (VIP), and somatostatin are involved in signal transmission for this system.

***Right vagus** runs posterior to stomach and gives off **Criminal nerve of Grassi**. If undivided during vagotomy → recurrent ulcers.*

LYMPHATIC DRAINAGE

Sixteen lymph node stations, grouped by location and level of cancer extension, are defined. Stations incorporate specific nodal basins along the perigastric (lesser and greater curvature), left gastric artery, common hepatic artery, celiac trunk, splenic hilum, splenic artery, hepatoduodenal ligament, mesenteric root, para-aortic, and paracolic regions. The locations of the nodes help guide lymphadenectomy during gastric resection for cancer.

Extent of lymphadenectomy during gastric resection–

D1: Perigastric nodes (greater and lesser curve)
- *Stations 2, 4, 6–Greater curve*
- *Stations 1, 3, 5–Lesser curve*

D2: Nodes around left gastric artery, common hepatic artery, celiac axis, splenic hilum, splenic artery

D3: Hepatoduodenal ligament and mesenteric root nodes

D4: Para-aortic and paracolic nodes

Gastrointestinal Hormones

A number of gastrointestinal (GI) hormones are present and critical for the interactions between organs as well as for independent organ function (see Table 5-2).

Gastric Physiology

Stomach secretes up to 1500 mL daily during fasting and up to 1000 mL after meals. Fluid composition varies with food intake, but general components include high levels H^+ and Cl^- as well as Na^+, K^+, HCO_3^-, IF, mucous, and digestive enzymes (eg, pepsinogen).

Gastric Acid Secretion

Gastric acid secretion by the parietal cells is stimulated by histamine, gastrin, and acetylcholine (see Table 5-3). HCl release is inhibited by secretin, prostaglandins (eg, PGE2), and somatostatin. **Somatostatin and PGE_2 inhibit the cyclic adenosine monophosphate (cAMP) pathway.** H^+ is driven extracellularly via the H^+-K^+ ATPase pump.

A basal level of HCl secretion is maintained by histamine and acetylcholine. Meal-induced HCl release occurs in three phases:

- **Cephalic:** Sight, smell, or thought of food stimulates vagally mediated release of acetylcholine and ultimately, the release of HCl, pepsinogen, and gastrin.
- **Gastric: Responsible for the majority of HCl release.** As food enters the stomach, gastric distention (vagally-mediated) and the presence of amino acids and peptides (gastrin-mediated) stimulate HCl release.
- **Intestinal:** Begins as chyme enters duodenum and continues until the proximal SI is empty. Mechanism of HCl release is not clear.

Motility of the Stomach

As food enters the stomach, the vagus stimulates **receptive relaxation**, whereby smooth muscle is inhibited, and the proximal stomach relaxes to accommodate and store the bolus. Slow, sustained contractions drive the bolus into the distal stomach where mixing and grinding occurs. At this point, small portions pass through the pylorus. Larger clusters remain in the stomach and ultimately enter the duodenum in response to the migrating myoelectric complex (MMC) (see Chapter 6).

TABLE 5-2. Gastrointestinal Hormones

Hormone	Source	Stimulating Factors	1° Functions
Gastrin	**Antrum,** duodenum (G cells).	Peptides, amino acids, free fatty acids, vagal stimulation.	Stimulates gastric acid (HCl), pepsinogen, pancreatic enzyme secretion. Stimulates lower esophageal sphincter (LES). Relaxes pyloric sphincter. Trophic effects on GI mucosa.
CCK	**Duodenum,** jejunum, ileum (I cells).	Fatty acids, amino acids, HCl.	Stimulates gallbladder contraction/emptying, sphincter of Oddi relaxation, pancreatic enzyme release. Inhibits gastric emptying.
Secretin	Duodenum (S cells).	HCl.	Stimulates pancreaticobiliary HCO_3^- and H_2O secretion. Inhibits gastric acid secretion.
Gastrin-releasing peptide (bombesin)	Neurons of antral and small intestine (SI) mucosal cells.	Vagal stimulation.	**Stimulates** release of all GI hormones (except secretin). Stimulates GI motility.
Somatostatin	**Antrum,** pancreatic islets, throughout intestine (D cells).	Fat, protein, HCl, glucose, CCK, gastrin.	**Inhibits** release of all GI secretions/hormones. Modulates glucagon and insulin. Inhibits GI motility.
Motilin	Duodenum.	Alkaline pH.	Stimulates gastric activity. Regulates gastric emptying.
Gastric inhibitory polypeptide	Duodenum, proximal jejunum (K cells).	Bombesin-like peptides, fats.	**Stimulates insulin secretion.** Inhibits gastric acid secretion.
VIP	Neurons of enteric nervous system.	Enteric nervous system.	Stimulates vasodilation, smooth muscle relaxation, intestinal secretion, bile secretion. Inhibits gastric secretion. Inhibits gastric acid secretion. Inhibits GI motility.
Substance P	Neurons of all layers of gut wall.		Modulates gut smooth muscle.

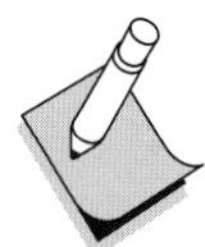

Histamine-induced ↑ HCl–
Activated adenylate cyclase →↑ cAMP → PKA activation

TABLE 5-3. Gastric Acid Release Stimulators

MEDIATOR	SOURCE	MECHANISM OF RELEASE
Acetylcholine	Vagus nerve	Inositol phospholipid (IP_3) activation →↑ **intracellular Ca^{2+}** → protein kinase C (PKC) activation.
Gastrin	G cells	Inositol phospholipid (IP_3) activation →↑ **intracellular Ca^{2+}** → PKC activation.
Histamine	ECL cells	Activated adenylate cyclase →↑ **cAMP** → **protein kinase A (PKA) activation.**

1° digestive role of the stomach–
Regulation of gastric contents entering the duodenum

Etiologies of stress gastritis–**3 S's** of Stre**SS**:
Sepsis
Shock
Severe Burn

▶ CLINICAL SCIENCE

Gastritis

DEMOGRAPHICS/RISK FACTORS

Inflammation of the stomach due to a number of inflammatory, infectious, and chemical causes. Causes, signs, symptoms, and treatment are type specific (see Table 5-4).

A 37-year-old man presents with a 2-month history of gnawing epigastric pain relieved by eating. He is found to be mildly anemic; an RUQ ultrasound is negative for cholelithiasis. An upper endoscopy reveals a duodenal ulcer. Mucosal biopsies are performed; a rapid urease assay is positive. What is the appropriate management for his peptic ulcer disease (PUD)? Treat with a 2-week course of lansoprazole, metronidazole, and amoxicillin. Repeat a urease breath test after completion of therapy to confirm eradication of *Helicobacter pylori.*

Peptic Ulcer Disease

DEMOGRAPHICS/RISK FACTORS

Involves mucosal erosions of the stomach and duodenum. Diagnosed in about 1.8% of the U.S. population annually. Gastric ulcers occur predominantly in men aged 40-60 years, while duodenal ulcers tend to occur in a younger population aged 25-40 years of age. Major causes include excessive HCl secretion (particularly in the setting of compromised mucosal barrier; eg, Zollinger-Ellison syndrome [ZES]), *H. pylori* infection, stress, chemical ingestion, and use of NSAIDs, tobacco, or alcohol.

TYPES

Differentiated by location.

- **Gastric:** About 60-90% are associated with *H. pylori* infection. NSAID ingestion contributes more to gastric disease than to duodenal disease. Must

TABLE 5-4. Types of Gastritis

Type	Etiologies	Signs/Symptoms	Diagnosis	Treatment
Erosive	Toxic substances (nonsteroidal anti-inflammatory drugs [NSAIDs], alcohol, drugs)	Abdominal pain, upper GI (UGI) bleeding, perforation (rare)	Endoscopy	Remove causative agents. Anti-acid therapy with H^+-pump inhibitor (PPI) or H_2-blocker, vagotomy with pyloroplasty for severe cases.
Alkaline reflux	Alkaline bile refluxes into the stomach → irritation and mucosal inflammation. Common after pyloroplasty or Billroth II.	Postprandial abdominal pain, often severe	Endoscopy with biopsy	Reconstruction with Roux-en-Y gastrojejunostomy
Stress- or central nervous system (CNS) injury-related≥	Sepsis, shock, burns involving > 30% total body surface area (TBSA; **Curling's ulcer**) → mucosal ischemia. Central nervous system tumor/trauma (**Cushing's ulcer**) →↑ gastrin, HCl hypersecretion	UGI bleeding	Endoscopy with or without biopsy	IV-fluid resuscitation, anti-acid therapy
Pernicious anemia	Vitamin B_{12} deficiency.	Weight loss, megaloblastic anemia	Endoscopy with biopsy	Administer IF. If severe, total gastrectomy with parenteral vitamin B_{12} administration

always rule out an **ulcerated gastric adenocarcinoma.** Subtypes are summarized in Table 5-5. Type I lesions are associated with blood type A; types II-IV are associated with blood type O.

- **Duodenal: Most common type.** About 90% of cases occur in the setting of *H. pylori* infection.

Type **I** gastric ulcers are **#1:**
Most common.
Associated with blood type A (**I**[st] letter of alphabet).
Type **II** gastric ulcers
2 types of ulcers: Gastric and duodenal.

Signs/Symptoms

Most commonly associated with burning epigastric abdominal pain that, unlike pancreatitis pain, does not radiate. **Food tends to exacerbate gastric ulcer pain,** while it tends to **relieve duodenal ulcer pain**. Complications include bleeding with or without hematemesis or melena (can involve the **GDA**), obstruction, or perforation (commonly **posterior**). Massive hemorrhage can be associated with hemodynamic instability; perforation may be associated with severe epigastric pain, hemodynamic instability, and peritoneal signs.

Diagnosis

UGI contrast study is the most cost-effective diagnostic test. UGI endoscopy is more expensive but allows for obtaining a biopsy, particularly when cancer

Perforations occur posteriorly. Hemorrhage involves the GDA.

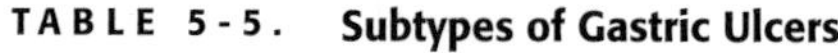

TABLE 5-5. Subtypes of Gastric Ulcers

TYPE	LOCATION	ETIOLOGY
Type I	Distal portion of lesser curvature	Nl / ↓ HCl
Type II	Distal portion of lesser curvature. **Associated with duodenal ulcer**	↑ HCl
Type III	Prepyloric or pyloric	↑ HCl
Type IV	Proximal portion of lesser curvature	Nl / ↓ HCl
Type V (medication-induced; eg, NSAIDs)	Anywhere	Nl HCl

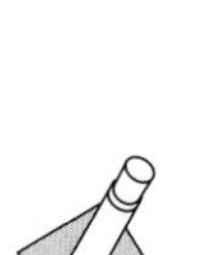

General rule for PUD surgeries–
The smaller, less anatomically altering the procedure (eg, HSV) → ↓ morbidity/mortality and ↑ ulcer recurrence.

must be ruled out. All patients should have an *H. pylori* assessment: serology and endoscopy with biopsy (including rapid urease assay, histology, culture).

TREATMENT

Mainstay is avoidance of causative agents including cessation of NSAIDs and eradication of *H. pylori* infection (ie, triple therapy with a PPI and two antibiotics, usually two of the following: clarithromycin, amoxicillin, or metronidazole). Acid-blocking therapy with a PPI or H_2-blocker should be initiated. Surgery is indicated for refractory or recurrent disease or for complications (eg, perforation, obstruction, uncontrollable bleeding). Specific surgical options are summarized in Table 5-6. **All gastric ulcers must be biopsied to rule out gastric adenocarcinoma.**

A 25-year-old man presents with intermittent, burning epigastric pain. He endorses longstanding diarrhea and unintentional weight loss. His past medical history is significant for nephrolithiasis. Labs reveal hypercalcemia, anemia, and serum gastrin = 1350 pg/mL. What is this patient's likely diagnosis? Management? The patient likely has multiple endocrine neoplasia I (MEN-1) syndrome. Consider four gland parathyroidectomy with autotransplantation for his hyperparathyroidism. Treat his gastrinoma medically with PPIs.

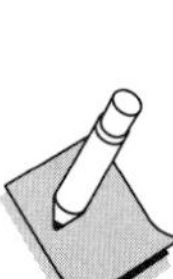

Postvagotomy syndromes–
Diarrhea: Explosive, bilious diarrhea not associated with food intake. Treat with cholestyramine or if refractory, reverse-segment jejunal interposition.
Gastric atony: Inability to empty solids from stomach. Treat with promotility agents (eg, erythromycin, metoclopramide).

Zollinger–Ellison Syndrome

Rare disorder caused by gastrin-secreting tumor (ie, gastrinoma). Approximately 65% are malignant and half are multiple; up to 25% occur in the setting of MEN-1 syndrome. Gastric acid hypersecretion results in severe, intractable, and often multiple ulcers. Diarrhea, weight loss, steatorrhea, and signs of MEN-1 syndrome may be present. Diagnosis is confirmed with **serum gastrin levels > 1000 pg/mL and an ↑ in serum gastrin level > 200 pg/mL after a secretin challenge.** Endoscopy will reveal mucosal hypertrophy and an ulcer, commonly at the proximal duodenum. Localize lesion with abdominal CT or MRI, endoscopic ultrasound, or an **octreotide scan**. The lesion will usually be located at the **gastrinoma triangle**: pancreatic neck, porta hepatis, and third portion of

TABLE 5-6. Surgical Options for PUD

Types	Indications	Gastric Effects	Advantages	Disadvantages
Truncal vagotomy, pyloroplasty	Gastric or duodenal ulcers	↑ Liquid emptying rate	Quick and technically easy. Good for unstable patients	Diarrhea, dumping. 10% recurrence
Truncal vagotomy, antrectomy	Gastric or duodenal ulcers	↑ Liquid emptying rate	**Lowest recurrence rate** (0-2%)	Diarrhea, dumping. Requires reconstruction. **1% mortality**
Highly selective vagotomy (HSV)	Gastric or duodenal ulcers (except type III)	Nl / ↑ liquid emptying rate. Unlike solid emptying after truncal vagotomy, post-HSV solid emptying is nl. ↓ Receptive relaxation, ↑ satiety	Preservation of pyloro-antral function	Not effective for type III ulcers. 15-20% recurrence
Subtotal gastrectomy	Intractable pain, bleeding, perforation, obstruction	↑ Liquid emptying rate. Early satiety, gastroesophageal reflux disease (GERD)	**Curative.** Prevents development of malignancy	Requires reconstruction

the duodenum. Medical therapy includes PPIs. Surgical resection is indicated for isolated duodenal wall lesions identified on preoperative imaging studies and is generally avoided in patients with MEN-1.

Clinical triad of ZES–

Hypersecretion of HCl

Severe PUD

Gastrinoma

Dieulafoy's Lesion

Large, tortuous, submucosal artery usually in the proximal stomach. Pulsations cause ulceration of the overlying mucosa, leading to intraluminal bleeding. Endoscopy is diagnostic and therapeutic (eg, electrocoagulation, photocoagulation, sclerotherapy, band ligation, clipping); embolization may also be effective. Open or laparoscopic surgery can be performed with wedge resection of the offending area if nonsurgical therapies fail.

Non-ZES causes of hypergastrinemia–

Gastric outlet obstruction

Anemia (pernicious)

PPI

Gastritis (atrophic)

Antrum (retained/excluded)

Renal failure

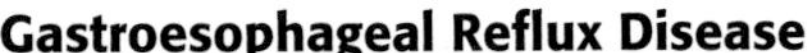

Gastroesophageal Reflux Disease

Demographics/Risk Factors

Most common pathology of the esophagus affecting people of all ages. Due to the transient or permanent loss of the gastroesophageal barrier (ie, LES) with subsequent retrograde flow of gastric contents into the esophagus. Risk factors include ↑ gastric pressures (eg, pregnancy, obesity), motility disorders that disrupt LES tone (eg, scleroderma), hiatal hernias, disorders that ↑ gastric acid production (eg, ZES), and tobacco, alcohol, or caffeine use.

Signs/Symptoms

Commonly associated **substernal heartburn**. Can also result in dysphagia (due to stricture), laryngitis, sinusitis, chronic otalgia, wheezing, or hoarseness. Children present with vomiting, coughing, halitosis, or inconsolable crying.

DIAGNOSIS

Generally a clinical diagnosis. If a patient fails to improve with medical management, has atypical symptoms, or is considered for an antireflux procedure, workup includes upper endoscopy with biopsy (assess for Barrett's strictures, LES locations), esophageal manometry (assess LES pressure; resting pressure < 6 mm Hg suggests GERD), and 24-hour pH probe monitoring. **In order to diagnose pathologic GERD, pH monitoring must assess: longest reflux episode, number of episodes and number of episodes ≥ 5 minutes, total time during which pH < 4, and total upright and supine time during which pH < 4.**

TREATMENT

Medical management is first-line and includes H_2-blockers or PPIs, avoidance of causative factors, head of bed elevation, small, frequent meals, and avoidance of meals before sleeping. **Surgery is indicated for suspected or proven malignancy, gastric necrosis, gastric obstruction, severe hemorrhage, or perforation.** Relative indications include failure of medical management, presence of paraesophageal hernia, or the presence of GERD-induced complications. **Nissen fundoplication** (open or laparoscopic) is the most commonly performed operation for GERD and involves a 360° wrap. Other fundoplications include the **Toupet** (180° wrap) and **Belsey Mark IV** (270° wrap, performed through the chest). If esophageal lengthening is needed, perform a Collis gastroplasty. Complications from antireflux procedures include **pneumothorax (most common)**, wrap herniation, gas-bloat syndrome, perforation, and hemorrhage (eg, splenic laceration).

Gastric Adenocarcinoma

DEMOGRAPHICS/RISK FACTORS

Most common form of gastric cancer. Second most common cancer worldwide and tenth most common in the United States. Wide geographic variability with particularly high rates in Japan and South America. Other risk factors include male gender, blood type A, age (peak incidence in seventh decade), chronic inflammation (eg, pernicious anemia, *H. pylori* infection), tobacco use, low socioeconomic status, and family history of gastric cancer.

TYPES

Intestinal type has a glandular histology and occurs in older patients, in the distal stomach, and in association with *H. pylori* infection and atrophic gastritis. Diffuse type tends to occur in younger patients, in the proximal stomach, and has a much more extensive submucosal, transmural, and metastatic pathology. **Signet ring cell** cancer has a particularly aggressive histology. **Linitis plastica** is a diffuse neoplasm involving the entire stomach to give a "leather bottle" appearance.

SIGNS/SYMPTOMS

Most common symptoms are **weight loss, early satiety**, and vague, constant epigastric pain. Indigestion, hematemesis or melena, anemia, or a palpable epigastric mass might also be present. Characteristic lymphadenopathy may be present.

DIAGNOSIS

Upper endoscopy with multiple biopsies localizes the lesion and confirms the diagnosis. CT of the abdomen and pelvis identifies metastatic disease; endoscopic ultrasound is useful for staging. Diagnostic laparoscopy with peritoneal fluid cytology can help detect liver lesions or peritoneal nodules not visualized on radiographs.

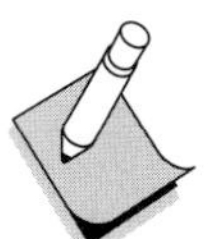

Characteristic lymphadenopathy and metastases of gastric cancer–

Virchow's: Right supraclavicular lymph node.

Sister Mary Joseph's: Periumbilical lymph node.

Blumer's shelf: Peritoneal lymph nodes (palpable on rectal examination).

Krukenberg tumor: Ovarian metastasis.

TREATMENT

Surgical resection with a 6-cm resection margin is the only potentially curative therapeutic modality. Neoadjuvant chemotherapy is sometimes used for locally advanced tumors; adjuvant chemotherapy with or without radiation is commonly used for node + cancers or more advanced T stage tumors. Resection type is based on tumor location:

- Proximal lesion: Total gastrectomy is preferred. Proximal gastric resection is associated with ↑ morbidity and mortality.
- Distal lesion: Subtotal gastrectomy with - margins is preferred over total gastrectomy.

For metastatic disease, palliative options include endoscopic dilation, stent placement, and surgical bypass.

Postgastrectomy syndromes are common complications of gastric resection (see Table 5-7).

STAGING/OUTCOME

Tumor, node status, metastasis (TNM) categories include

- T: T1 (invades lamina propria or submucosa), T2 (invades muscularis propria or subserosa), T3 (invades serosa), T4 (invades adjacent structures)
- N: N0 (- regional lymph nodes), N1 (1-6 + regional lymph nodes), N2 (7-15 + regional lymph nodes), N3 (> 15 + regional lymph nodes)
- M: M0 (metastatic disease absent), M1 (metastatic disease present)

Staging includes

- Stage I: T1N0-1M0 or T2N0M0
- Stage II: T1N2M0 or T2N1M0 or T3N0M0
- Stage III: T2N2M0 or T3N1-2M0 or T4N0M0
- Stage IV: T4N1-3M0 or T1-3N3M0 or Any T, any N, M1

Outcome is generally dismal with a 5-year survival of 10-20%. Recurrence often occurs in the setting of locoregional failure and peritoneal dissemination. Patients should have an exam, labs, and CXR every 4 months for the first year, every 6 months for the second year, and annually thereafter. CT of abdomen and pelvis with upper endoscopy should be performed at regular intervals.

Gastrointestinal Stromal Tumors

DEMOGRAPHICS

Submucosal, mesenchymal tumors arising from **interstitial cells of Cajal**. Most common in the stomach. Contain a gain of function **tyrosine kinase mutation** (usually the ***KIT*** proto-oncogene). Slightly more common in men during the seventh decade of life.

TABLE 5-7. Postgastrectomy Syndromes

SYNDROME	SIGNS/SYMPTOMS	TREATMENT
Dumping, early	Explosive diarrhea, abdominal pain, nausea, vomiting, ↑ HR, syncope, diaphoresis within **20-30 minutes of eating**. Caused by rapid passage of high osmolarity food from stomach to SI → H_2O shift into SI lumen.	Small meals with high protein/low simple carbohydrates, supine position after eating, octreotide. For refractory cases, conversion of Billroth to Roux-en-Y or reversed intestinal segment.
Dumping, late	Same symptoms as above. Occurs **2-3 hours** after eating. Due to hyperactive insulin release → hypoglycemia after a glucose load.	
Afferent loop syndrome*	Partial obstruction of afferent limb → postprandial pain and fullness, bilious, projectile vomiting (without food). Caused by ↑ afferent loop pressure (mechanical obstruction with ↑ GI secretion).	Conversion of Billroth II to Billroth I or to Roux-en-Y with vagotomy.
Efferent loop syndrome	Obstruction of efferent limb → abdominal pain, bilious vomiting, distention.	Exploration with reduction of internal hernia, closure of mesenteric defect.
Alkaline reflux gastritis*	Severe epigastric pain with bilious vomiting and weight loss caused by reflux of alkaline material into stomach and esophagus.	Conversion to Roux-en-Y anastomosis, isoperistaltic jejunal interposition. Often combined with distal gastrectomy, vagotomy.
Roux syndrome	Epigastric pain, vomiting, weight loss due to abnormal gastric emptying. **Abnormality in motility,** not a mechanical obstruction.	Promotility agents. Gastrectomy to ↓ gastric remnant size.
Retained antrum	Results in postoperative gastritis and ulcers due to ↑ HCl secretion. Retained antral mucosa in duodenal stump is continually bathed in alkaline secretions, which stimulates large, unchecked gastrin release.	Confirm with technetium scan. H_2-blockade or PPI. If refractory, excise retained tissue or convert to Billroth I.

*Afferent loop syndrome and alkaline reflux gastritis are more common after Billroth II reconstructions.

SIGNS/SYMPTOMS

Commonly present with epigastric pain, indigestion, and **GI bleeding** (eg, hematemesis, melena).

DIAGNOSIS

Upper endoscopy, CT scan of abdomen, and endoscopic ultrasound can identify a mass suspicious for gastrointestinal stromal tumor (GIST). UGI contrast radiography demonstrates a smooth, round filling defect. **KIT+ immunohistochemical staining** confirms diagnosis.

TREATMENT

Nonmetastatic disease should be treated with en bloc resection with - margins; **lymph node dissection is not indicated.** For metastatic, unresectable, or recurrent tumors, administer **imatinib mesylate (a tyrosine kinase inhibitor)** and then perform resection if complete excision is possible. Five-year survival is ~55%. Gastric GIST has best survival.

Gastric Lymphoma and Gastric MALToma

Most common site for 1° GI lymphoma. Most common in elderly men. Often present with anemia, early satiety, pain, weakness, and fatigue. Staging is important to rule out systemic disease. Treat with **chemoradiation** as the addition of **surgical resection does not improve survival**. Gastric MALTomas are non-Hodgkin lymphomas associated with ***H. pylori***; treat early stage MALTomas with eradication of *H. pylori* infection.

A 48-year-old woman presents 4 days after laparoscopic Roux-en-Y gastric bypass with abdominal pain and bloating. She is tachycardiac and has a distended abdomen with rebound tenderness and guarding. A CT scan of the abdomen reveals distention of the distal gastric segment and biliopancreatic limb. What is the correct next step for this patient? IV-fluid resuscitation and immediate reoperation. Patient has most likely developed an internal hernia and requires re-exploration to prevent strangulation and rupture of the gastric staple line.

Morbid Obesity

DEMOGRAPHICS/RISK FACTORS

About 5% of the adult U.S. population is morbidly obese. The incidence of childhood obesity is also increasing.

Mortally obese—

> 100 lb overweight and at serious risk for many obesity-related disorders.

GRADES OF OBESITY

Grades include

- Grade I (overweight): Body mass index (BMI) 25-29.9 kg/m^2
- Grade II (obese): BMI > 30 kg/m^2
- Grade III (morbidly/severely obese): BMI > 40 kg/m^2

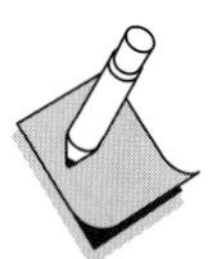

Metabolic syndrome–

Type II DM

Glucose intolerance

Dyslipidemia

HTN

Signs/Symptoms

Associated with obesity-related disorders including osteoarthritis, degenerative joint disease, hyperlipidemia, obstructive sleep apnea, HTN, diabetes mellitus (DM), asthma, and GERD.

Diagnosis

Clinical diagnosis. Assess BMI and history of failed weight loss attempts.

Treatment

Nonsurgical weight loss plans have limited success (≤ 3% have significant weight loss with medical therapy alone). Surgical options may be performed open or laparoscopically and are summarized in Table 5-8.

Indications for bariatric surgery–

- *BMI > 40 kg/m² or > 35 kg/m² with a comorbid condition that is worsened by obesity (eg, HTN, DM, high cholesterol, osteoarthritis)*
- *Psychiatric stability*
- *Documented failed attempt at dietary weight loss*
- *Complete understanding of operation and its risks and benefits*

TABLE 5-8. Bariatric Operations

Procedure	Technique	Results	Complications
Laparoscopic adjustable gastric banding (restrictive)	Placement of band via pars flaccida technique. Subcutaneous port allows for band adjustment.	50-60% excess weight lost by 5 years. Good resolution of comorbidities.	Slippage, erosion, wound infection, port complication, gastric/esophageal perforation.
Roux-en-Y gastric bypass (restrictive, malabsorptive)	Division of stomach into proximal gastric pouch, gastrojejunostomy and distal enteroenterostomy with 80-150 cm Roux limb (longer is better for ↑ BMI). **Close mesenteric defects to prevent internal hernias.**	58-62% excess weight loss by 5 years. Excellent resolution of comorbidities.	Hemorrhage, anastomotic leak, pulmonary embolism (PE), small bowel obstruction (SBO), stenosis, wound infection, internal hernia, marginal ulceration.
Biliopancreatic diversion (malabsorptive)	Distal hemigastrectomy, proximal gastric pouch with gastroileostomy, distal ileo-ileostomy 50-100 cm from ileocecal valve.	65-75% excess weight loss by 5 years. Excellent resolution of comorbidities.	Hemorrhage, leak, PE, SBO, wound infection, bloating, postcibal syndrome, marginal ulceration, protein-calorie malnutrition.
Duodenal switch (malabsorptive)	Greater curvature sleeve gastrectomy, end-to-side duodeno-ileostomy, ileo-ileostomy 100 cm proximal to ileocecal valve.	65-75% excess weight loss by 5 years. Excellent resolution of comorbidities.	Protein-energy malnutrition, hemorrhage, leak, PE, stenosis, anemia, wound infection.

▶ SAMPLE QUESTIONS

What GI hormones are involved in the regulation of insulin release?	Gastric inhibitory peptide, CCK.
What pathway is involved in vagally-mediated parietal cell stimulation? Histamine-mediated?	Vagus: IP_3 activation →↑ intracellular Ca^{2+} → PKC activation. Histamine: Activated adenylate cyclase →↑ cAMP → PKA activation.
A 69-year-old man is diagnosed with gastric adenocarcinoma. What are the most common symptoms?	Weight loss, early satiety, abdominal pain.
A 55-year-old woman is found to have PUD without ↑ HCl secretion. What types of gastric ulcers may be present?	Types I or IV.
What type of gastric ulcer is often not responsive to highly selective vagotomy?	Type III.
A 30-year-old male has GERD and has failed medical therapy. What is the test of choice to confirm and quantify the degree of reflux?	Twenty-four hour pH monitoring. Assess the longest reflux episode, number of episodes, number of episodes ≥ 5 minutes, total time in which pH < 4, and total upright and supine time in which pH < 4.
What risks are associated with laparoscopic Nissen fundoplication for GERD?	Pneumothorax (most common), bleeding (splenic laceration), perforation (esophageal, stomach), dysphagia, gas-bloat syndrome.
What technique is used for laparoscopic band placement during which the gastrohepatic ligament is divided, a plane between the right diaphragmatic crus, and the overlying fat pad is dissected?	Pars flaccida technique.
A 50-year-old female with chronic NSAID use presents with hemodynamic instability, peritonitis, and free air under the diaphragm. She is found to have a perforated gastric ulcer of the body. What is the correct surgical management?	Biopsy the ulcer to rule out malignancy. Perform a distal gastrectomy.
What is the strongest layer of the GI tract wall?	Submucosa.

A 60-year-old female has + peritoneal cytology for gastric adenocarcinoma. Is her disease considered stage IV?	No. Positive peritoneal cytology without gross metastases does not constitute stage IV disease for gastric adenocarcinoma.
A 35-year-male has a submucosal gastric lesion. What mutation is most commonly associated with this lesion?	*KIT* protooncogene mutation is most common mutation found in GISTs.

CHAPTER 6

Liver, Biliary System, and Spleen

Yanghee Woo, MD
Reviewed by Warren D. Widmann, MD

▶ BASIC SCIENCE

Embryology

Between the third and fourth weeks of embryogenesis, the liver primordium and bile duct arise from the ventral (endodermal) outgrowth of the foregut. Rapidly proliferating cells of the liver primordium penetrate the septum transversum to become the liver bud early in the fifth week. Kupffer cells, hepatic stroma, and hepatic vessels arise from the septum transversum (mesoderm). A small ventral outgrowth of the bile duct forms the gallbladder and the cystic duct. By the ninth week, the liver accounts for 10% of the fetus' total body weight; at birth it accounts for only 5%. The spleen primordium is a proliferation of the mesenchymal cells in the dorsal mesogastrium appearing in the fifth week.

Anatomy

MACROSCOPIC ANATOMY OF THE LIVER

There are two main classification systems (see Figure 6-1):

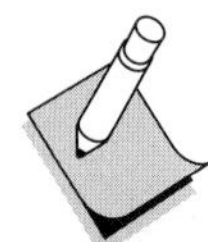

Hepatic lobe-segment correlations–

Caudate lobe → Segment I

Left lobe → Segments II, III, IV

Right lobe → Segments V, VI, VII, VIII

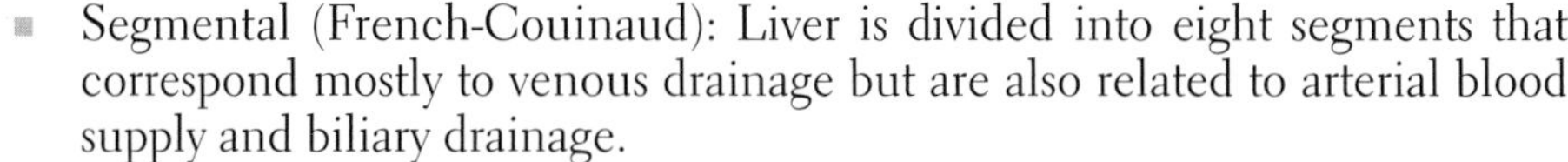

- Segmental (French-Couinaud): Liver is divided into eight segments that correspond mostly to venous drainage but are also related to arterial blood supply and biliary drainage.
- Lobar (American): Two main lobes (right and left) are divided by the interlobar fissure (**Cantlie's line**), which runs from the left side of the gallbladder fossa to the inferior vena cava (IVC). The caudate lobe is distinct from the right and left lobes because its venous drainage is directly into the vena cava.

MICROSCOPIC ANATOMY OF THE LIVER

Hepatocytes perform major metabolic and excretory functions. The **acinar unit** is the functional unit of the liver. Components include the biliary ductule, hepatic arteriole, and portal venule (afferent). Zones are defined relative to O_2 and solute concentration gradients: Zone 1 is located closest to the portal triad (**least susceptible to ischemic insult**, but **most susceptible to toxic or chemical injury**), while the peripheral zone 3 is adjacent to the terminal hepatic

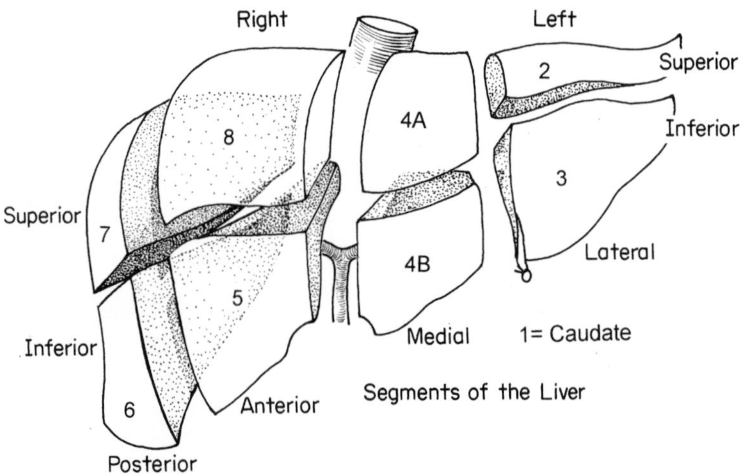

FIGURE 6-1. Anatomy of the liver.

(Reproduced, with permission, from Zollinger RM Jr, Zollinger RM Sr. *Zollinger's Atlas of Surgical Operations*, 8th ed. New York: McGraw-Hill, 2003:219.)

vein (**most susceptible to ischemic injury**). Kupffer cells are macrophages and are involved in phagocytosis.

Normal size for the CBD is < 5 mm for a patient < 50 years old. Size can increase 1 mm/decade after 50 years of age. The CBD is normally enlarged up to 12 mm following cholecystectomy.

MACROSCOPIC ANATOMY OF THE BILIARY SYSTEM

Bile duct anatomy is summarized in Figure 6-2. Bile is secreted into the bile canaliculi and travels through intrahepatic ductules, which eventually form the right (drains segments V, VI, VII, VIII) and left (drains segments II, III, IV) hepatic ducts. Bile from the caudate lobe usually drains into the left hepatic ductal system. Bile is concentrated and stored in the gallbladder, located on the undersurface of liver segments IV and V. Normal gallbladder wall thickness is < 4 mm.

There is controversy over whether the **ducts of Luschka** are accessory bile ducts that drain bile from the liver bed directly to the gallbladder or whether they are drainage ducts running from subsegments of the liver along the gallbladder bed to join the cystic duct or common bile duct (CBD). **They are often implicated as a source of postoperative bile leaks when correct operative**

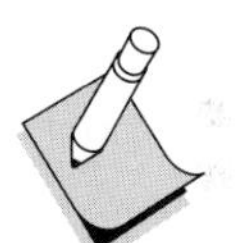

Ducts of Luschka are implicated as a common source of postcholecystectomy biliary leaks that are not caused by injury to the major ducts or by failure to close the cystic duct stump. They are rarely visualized on intraoperative cholangiograms.

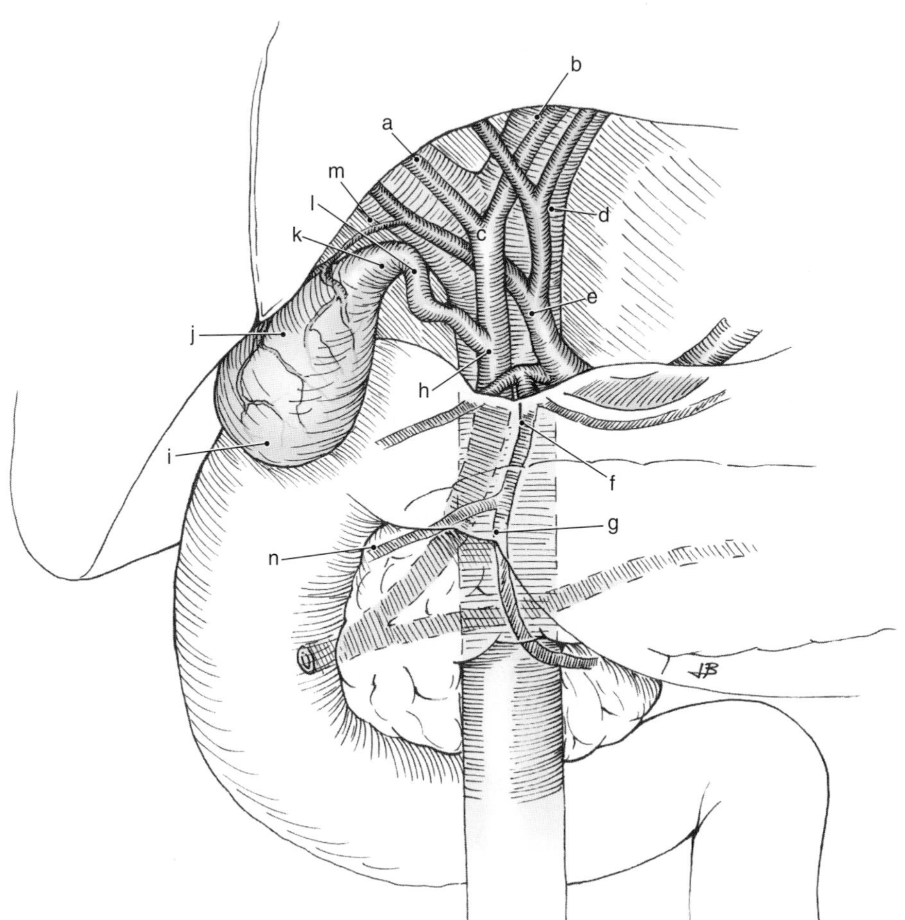

FIGURE 6-2. Anterior aspect of the biliary anatomy. a. Right hepatic duct. b. Left hepatic duct. c. Common hepatic duct. d. Portal vein. e. Hepatic artery. f. Gastroduodenal artery. g. Right gastroepiploic artery. h. Common bile duct. i. Fundus of the gallbladder. j. Body of the gallbladder. k. Infundibulum. l. Cystic duct. m. Cystic artery. n. Superior pancreaticoduodenal artery. Note the situation of the hepatic bile duct confluence anterior to the right branch of the portal vein, and the posterior course of the right hepatic artery behind the common hepatic duct.

(Reproduced, with permission, from Brunicardi FC, et al. *Schwartz's Principles of Surgery*, 8th ed. New York: McGraw-Hill, 2005:1188.)

techniques have been followed. After completing a cholecystectomy, one should search for such ducts and correct leaks with sutures or clips.

Important biliary anatomic relationships–
HA lies anterior to the PV and medial to the CBD.

Microscopic Anatomy of the Biliary System

Layers of the gallbladder include the mucosa, muscularis, subserosa, and serosa. There is **no submucosa**. The mucosa is composed of **columnar epithelium** specialized for absorption of H_2O with resultant concentration of the hepatic bile. **Rokitansky–Aschoff** sinuses form from the invagination of the epithelium through the fibromuscular layer as a result of inflammation and ↑ intraluminal pressure in the gallbladder (eg, cholangitis, acute cholecystitis).

Replaced right HA exists in 17% of patients and comes off the superior mesenteric artery (SMA) to run lateral to the CBD.

Macroscopic Anatomy of the Spleen

Located in the left upper quadrant of the abdomen and secured by the parietal peritoneum. Anatomic relationships include:

- Attachment to the greater curvature of the stomach by the **gastrosplenic ligament**, in which the short gastric vessels (from the splenic artery and vein) travel.
- Attachment to the left kidney by the **splenorenal ligament**, which in the absence of portal HTN, is usually avascular.

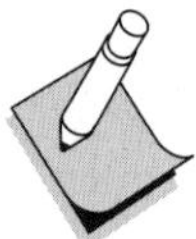

Replaced left HA occurs in 10% of patients and usually comes off of the splenic or left gastric artery.

Microscopic Anatomy of the Spleen

Functionally divided into red and white pulp, which function as a filter for all foreign matter in the blood stream (see Table 6-1).

Blood Supply of the Liver

Inflow blood supply comes from the portal vein (PV) and the hepatic artery (HA). PV is formed by splenic and superior mesenteric veins. HA branches off the celiac as the common HA and ultimately becomes the proper HA, giving off the left HA and the right HA. Cystic artery usually branches off the right HA. PV and HA each contribute 50% of the O_2 supply to the liver, but the PV carries 75% of the total blood flow to the liver.

Hepatic venous drainage occurs via three hepatic veins (HV) that drain into the IVC: left HV (segments II, III, superior IV), middle HV (segments V, inferior IV), and right HV (segments VI, VII, VIII).

The caudate lobe has its own blood supply from the right and left PVs and HAs. Separate HVs drain the caudate lobe directly into the IVC. Thus, in Budd-Chiari syndrome, the caudate lobe is typically spared.

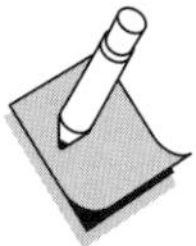

Most liver tumors are supplied primarily by the HA. This is true for both 1° liver tumors and for metastatic tumors of the liver.

TABLE 6-1. Differences in Splenic Red and White Pulp

	Red Pulp	White Pulp
% Splenic Composition	85%	15%
Specific Cell Types	Mononuclear phagocytes.	Lymphoid cells, mostly B cells.
Specific Function	Clearing of nucleated remnants from immature red blood cells (RBC), clearing of damaged or dead RBC.	Clearing of bloodborne antigens: bacteria without preexisting antibodies, poorly opsonized bacteria, foreign particles, cellular debris.

The middle HV converges with the left HV before entering the IVC in 80% of cases. The remaining 20% drain directly into the IVC.

Blood Supply of the Biliary System

Cystic artery (from the right HA) and vein (drains into the right PV) are the blood vessels of the gallbladder. However, the cystic vein is usually absent, and venous drainage is through multiple surface veins that drain directly into the liver bed.

Blood Supply of the Spleen

Splenic artery, left gastroepiploic artery, and short gastric arteries provide arterial blood flow to the spleen. Splenic vein courses posterior and inferior to the splenic artery and drains into the PV.

Innervation of the Liver

Sympathetic fibers arise from T7-T10. Parasympathetic innervation arises from the right and left vagus nerves. These synapse with the peripheral nerve fibers that run anterior and posterior to the HA.

Lymphatic Drainage of the Liver

Hepatic lymphatics begin in the perisinusoidal spaces of Disse and in the clefts of Mall. They then drain to the porta hepatis → cisterna chili → thoracic duct. Thus, **lymph flows in the opposite direction of PV blood** and does not follow HV flow.

Pathophysiology of ascites— *↓ Permeability of the sinusoidal epithelial cells alters lymphatic drainage → ascites.*

Physiology of the Liver

Functions include antigen clearance, hemoglobin (Hgb) degradation, detoxification, bile production, protein synthesis, nutrient storage, and glucose, lipid, and protein metabolism.

Antigen Clearance

Reticuloendothelial system (including Kupffer cells) are involved in phagocytosis of antigens as they enter the liver parenchyma.

Hemoglobin Degradation

Hgb degradation involves iron recycling and heme metabolism. Heme is converted to **biliverdin** and ultimately to **bilirubin**. Free, unconjugated bilirubin undergoes glucuronidation (**glucuronyl transferase**) to the conjugated, H_2O-soluble form that is excreted.

P-450 system is described in further detail in Chapter 3.

Detoxification

Liver converts hydrophobic compounds to hydrophilic conjugates to be secreted. Phase I reactions involve oxidation (via the cytochrome P-450 system), reduction, hydroxylation, or hydrolysis to expose functional groups. Phase II reactions involve conjugation to alter solubility.

Bile Production

Bile is the exocrine secretion of the liver; ~1 L is secreted daily. Composed of 1° bile acids (eg, **cholic** and **chenodeoxycholic acids**), 2° bile acids (eg, deoxycholic, lithocholic, ursodeoxycholic acids), bilirubin, phospholipids (primarily

Factor VIII, made primarily by endothelial cells, is made to some degree by the liver. Following successful liver transplantation in patients with hemophilia A, normal levels of Factor VIII can be found.

LIVER, BILIARY SYSTEM, AND SPLEEN

lecithin), cholesterol, H_2O, and electrolytes. Rate limiting enzyme in bile acid production is **cholesterol 7α-hydroxylase.** Bile salts are absorbed at the terminal ileum via the Na^+-dependent bile salt transporter and returned to the liver via the **enterohepatic circulation**.

PROTEIN SYNTHESIS

Responsible for production of a number of plasma proteins including coagulation factors (eg, Factors I, II, V, VII, IX, X, XI, antithrombin III, protein C, protein S), complement factors, and a number of acute phase proteins (eg, transferrin, albumin, C-reactive protein, ceruloplasmin, fibrinogen, haptoglobin).

NUTRIENT STORAGE

Stores **glycogen**, triglycerides, vitamin B_{12}, iron, copper, and fat-soluble vitamins.

GLUCOSE, LIPID, AND PROTEIN METABOLISM

Source of a number of metabolic pathways, including:

- Glucose synthesis: Glycogenolysis, gluconeogenesis.
- Glycogenesis.
- Lipogenesis (from amino acids, glucose).
- Deamination and transamination of amino acids.
- Conversion of ammonia to urea (urea cycle).
- Production of nonessential amino acids.

► CLINICAL SCIENCE

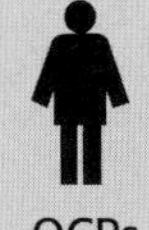

A 35-year-old female who takes oral contraceptive pills (OCPs) presents with right upper quadrant (RUQ) pain. Workup reveals a 3-cm lesion in the liver consistent with hepatic adenoma. What is the treatment? Stop OCPs and observe. If the lesion becomes > 4 cm or if symptoms persist, resection is indicated.

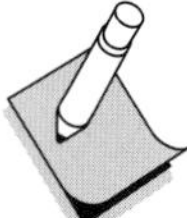

Kasabach–Merritt syndrome *–Consumption thrombocytopenia related to hepatic hemangiomata. Can lead to disseminated intravascular coagulation (DIC).*

Benign Liver Lesions

Common benign liver lesions are summarized in Table 6-2.

Liver Abscesses

Include bacterial (pyogenic), amebic, and fungal types (see Table 6-3). Fungal abscesses are rare (< 10%), and most commonly caused by *Candida* species.

Hydatid Cysts

Results from infection with the parasite ***Echinococcus granulosum.*** Rare in the United States; more prevalent in areas in which sheep are raised (eg, South America, Southern Europe). Dogs (1° host) shed the parasite in the stool, which then infects humans (intermediate hosts). Cysts can develop anywhere in the body but have a predilection for the **right lobe of the liver**. May be associated with RUQ pain, hepatomegaly, or obstructive symptoms (eg, jaundice, pruritus). If cyst leaks or ruptures, may be associated with allergic symptoms ranging from wheezing to shock. Labs may

TABLE 6-2. Benign Liver Lesions

	Hemangioma	Focal Nodular Hyperplasia	Adenoma
Demographics/ Risk Factors	**Most common benign liver tumor**. Not related to OCP use.	More common in women. Average age of diagnosis = 35 years. **Not related to OCP use.**	Reproductive-aged women who use **OCPs**.
Signs/ Symptoms	Usually asymptomatic and found incidentally.	Usually asymptomatic.	75% present with **abdominal pain**.
Diagnosis	Contrast-enhanced CT, MRI **(T2-bright)**.	MRI, CT are superior. CT shows hypervascular mass with **hypodense stellate scar. "Hot"** on ^{99}Tc-macroaggregated albumin scan. Biopsy shows hepatocytes and bile ducts.	MRI, CT (lacks central scar). **"Cold"** on ^{99}Tc-macroaggregated albumin scan. Biopsy shows hepatocytes.
Management	If asymptomatic, observe. Enucleation or lobectomy if + symptoms or if uncertain diagnosis. Radioablation or embolization of the HA for poor surgical candidates.	If asymptomatic, observe with serial CT scans. If symptomatic, resect.	Discontinue OCPs. If < 4 cm, observe, as lesion may regress. If > 4 cm, resect due to **risk of rupture** and **malignant degeneration**.
Complications	Rupture (rare) → hemorrhagic shock. May act like an atriovenous fistula → cardiac hypertrophy, congestive heart failure.	No potential for malignant degeneration. Low chance of rupture.	**25% chance of rupture/ hemorrhage**. Rare malignant degeneration.

show eosinophilia, + **indirect agglutination** (85%), or + complement fixation test. Abdominal CT demonstrates **calcified ectocyst and endocyst**. Treat with preoperative **albendazole or mebendazole** followed by complete surgical removal (including cyst wall). Intraoperative aspiration followed by injection of hypertonic saline may be performed as an adjunct with surgical removal. During surgery, wall off the area from the rest of peritoneal cavity to prevent accidental spillage and seeding as well as anaphylactic reactions. Percutaneous aspiration is rarely used as leaks can cause anaphylactic shock.

Natural history of hydatid cysts–

Expansion → rupture → spread of infection → anaphylaxis → death

Primary Sclerosing Cholangitis

Demographics/Risk Factors

Includes cholestasis and fibrotic strictures of the intrahepatic and extrahepatic biliary tree. Most commonly affects men in their third to fourth decades. **Autoimmune disease** found in association with **ulcerative colitis** (UC), HLA B8, HLA DR3, retroperitoneal fibrosis, insulin-dependent diabetes mellitus (DM), Grave's disease, Sjögren's syndrome, Riedel's thyroiditis, autoimmune pancreatitis, and myasthenia gravis.

TABLE 6-3. Liver Abscesses

	Bacterial Abscesses	Amebic Abscesses
Demographics/risk factors	**Most common type in United States** (80%). Causes include hematogenous spread from intra-abdominal infection (**diverticulitis, appendicitis**) or ascending biliary infection (cholangitis), direct extension from intraperitoneal infection, stent placement/manipulation, trauma. **Most common organisms include *Staphylococcus aureus*, gram negative rods (*Escherichia coli, Klebsiella*) and anaerobes (*Bacteroides fragilis*).**	Most common cause worldwide. Primary infection occurs in colon and spreads to the liver via the PV. Caused by the ***Entamoeba histolytica.*** Most commonly presents as a **single abscess in the right lobe.**
Signs/symptoms	**Fever**, chills, sweating, nausea, vomiting, anorexia, weight loss, liver tenderness/enlargement, **jaundice.**	**Fever, RUQ pain,** chills, sweating, hepatomegaly, **antecedent diarrhea (25%). Jaundice is rare.** The abscess content is described as **"anchovy paste."**
Diagnosis	Leukocytosis, + blood cultures (40%). Confirm with CT or ultrasound. On CT, abscess is **hypodense** relative to liver; wall will enhance with IV contrast.	Leukocytosis, abnormal liver function tests (LFTs), + ***Entamoeba histolytica* serology (90%).** Positive stool culture present only 15% of time. Cultures of abscess are usually sterile. Radiographic findings similar to bacterial.
Management	IV antibiotics (2 weeks) followed by oral antibiotics (1 month), CT- or ultrasound-guided aspiration/drain placement. Surgical and percutaneous drainages have equivalent success. If multiple abscesses are present, prolonged antibiotic treatment is necessary.	**Metronidazole.** Percutaneous or surgical drainage is reserved to cases that fail antibiotic therapy or have complications (eg, bacterial superinfection).

Signs/Symptoms

Intermittent jaundice, fatigue, weight loss, **pruritus,** and abdominal pain. More than 50% of patients are symptomatic at time of diagnosis. The disease has a highly variable clinical course with periods of remissions and exacerbations. May cause cirrhosis or **cholangiocarcinoma** (up to 20% of primary sclerosing cholangitis [PSC] cases).

Diagnosis

↑ Alkaline phosphatase and bilirubin. Endoscopic retrograde cholangiopancreatography (ERCP) will demonstrate **multiple dilatations and strictures of both the intra- and extra-hepatic biliary tree.** Liver biopsy can help determine the degree of hepatic fibrosis and the presence of cirrhosis.

Treatment

No effective treatment or cure exists. Endoscopic or percutaneous dilation and stenting of biliary strictures may provide temporary relief of symptoms. In patients without significant hepatic fibrosis or cirrhosis, surgical resection of the extrahepatic biliary tree with hepaticojejunostomy may offer a more lasting relief of symptoms. Liver transplantation is the only option for patients with PSC and advanced liver disease. After transplantation, 10-20% of patients will have recurrent disease. Colectomy in cases associated with UC does not alter course of PSC.

ERCP and liver biopsy confirm the diagnosis of PSC. Must rule out cholangiocarcinoma.

Cirrhosis

Demographics/Risk Factors

Chronic inflammation → hepatocyte destruction and regeneration → fibrosis → portal HTN. Causes include alcohol **(most common in the United States)**, hepatitis B virus (HBV), hepatitis C virus (HCV, **most common worldwide)**, prolonged cholestasis, metabolic disorders (eg, Wilson's disease, α1-antitrypsin), or autoimmune disease.

AST and ALT > 3 times normal → chronic liver disease

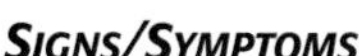

Signs/Symptoms

Nonspecific symptoms include weight loss, malaise, and weakness. Exam may reveal spider angiomata, palmar erythema, gynecomastia, testicular atrophy, caput medusae, fetor hepaticus, splenomegaly, jaundice, altered mental status, asterixis, or ascites.

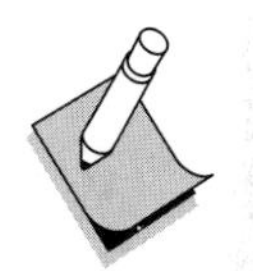

ALT/AST > 2 → Alcoholic cirrhosis

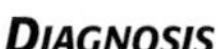

Diagnosis

Labs may reveal anemia (caused by bleeding, nutritional deficiencies, bone marrow depression, hemolysis), thrombocytopenia, ↑ prothrombin time (PT) and international normalized ratio (INR), and ↑ aspartate aminotransferase (AST) or alanine aminotransferase (ALT). Liver biopsy can confirm the presence of cirrhosis and help establish a cause. **Child-Pugh classification helps determine the extent of cirrhosis and predict operative mortality** (see Table 6-4).

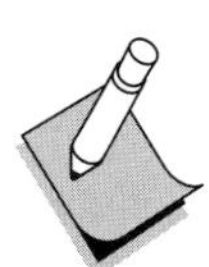

The synthetic function of the liver is best assessed by PT.

TABLE 6-4. Child-Pugh Classification of Cirrhosis

	Class		
	A	**B**	**C**
Ascites	None	Minimal, controlled	Moderate-severe
Neurologic disorder	None	Minimal, controlled	Moderate-severe (coma)
Serum bilirubin (mg/dL)	< 2	2-3	> 3
Serum albumin (g/dL)	> 3.5	2.8-3.5	< 2.8
PT (↑ in sec) INR	1–3 < 1.7	4–6 1.7–2.2	> 6 > 2.2
Operative mortality	10%	30%	70%

(Adapted, with permission, from Brunicardi FC, et al. *Schwartz's Principles of Surgery*, 8th ed. New York: McGraw-Hill, 2005:1154.)

Child-Pugh classification of cirrhosis–**ProBAAN:**
Prothrombin
Bilirubin
Albumin
Ascites
Neurologic disorder

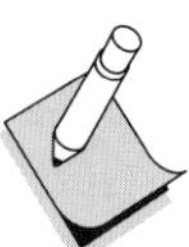

Collaterals between the short gastric veins to the azygous system result in esophageal varices.

TREATMENT

Treat the symptoms and complications of cirrhosis.

- Ascites: Diuresis (eg, spironolactone, furosemide), large-volume paracentesis (for symptomatic relief), peritoneal-jugular shunts (for ascites refractory to medical management).
- Spontaneous bacterial peritonitis: Acute infection of peritoneal fluid that commonly presents with fever and abdominal pain. Most commonly caused by enteric pathogens (***E. coli*—most common**); **suspect other etiologies if polymicrobial flora found on culture.** Confirm diagnosis > 250 PMN/μL in ascitic fluid that is culture +. Treat with third generation cephalosporins (eg, **cefotaxime**).
- Portal HTN: Discussed below. Results in complications including ascites and esophageal varices. Variceal bleeding associated with 33% mortality with first episode and 50% mortality with rebleeds. Treat with endoscopy and rubber band ligation or sclerotherapy, vasopressin or octreotide, and transjugular intrahepatic portasystemic shunting (TIPS; for refractory cases).
- Liver failure: Requires liver transplantation (see Chapter 20).

Portal Hypertension

DEMOGRAPHICS/RISK FACTORS

Defined as an abnormal ↑ PV pressure (ie, **portal pressure gradient > 12 mm Hg**). Obstruction blocks portal flow → ↑ PV pressure → vasoconstriction → vasodilation and ↑ splanchnic inflow → development of collaterals develop between portal and systemic circulations (eg, coronary, umbilical, retroperitoneal, hemorrhoidal, short gastric veins). In some cases there can be hepatofugal PV flow (ie, blood flow in the PV is reversed, and blood flows **out** from the liver).

TYPES

Obstruction may be presinusoidal, sinusoidal, or postsinusoidal (see Figure 6-3).

Budd–Chiari syndrome involves **occlusion of the major hepatic veins** resulting in postsinusoidal portal HTN. More common in women, particularly

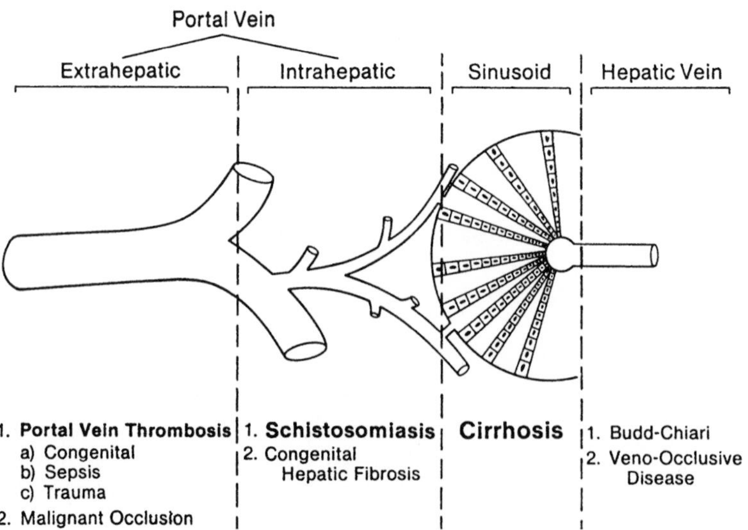

FIGURE 6-3. Etiologies of portal hypertension.

(Reproduced, with permission, from Zinner MJ, Ashley SW. *Maingot's Abdominal Operations*, 11th ed. New York: McGraw-Hill, 2007:833.)

those with **hypercoagulable states** (see Chapter 2). Signs and symptoms can include RUQ pain, jaundice, ascites, hepatosplenomegaly, and complications from portal HTN. After diagnosis is confirmed, patient should be **anticoagulated**. Portacaval shunting may help depending on IVC pressure; porta-atrial shunting may be necessary. TIPS is not an effective treatment. The caudate lobe is spared in most cases and enhances on isotope liver scans.

SIGNS/SYMPTOMS

Similar to cirrhosis. Common complications include ascites, esophageal varices, and liver failure (see Figure 6-4).

DIAGNOSIS

Confirm diagnosis with transcutaneous liver Doppler ultrasound to characterize parenchyma and blood flow patterns. Laboratory tests to confirm source of cirrhosis are necessary (eg, HCV and HBV titers).

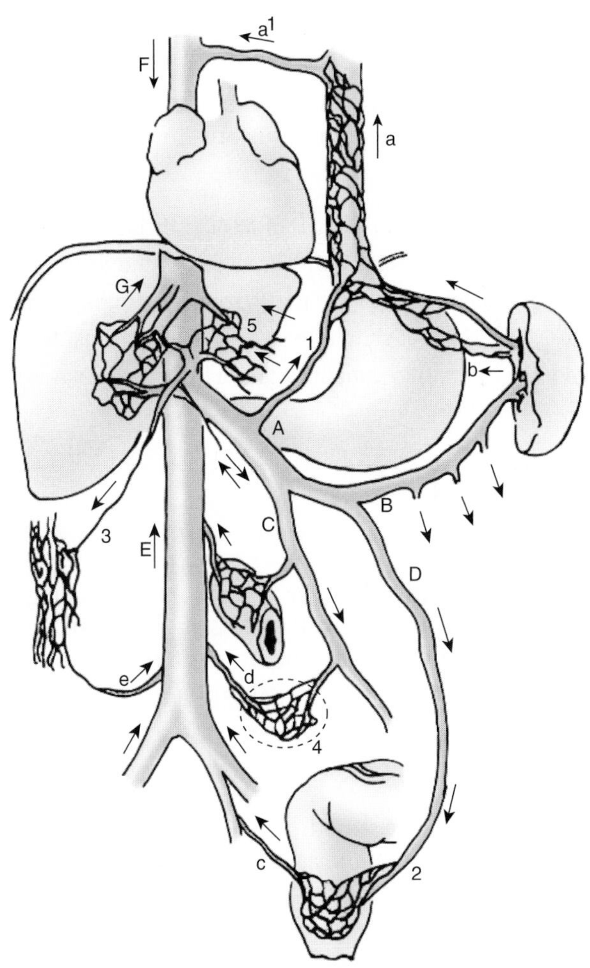

FIGURE 6-4. Intra-abdominal venous flow pathways leading to engorged veins (varices) from portal hypertension. 1, coronary vein; 2, superior hemorrhoidal veins; 3, paraumbilical veins; 4, veins of Retzius; 5, veins of Sappey; A, portal vein; B, spienic vein; C, superior mesenteric vein; D, inferior mesenteric vein; E, inferior vena cava; F, superior vena cava; G, hepatic veins; a, esophageal veins; a[1], azygos system; b, vasa brevia; c, middle and inferior hemorrhoidal veins; d, intestinal; e, epigastric veins.

(Reproduced, with permission, from Brunicardi FC, et al. *Schwartz's Principles of Surgery*, 8th ed. New York: McGraw-Hill, 2005:1155.)

TREATMENT

Treatment can include surgical shunting or liver transplantation.

- Surgical shunt: Indicated for patients with relatively well-preserved liver function (ie, Child-Pugh classes A and B) who may require liver transplant in the future (> 1 year). Types include portacaval and mesocaval shunts.
- Liver transplantation: Details described in Chapter 20. The **Model for End-stage Liver Disease (MELD) score** is used by the transplant community to prioritize patients.

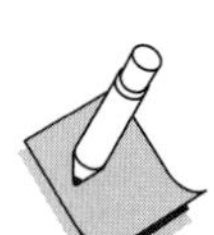

Sinistral portal HTN– *Caused by splenic vein thrombosis, typically resultant from pancreatitis. Results in gastroesophageal varices without main PV HTN. Typically patients have preserved liver function, but bleeding may occur. Treatment includes splenectomy.*

LIVER, BILIARY SYSTEM, AND SPLEEN

Portal Vein Thrombosis

Involves occlusion of the PV. In childhood, often caused by umbilical vein catheterization. Liver function is generally well-preserved, but some cases might require portacaval shunting. There is no role for TIPS. Cases in adults can be caused by malignancy (eg, hepatocellular carcinoma [HCC]), cirrhosis (resulting in low hepatopetal flow), hypercoagulable states, dehydration, and infection (eg, schistosomiasis). May be asymptomatic and diagnosed incidentally but can be associated with splenomegaly or hemorrhage. Diagnosis can be confirmed with duplex Doppler ultrasound, CT angiography (CTA), or MR angiography (MRA). Treatment includes long-term anticoagulation and possibly clot lysis via transhepatic infusions through the PV.

> A 50-year-old man with a history of HBV is incidentally found to have a hepatic mass. α-fetoprotein (AFP) is elevated; the lesion is confirmed to be HCC. In addition to staging the lesion, what other factors will determine resectability? The patient's Child-Pugh classification must be determined as resection is generally limited to patients with Child-Pugh class A or B cirrhosis.

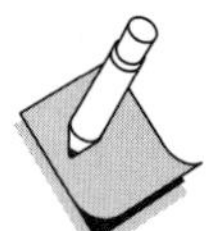

The vast majority of liver masses are metastatic lesions. However, 1 in 20 of malignant liver tumors are HCC. Therefore, lesions in the liver require a cancer workup to localize the 1° lesion.

Hepatocellular Carcinoma

DEMOGRAPHICS/RISK FACTORS

Most common cancer worldwide with > 1 million cases diagnosed annually. More common in men as age ↑. Risk factors include HBV (**most common cause worldwide**), HCV, alcohol, hemochromatosis, α1-antitrypsin deficiency, PSC, hepatic adenoma, steroid use, and exposure to aflatoxins or pesticides.

SIGNS/SYMPTOMS

May be asymptomatic or present with vague RUQ pain and weight loss. On exam, hepatomegaly, palpable mass, ascites, jaundice, or encephalopathy may be present.

DIAGNOSIS

Typically associated with **serum AFP > 500 ng/dL**. Lesion can be visualized with ultrasound (during workup for cirrhosis or portal HTN), abdominal CT, or MRI. If AFP is nondiagnostic and the patient is not a surgical candidate, perform fine needle aspiration with cytology to confirm diagnosis. If the patient is a surgical candidate, perform exploratory laparotomy with or without biopsy. CXR, chest CT, and bone scan should be performed to rule out metastatic disease.

TREATMENT

Preferred treatment is partial hepatectomy in Child-Pugh class A and B patients. Neoadjuvant chemoradiation or adjuvant chemotherapy may be indicated for some patients. Transplantation may be possible for patients with a **tumor < 5 cm, < 3 tumors, and with no PV or IVC involvement**. Only 15–20% of cases are amenable to surgical resection because of tumor multicentricity, extensive involvement of both lobes of liver, PV invasion, or lymphatic metastases. Patients who do not qualify for surgery may receive HA embolization or tumor cryotherapy, radio-ablation, or ethanol injection.

STAGING/OUTCOME

Staging is determined by number of tumors, size of tumors, and vascular invasion. Overall survival is poor; 5-year survival for all comers is < 30%.

Cholangiocarcinoma

Cancer of the intra- or extra-hepatic bile ducts. Associated with **PSC**, ***Clonorchis sinensis***, UC, choledochal cysts, and chronic bile duct infection. Usually affects elderly males who present with painless jaundice, weight loss, pruritus, or cholangitis. Labs will be consistent with biliary obstruction: ↑ alkaline phosphatase, ↑ bilirubin, and ↑ γ-glutamyl transpeptidase (GGT); transaminases will be normal. Confirm diagnosis with ERCP and MRI. Treatment depends on the location of tumor in the bile duct:

- Upper 1/3: **Most common.** Usually unresectable, but if amenable, attempt resection of the affected liver lobe and bile duct
- Middle 1/3: Hepaticojejunostomy
- Lower 1/3: Whipple procedure.

Median survival is 12-59 months after resection with an overall 5-year survival of 20-42%.

Klatskins tumor—*Cholangiocarcinoma at the junction of the right and left hepatic ducts.*

Disorders of the Gallbladder

Gallstone types include

- Cholesterol: **Most common type in United States.** Due to failure of cholesterol and Ca^{2+} salts to remain in solution as a result of an imbalance of cholesterol, lecithin, and bile acids.
- Pigmented: Black stones are caused by precipitation of unconjugated bilirubin with Ca^{2+} → calcium bilirubinate. Found in association with **hemolysis**, cirrhosis, **chronic TPN**, and **ileal resections.** Brown stones are related to chronic biliary infections, most commonly *E. coli*.

Gallstone-related diseases includes biliary colic, acute cholecystitis, choledocholithiasis, and acute cholangitis (see Table 6-5).

Complications from gallstone disease include:

RUQ ultrasound is the imaging study of choice for gallstone-related diseases.

- **Gallstone pancreatitis:** Caused by obstruction of the pancreatic duct by a stone. Responsible for about one-third of acute pancreatitis cases (see Chapter 7). Though timing of cholecystectomy is controversial, ERCP with sphincterotomy and stone extraction is indicated for choledocholithiasis and cholangitis. More than 90% of patients pass the offending stone spontaneously.
- **Gallstone ileus:** Affects < 1% of patients with gallstones. Found in ~25% of cases of small bowel obstruction (SBO) in elderly patients who do not have hernias or adhesions. Presents with signs and symptoms of SBO

TABLE 6-5. Gallstone-Related Diseases

	Biliary Colic	Acute Cholecystitis	Choledocholithiasis	Acute Cholangitis
Definition	Pain caused by **transient obstruction of the cystic duct** by a gallstone.	**Gallbladder inflammation** usually caused by gallstone obstruction of the cystic duct.	Gallstones in the **CBD.**	**Bacterial infection** of the biliary tract.
Signs/symptoms	Abrupt or transient, RUQ/epigastric pain. May be postprandial (typically fatty foods, but any foods can precipitate).	RUQ pain, + **Murphy's sign**, fever.	RUQ/epigastric pain, fever, chills, jaundice, acute pancreatitis.	**Charcot's triad:** Fever, RUQ pain, jaundice. **Reynold's pentad:** Charcot's triad plus hypotension, altered mental status.
Diagnosis	Gallstones found on RUQ ultrasound.	Nl LFTs, white blood cell (WBC) count 12–15 K/μL. RUQ ultrasound = **gallstones, gallbladder wall thickening (> 4 mm), pericholecystic fluid, + sonographic Murphy's sign.**	↑ Alkaline phosphatase/ GGT. RUQ ultrasound = dilated CBD > 8 mm. Stones not well visualized if in distal duct.	Perform RUQ ultrasound. Nl biliary tree or dilated CBD (> 8 mm) without a clear CBD stone does not rule out cholangitis.
Management	Avoidance of inciting factors. Elective cholecystectomy indicated for symptomatic patients without serious comorbidities.	IV antibiotics, cholecystectomy, percutaneous cholecystostomy tube in seriously ill patients.	ERCP with sphincterotomy for patients with previous cholecystectomy or preoperative CBD clearance. Laparoscopic cholecystectomy with intraoperative cholangiogram if preoperative clearance was not achieved.	Supportive therapy with aggressive fluid resuscitation, electrolyte correction, broad spectrum IV antibiotics, pain control. Timely ductal drainage: ERCP, sphincterotomy, and stone extraction.

(see Chapter 9) after a gallstone enters the intestine via a **cholecystoduodenal fistula** and lodges in the terminal ileum typically 1–2 ft proximal to the ileocecal valve. Abdominal radiographs demonstrate signs of SBO; a stone and air in the biliary tree might be visible. Treat with surgical removal of the stone via a proximal, longitudinal enterotomy with transverse closure after running the small bowel to exclude other in-transit stones. In very stable patients consider closure of the fistula and cholecystectomy.

Gallbladder Adenocarcinoma

Rare cancer found in up to 1% of gallbladder specimens. Most commonly affects women with ↑ age. Associated with chronic gallbladder inflammation (eg, **gallstones**, infection) and may be found in association with **porcelain**

gallbladder (ie, diffuse deposition of Ca^{2+} in the gallbladder wall). Patients are usually asymptomatic or have symptoms similar to biliary colic that persist for an extended time. Diagnosis is confirmed with ultrasound, abdominal CT, or MRI and magnetic resonance cholangiopancreatography (MRCP). Resection is indicated for amenable cases. For cases **incidentally found after cholecystectomy and with - margins (no extension through the gallbladder wall), no further treatment is necessary.** However, all other resectable cases require en bloc resection of the gallbladder and underlying liver to a depth of 2 cm as well as regional lymphadenectomy. Endoscopic stenting may be used for palliation. Overall 5-year survival is poor (~5%).

> A 35-year-old male presents with a shattered spleen after an MVC. He is hemodynamically unstable and is taken emergently to the OR where a splenectomy is performed. What postoperative vaccines are indicated?
> *Pneumococcus, meningococcus, Haemophilus influenzae.*

Splenectomy

Common indications for splenectomy include:

- Traumatic injury: In adults, perform for hemodynamic instability, > 2 units of packed red blood cells (PRBC) transfusion or persistent decline in Hgb, peritonitis, or significant intra-abdominal blood. **In children, the threshold to perform splenectomy is 40 mL/kg transfused blood or instability.**
- Hodgkin's disease: Splenectomy was formerly necessary for staging of patients, particularly those without evidence of nodal or hepatic disease. Currently, splenectomy is rarely done unless staging will influence treatment.
- Hematologic disorders: Myeloproliferative disorders, refractory idiopathic thrombocytopenic purpura or thrombotic thrombocytopenic purpura, hereditary spherocytosis, and thalassemia major.

Postsplenectomy complications include pancreatic leak, abscess, left pleural effusions, infection (particularly with encapsulated organisms), thrombocytosis, and splenic vein and PV thromboses.

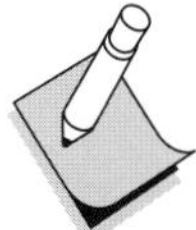

Splenosis–
Benign implantation of splenic tissue following splenic rupture. May retain function and clear particulate matter from RBCs with resultant normal blood smear.

Postsplenectomy vaccines–
Pneumococcus
Meningococcus
H. influenzae

▶ SAMPLE QUESTIONS

What percent of patients have replaced right HA? Left HA?	Replaced right HA: 17%. Replaced left HA: 10%.
Where does the clearing of damaged or dead blood cells occur in the spleen?	By mononuclear phagocytes in the red pulp of the spleen.
Under which segments of the liver do you expect to find the gallbladder?	Segments IV and V.
A 72-year-old woman presents with biliary obstruction. What medical factors necessitate preoperative percutaneous drainage?	Presence of cholangitis, immunosuppression, renal insufficiency, coagulopathy.
A 68-year-old male with recent travel to Mexico presents with 3 days of diarrhea, RUQ pain, fevers, and chills. For which organism will his serology test +? In what percentage of patients will there be + findings in the patient's stool?	Serology will be + for *Entamoeba histolytica* 90% of the time in patients with amoebic liver abscess. Stool amoeba will be found in 15% of cases.
A 40-year-old man UGI bleed from esophageal varices. What medications may be used?	Vasopressin, octreotide.
A 79-year-old alcoholic with Child-Pugh class C cirrhosis presents with intermittent RUQ pain for the past 2 days. Each episode lasts 4-6 hours. His evaluation reveals a WBC = 12 K/μL. An ultrasound shows gallstones without gallbladder wall thickening, pericholecystic fluid, or sonographic Murphy's sign. How should you manage this patient?	Nonoperative medical management of his biliary colic. His operative mortality risk is 70%.
A 25-year-old female with protein C deficiency presents with the acute onset RUQ pain and jaundice. Her evaluation reveals occlusion of her hepatic veins at the level of her IVC. What syndrome does she have? What is the immediate first treatment?	Budd-Chiari syndrome. First-line therapy is anticoagulation.
A 75-year-old female presents with RUQ pain, jaundice, and fever. She has a WBC = 16 K/μL with a left shift. If left untreated, what other symptoms will she develop? What is the next step in management?	If her cholangitis is left untreated, she may develop Reynold's pentad: Charcot's triad plus hypotension and altered mental status. Treat her aggressively with fluid resuscitation, broad spectrum IV antibiotics. Perform timely ERCP with sphincterotomy and stone extraction.

CHAPTER 7

Pancreas

Janivette Alsina, MD, PhD
Reviewed by Cristina R. Ferrone, MD

▶ BASIC SCIENCE

Pancreas divisum is the most common congenital anomaly of the pancreas.

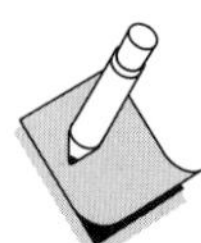

Pancreatic congenital anomalies–
Failure to fuse → pancreatic divisum. Treat with sphincterotomy and cholecystectomy.
Failure of the ventral bud to rotate → annular pancreas. Treat with duodenojejunostomy.
See Chapter 19 for additional details.

Embryology

The pancreas develops from the endoderm of the primitive gut. Two endodermal buds (ventral and dorsal) fuse to form the structures of the pancreas (see Table 7-1). The smaller ventral bud (from the hepatic diverticulum) gives rise to the proximal pancreatic structures: proximal main pancreatic duct (Wirsung's), uncinate process, common bile duct (CBD), and parts of the head. The dorsal bud (from the duodenum) gives rise to the accessory pancreatic duct (Șantorini's), remainder of the pancreatic head, and the pancreatic body and tail.

Anatomy

Macroscopic Anatomy

Retroperitoneal structure with anatomic segments including the head, neck, uncinate process, body, and tail. Important anatomic relations to the inferior vena cava (IVC; posterior to head), splenic artery and vein (posterior to body and tail), and superior mesenteric artery (SMA), superior mesenteric vein (SMV), and portal vein (PV; posterior to neck and medial to the uncinate process) are depicted in Figure 7-1.

The main pancreatic duct merges with the CBD to form a common channel, which empties into the duodenum at the ampulla of Vater. For patients with pancreatic divisum, a lesser papilla draining the dorsal duct of Santorini may be located proximal to the ampulla.

Microscopic Anatomy

Histologically divided into endocrine and exocrine compartments.

- **Endocrine pancreas:** Composed of hormone-producing cells that comprise the islets of Langerhans. Include **α cells** (secrete glucagon), **β cells** (secrete insulin), **δ cells** (secrete somatostatin), **PP cells** (secrete pancreatic polypeptide, PP), and **G cells** (secrete gastrin).
- **Exocrine pancreas:** About 85% of the pancreatic mass. Composed of pancreatic lobules that include acinar and ductal cells.
  - Acinar cells secrete digestive enzymes including lipase, amylase, phospholipase A2, and trypsinogen. Amylase and lipase are secreted as active enzymes, while phospholipase A2 and the peptidases (eg, trypsinogen, chymotrypsinogen) are secreted as proenzymes that are activated in the duodenum by enterokinase.

TABLE 7-1. Embryonic Origins of Adult Pancreatic Structures

Embryologic Structure	Adult Structures
Ventral pancreatic bud	CBD, proximal main pancreatic duct (Wirsung's), uncinate process, inferior portion of the head of the pancreas.
Dorsal pancreatic bud	Superior portion of the head of the pancreas, body and tail of the pancreas, accessory pancreatic duct (Santorini's).

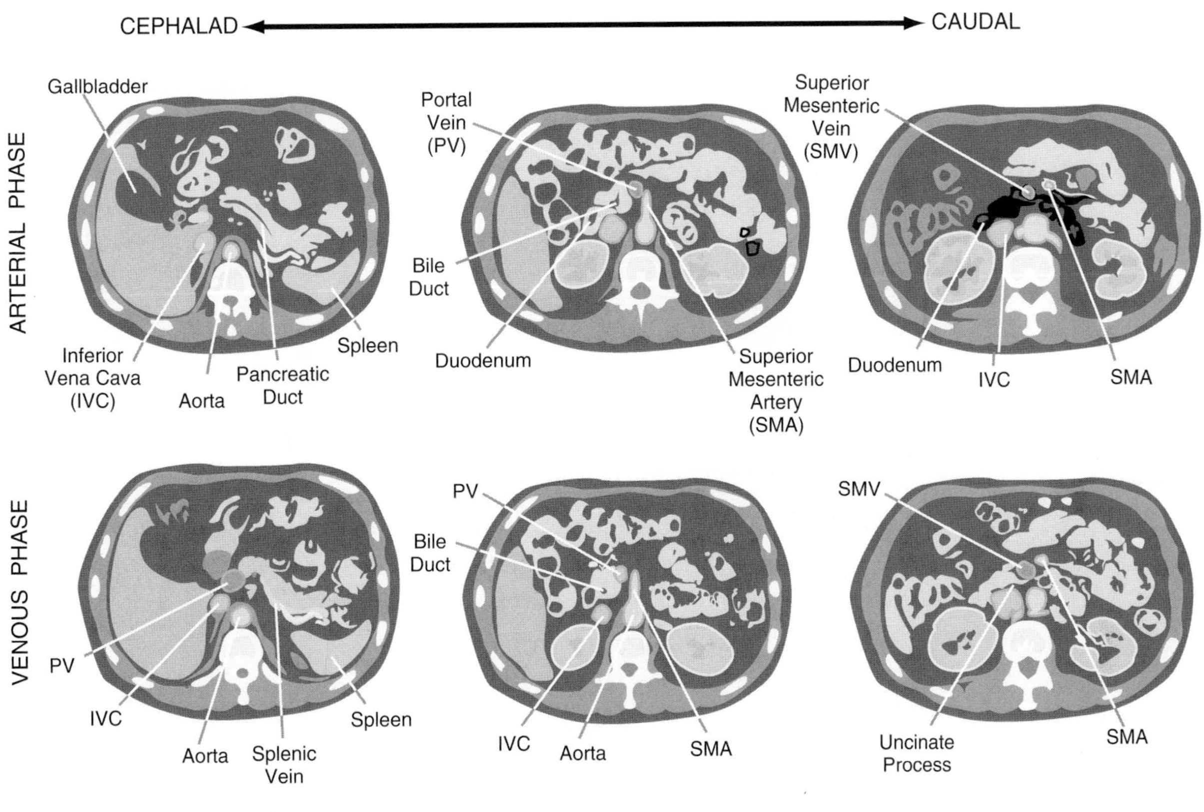

FIGURE 7-1. Pancreatic anatomy.

(Reproduced, with permission, from Brunicardi FC, et al. *Schwartz's Principles of Surgery*, 8th ed. New York: McGraw-Hill, 2005:1222.)

- Ductal cells secrete HCO_3^-.
- Exocrine cells have receptors for secretagogues produced in the gastrointestinal (GI) tract including secretin (from the duodenum and jejunum, in response to low pH), acetylcholine (from vagus nerve), gastrin (from the antral cells in the stomach), substance P, and cholecystokinin (CCK; from the enteroendocrine of the duodenum and jejunum).

BLOOD SUPPLY

Arterial supply to the pancreas derives from branches of the celiac axis and SMA:

- The head is supplied by the SMA and by the superior and inferior pancreaticoduodenal branches of the gastroduodenal artery (GDA).
- The body of the pancreas is supplied by branches from the splenic artery.
- The tail of the pancreas is supplied by branches from the dorsal pancreatic, splenic, and gastroepiploic arteries.

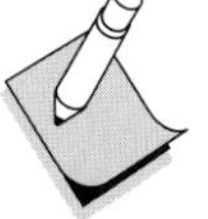

GDA is a branch of the common hepatic artery, which comes off the celiac trunk.

Venous drainage parallels the arterial supply with the superior veins draining directly into the **PV**. The inferior veins drain into the **inferior mesenteric vein**. The body and tail drain into the splenic vein.

INNERVATION

Densely innervated by fibers from the autonomic nervous system. Pancreatic secretion is stimulated in part by efferent fibers from the parasympathetic nervous system. Sympathetic innervation is primarily indirect and is involved in the regulation of blood flow to the exocrine pancreas.

TABLE 7-2. Pancreatic Enzymes and Target Substrates

Pancreatic Enzymes	Target Substrate(s)
Chymotrypsin, trypsin, elastase, carboxypeptidase	Proteins, peptides
Lipase, colipase, phospholipase	Fat, triglycerides, phospholipids
Amylase	Carbohydrates
Ribonuclease, deoxyribonuclease	Ribonucleic acids

Lymphatic Drainage

Drainage basins include the pancreaticoduodenal nodes (head), pancreaticosplenic nodes (neck, body, tail), and superior mesenteric nodes.

Pancreatic Physiology

Pancreas secretes ~500-1500 mL of pancreatic fluid daily. Secretion is controlled, in part, by CCK, secretin, and vagal stimulation. Fluid contains digestive enzymes, electrolytes, and small amounts of other proteins. Digestive enzymes make up ~95% of the pancreatic exocrine secretions and are responsible for the metabolism of protein, fats, carbohydrates, and ribonucleic acids (see Table 7-2). Secreted electrolytes (eg, Na^+, K^+, Ca^{2+}, HCO_3^-, Cl^-, sulfate, phosphate) ↑ the duodenal intraluminal pH to facilitate the activation and function of the digestive enzymes. HCO_3^- is secreted by ductal cells at concentrations much higher than those found in plasma (113 mEq/L versus 24 mEq/L), creating the **alkaline pancreatic fluid.**

Pancreatic hormones have specific functions and are regulated by interactions between the hormones, sympathetic nervous system, and nutrients that are sensed by the various pancreatic cell types (see Table 7-3).

TABLE 7-3. Pancreatic Regulation

Pancreatic Products	Secretion Stimulators	Secretion Inhibitors
Exocrine products	Secretin, CCK.	Somatostatin.
Endocrine hormones		
Insulin	Glucagon, glucose, amino acids, vagal and β-adrenergic input.	Insulin, somatostatin, α-adrenergic input.
Glucagon	Cortisol, growth hormone, amino acids, vagal and β-adrenergic input.	Insulin, somatostatin, α-adrenergic input.
Pancreatic polypeptide	Vagal input.	Unknown.
Somatostatin	Glucagon, glucose, amino acids.	Somatostatin, insulin.

Acinar-derived enzymes (eg, amylase, lipase, proteases) cleave carbohydrates, triglycerides, and peptides, respectively. Endocrine-derived hormones include

- **Insulin:** Made by β cells. Acts on the muscle, liver, and adipose tissue. Stimulates **anabolism** (eg, ↑ glycogenesis, ↓ gluconeogenesis, ↓ fatty acid breakdown, ↑ protein synthesis).
- **Glucagon:** Made by α cells. Acts on hepatocytes. Stimulates **catabolism** (ie, effects are the opposite of insulin).
- **Somatostatin:** Made by δ cells. Acts on multiple cell types. **Inhibits** GI hormone secretion, motility, and intestinal and pancreatic fluid secretion.
- **Pancreatic polypeptide:** Made by PP cells. Inhibits insulin and exocrine pancreas secretion.

Octreotide is a somatostatin analog. Indications for use include bleeding esophageal varices, inhibition of pituitary adenoma secretion, and carcinoid syndrome.

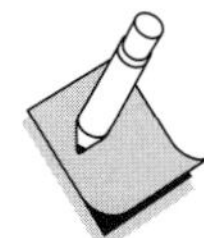

Functions of insulin and glucagon–
Insulin → anabolism → ↑ glycogenesis, ↓ gluconeogenesis, ↓ fatty acid breakdown, ↑ protein synthesis.
Glucagon → catabolism → ↓ glycogenesis ↑ gluconeogenesis, ↑ fatty acid breakdown, ↓ protein synthesis.

▶ CLINICAL SCIENCE

Acute Pancreatitis

DEMOGRAPHICS

Approximately 185,000 new cases annually with greater hospitalization rates for African Americans and males. Spectrum of disease includes mild, self-limiting pancreatitis, severe acute pancreatitis (ie, acute attack with complications), and severe necrotizing pancreatitis with multisystem organ failure. Develops as a result of autodigestion of the pancreas by pancreatic enzymes (eg, trypsin).

Eighty percent of acute pancreatitis in the United States is caused by gallstones or alcohol.

ETIOLOGIES

Include mechanical (eg, **gallstones**, post–endoscopic retrograde cholangiopancreatography [ERCP], duct obstruction, pancreatic divisum), metabolic (eg, **alcohol**, medications, hypercalcemia, hyperlipidemia), infectious (eg, cytomegalovirus [CMV], mumps), autoimmune (eg, systemic lupus erythematosus, polyarteritis nodosa), hereditary (eg, *PRSS1* and *SPINK1* mutations), and traumatic causes.

Drugs associated with acute pancreatitis–
steroids, diuretics (thiazides), immune-modulating drugs (azathioprine), antiretrovirals.

SIGNS/SYMPTOMS

Signs and symptoms may be nonspecific and can include epigastric or upper abdominal pain that can radiate to the back, nausea, vomiting, tachycardia, and fever. Severe, persistent, and symptomatic necrosis is associated with malaise, inability to tolerate an oral diet, and pain. Retroperitoneal bleeding (eg, flank ecchymosis [**Grey-Turner's sign**], periumbilical ecchymosis [**Cullen's sign**]) may be observed in severe cases but are not pathognomonic.

DIAGNOSIS

Labs might reveal ↑ white blood cell (WBC) counts, ↑ glucose, ↑ lactate dehydrogenase (LDH), ↑ aspartate aminotransferase (AST), ↑ amylase, and ↑ lipase. **Lipase is more sensitive and specific than amylase** for acute pancreatitis. **Contrast-enhanced abdominal CT confirms the diagnosis:** Peripancreatic fat stranding, fluid collections, and nonenhancing pancreatic parenchyma

TABLE 7-4. Ranson's Criteria

CRITERIA, ON ADMISSION	CRITERIA, WITHIN 48 HOURS OF ADMISSION
Age > 55 years	Blood urea nitrogen (BUN) ↑ > 5 mg/dL
Glucose > 200 mg/dL	Ca^{2+} < 8 mg/dL
WBC > 16 K/μL	Hematocrit (HCT) ↓ by > 10%
LDH > 350 IU/L	Base deficit > 4 mEq/L
AST > 250 IU/dL	PaO_2 < 60 mm Hg
	Fluid sequestration > 6 L

with gas (suggestive of necrosis) may be seen. If necrotizing pancreatitis is suspected, CT-guided aspiration can be used to differentiate between sterile and infected pancreatic necrosis, the latter requiring surgical debridement.

Pancreatic enzyme levels do not correlate with the severity of the disease or with outcome.

Ranson's criteria were created as a way to predict morbidity and mortality in patients admitted with acute pancreatitis (see Table 7-4). Each fulfilled criteria is assigned one point. Mortality risk is based on the number of points: 0-2 points = 2%, 3–4 points = 15%, 5-6 points = 40%, and 7–8 points = 100%. The Acute Physiology And Chronic Health Evaluation II (APACHE II) system is often used instead of Ranson criteria.

TREATMENT

Uncomplicated acute pancreatitis warrants conservative management with fluid resuscitation, NPO status, nasogastric tube (NGT) decompression, close monitoring of fluid balance, and pain control. Bowel rest with total parenteral nutrition (TPN) administration is indicated except in mild cases. Prophylactic antibiotics (eg, **imipenem** with or without antifungal coverage) are indicated for necrotizing pancreatitis. If gallstone pancreatitis is associated with obstructive choledocholithiasis or cholangitis, perform ERCP with sphincterotomy followed by cholecystectomy. Surgical treatment (eg, necrosectomy) is indicated for cases of infected necrotizing pancreatitis and symptomatic, organized pancreatic necrosis.

Chronic Pancreatitis

DEMOGRAPHICS/RISK FACTORS

Approximately 68,000 new cases diagnosed annually in the United States with a higher incidence among men and African Americans. Due to prolonged pancreatic inflammation → fibrosis and ductal obstruction → ↑ ductal pressures and ductal dilation. Changes are irreversible and lead to the loss of both exocrine and endocrine pancreatic function.

ETIOLOGIES

Include **alcohol abuse (most common)**, gallstones, obstruction (eg, tumor), pancreas divisum, autoimmune pancreatitis, and familial predisposition (eg, *SPINK1* or cystic fibrosis transmembrane conductance regulator [*CFTR*] mutations, familial hyperlipidemia).

Signs/Symptoms

Intermittent abdominal pain, weight loss, diabetes mellitus (DM; ie, endocrine insufficiency), and steatorrhea (ie, malabsorption or exocrine insufficiency).

Diagnosis

ERCP is the gold standard for the diagnosis of chronic pancreatitis. Look for irregular main duct, ductal dilation, and duct strictures.

Primarily a clinical diagnosis. Labs might reveal normal or ↑ amylase and lipase, ↑ alkaline phosphatase (if obstruction present), and ↑ blood glucose. CT might reveal a **dilated, calcified pancreatic duct** with areas of stenosis (ie, "chain of lakes" appearance). **ERCP** is the gold standard for the diagnosis; findings include **irregular main duct,** ductal dilation, and **duct strictures**.

Treatment

Avoid triggering factors (eg, alcohol), ensure pain control (nonsteroidal anti-inflammatory drugs [NSAIDs]), administer insulin if diabetic, and replace pancreatic enzymes (eg, pancrelipase) if exocrine-insufficient. Pancreatic stones are amenable to extracorporeal shock wave lithotripsy; strictures may be amenable to sphincterotomy and duct stenting.

Surgery is indicated for **intractable pain, suspected cancer, stenosis of the pancreatic duct, and obstruction of the duodenum or biliary tree.** Surgical procedures fall into three categories: Drainage, resection, or a combination of these. The choice of surgical procedure depends on the symptoms, diagnostic study results, and surgeon's experience.

- Duct of normal diameter: Pancreaticoduodenectomy (Whipple)
- Dilated duct: Longitudinal pancreaticojejunostomy (Puestow)
- Distal disease: Distal pancreatectomy
- Small duct with diffuse disease: Total pancreatectomy with autotransplantation of islet cells

Surgical treatment of chronic pancreatitis for pain control has very good outcomes: Up to 80% of patients have postoperative pain improvement.

Complications of chronic pancreatitis include pancreatic pseudocyst, pancreatic fistula, and obstruction of the duodenum or biliary tree.

Pancreatic Pseudocysts

During episodes of acute pancreatitis, some patients develop peripancreatic fluid collections with a **nonepithelialized** capsule. Majority resolve spontaneously within 4–6 weeks, but some become organized (ie, pseudocysts) particularly if chronic pancreatitis is present. Symptoms might include persistent abdominal pain and early satiety. Workup might reveal persistently ↑ amylase and lipase. Cyst fluid sampling shows **↑ amylase, normal carcinoembryonic antigen (CEA),** and **normal CA 19-9**. Management depends on the **presence of pain as well as the size and duration of the pseudocyst.** Must be differentiated from cystic neoplasms, congenital cysts, and retention cysts (which, unlike pseudocysts, have an epithelial lining). Cyst fluid analysis and imaging can help differentiate pseudocyst from cystic neoplasms (see Table 7-5). MRI is superior to CT in this differentiation. Treatment includes endoscopic, percutaneous, or surgical drainage. Consider surgical therapy if organized (> 6 weeks), if complications (eg, infection or rupture of pseudocyst, hemorrhage into nearby vascular structures, biliary obstruction, gastric outlet obstruction) are present, or if cancer is suspected.

Pancreatic pseudocysts are most commonly associated with alcoholic pancreatitis.

TABLE 7-5. Differences Between Pancreatic Pseudocysts and Cystic Neoplasms

DIAGNOSTIC TESTS	PANCREATIC PSEUDOCYSTS	IPMNS	MCNS
Imaging	Single cyst, no septations, absence of mass/nodularity inside cyst, + communication with main duct on ERCP/magnetic resonance cholangiopancreatography (MRCP).	Single or multiple lesions, +/– septations, +/– mass/nodularity inside cyst, + **communication with main duct** on ERCP/MRCP.	Single or multiple lesions, +/– septations, +/– mass/nodularity inside cyst, **no communication with main duct** on ERCP/MRCP.
Fluid analysis	↑ Amylase, nl CEA, nl CA 19-9.	↑ **Amylase**, nl/↑ CEA, nl/↑ CA 19-9.	↓ **Amylase**, nl/↑ CEA, nl/↑ CA 19-9.

Ovarian-like stroma is pathognomonic of MCNs.

IPMNs communicate with the main pancreatic duct; MCNs do not.

Cystic Neoplasms of the Pancreas

Intraductal papillary mucinous neoplasms (IPMNs) are an increasingly recognized entity characterized by mucin production, dilation of the pancreatic duct, and **communication with the main pancreatic duct**. Most commonly found in **men** and in the **head** of the pancreas. Lesions may be benign with minimal hyperplastic changes but can progress to invasive carcinoma. Invasive cancers are more commonly associated with main duct IPMNs; side branch IPMNs appear to have less malignant potential. Because of their malignant potential, **resection of main duct IPMNs is recommended.** Consider Whipple for lesions at the pancreatic head, distal pancreatectomy for tail lesions, and total pancreatectomy if multiple lesions are present throughout pancreas.

Mucinouscystic neoplasms (MCNs) are commonly found in **middle-aged females** and in the body or **tail** of the pancreas. Characterized by an **ovarian-like stroma** and a **lack of ductal communication**. Usually asymptomatic until large; often an incidental finding on imaging. Because of the risk for malignant progression, **surgical resection** (usually distal pancreatectomy) is recommended.

Solid pseudopapillary tumors are found primarily in **young women** in the third decade of life. Resection is indicated.

> A 55-year-old female presents with persistent epigastric pain radiating to the back. Her workup includes a CT scan that reveals a 3.5 cm mass at the head of the pancreas; her CA 19-9 is elevated. How is resectability determined? Assess for extrapancreatic disease and encasement or invasion of the celiac axis, hepatic artery, SMA, SMV, or PV.

Pancreatic Ductal Adenocarcinoma

DEMOGRAPHICS/RISK FACTORS

Approximately 37,000 new cases are diagnosed annually in the United States. Majority of patients succumb to disease within 1 year of diagnosis. Risk factors include age, African American race, **tobacco use**, chronic pancreatitis, DM, and family history (ie, hereditary cancer syndromes including familial multiple mole melanoma, hereditary breast-ovarian cancer syndrome, or hereditary pancreatitis-pancreatic cancer syndrome).

SIGNS/SYMPTOMS

Classic presentation is **painless jaundice**. Other symptoms include pain, weight loss, nausea, vomiting (because of gastric outlet obstruction), DM, exocrine insufficiency, acholic stools, pruritus, and dark urine. Signs include a palpable gallbladder (**Courvosier's sign**), palpable periumbilical metastatic disease (**Sister Mary Joseph's node**), migratory thrombophlebitis (**Trousseau's sign**), palpable left supraclavicular fossa node (**Virchow's node**), and palpable metastases on rectal examination (**Blumer's shelf**).

Liver metastases < 1 cm can be missed by CT scan.

DIAGNOSIS

Labs might reveal ↑ bilirubin, ↑ alkaline phosphatase, ↑ AST and ALT, and ↔ amylase and lipase. CEA and CA 19-9 may be ↑; **CA 19-9** is more specific than CEA. Imaging includes contrast-enhanced triple phase CT to determine stage and resectability of disease. Lesions are **hypoechoic** and may be associated with **pancreatic atrophy and distal ductal dilation**. Endoscopic ultrasound with fine needle aspiration can confirm diagnosis. ERCP may reveal the classic **double duct** sign (ie, CBD and pancreatic ductal dilatation) with two strictures (eg, CBD and pancreatic duct).

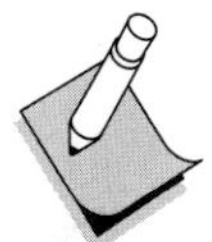

Characteristic ERCP findings–
Dilated pancreatic duct/CBD, 2 strictures → pancreatic ductal adenocarcinoma (PDAC).
Dilated pancreatic duct/CBD, 1 stricture → ampullary cancer.

TREATMENT

Treatment is based on resectability as determined by imaging and staging laparoscopy. Resectability is defined as **absence of extrapancreatic disease and no encasement or involvement of the celiac axis, hepatic artery (HA), SMA, SMV, or PV**. Resection type is based on location: Distal pancreatectomy for body and tail lesions or Whipple for lesions of the head and neck. Complications following Whipple include pancreatic fistulas, delayed gastric emptying, intra-abdominal abscesses, and wound infections.

Palliation is indicated for gastric outlet obstruction, biliary obstruction, and pain. Operative and nonoperative treatments exist:

- Operative interventions: Hepaticoduodenostomy or hepaticojejunostomy (for biliary drainage) and gastrojejunostomy with chemical splanchnicectomy of the celiac plexus.
- Nonoperative interventions: Endoscopic biliary decompression with polyethylene stents or metallic self-expanding gastroduodenal stents (relief of obstruction). Percutaneous, CT-guided celiac nerve blocks and oral analgesics (pain improvement).

Tumors of the body and tail of the pancreas are usually not detected at an early stage and are usually unresectable at time of diagnosis.

Neoadjuvant and adjuvant protocols for PDAC are still evolving. Chemoradiotherapeutic regimens (eg, gemcitabine, 5-fluorouracil [5-FU], and radiation) preoperatively or for palliation may yield a survival benefit.

STAGING/OUTCOMES

Tumor, node status, metastasis (TNM) categories include

- T: T_{is} (carcinoma in situ), T1 (limited to the pancreas and ≤ 2 cm in greatest dimension), T2 (limited to the pancreas and > 2 cm in greatest dimension), T3 (extends beyond the pancreas but without involvement of the celiac axis or SMA), T4 (involves the celiac axis or SMA)
- N: N0 (– regional lymph node), N1 (+ regional lymph nodes)
- M: M0 (metastatic disease absent), M1 (metastatic disease present)

Staging includes

- Stage 0: T_{is}N0M0
- Stage IA: T1N0M0

PANCREAS

- Stage IB: T2N0M0
- Stage IIA: T3N0M0
- Stage IIB: Any T, N1M0
- Stage III: T4, any N, M0
- Stage IV: Any T, any N, M1

Five-year survival is 10-20% though may be lower with larger tumor size (> 3 cm), + lymph nodes, perineural or perivascular invasion, + resection margins, or poorly differentiated histology.

A 35-year-old male collapses while walking to work. He is diaphoretic, tachycardiac, and his workup reveals a blood sugar of 35 mg/dL. What is the most appropriate management if a pancreatic source is suspected? Administer glucose. When he stabilizes, perform a CT scan with IV contrast, which will reveal a hypervascular lesion in the pancreas. Resection is indicated. Consider an octreotide scan to identify possible metastases.

Pancreatic Endocrine Tumors

Rare entities that may be functional or nonfunctional (see Table 7-6).

TABLE 7-6. Pancreatic Endocrine Tumors

Tumor	Cell of Origin/ Hormone	Distribution	Malignant Potential	Signs/Symptoms
Insulinoma	β cells/insulin	Evenly distributed through pancreas.	10% malignant.	**Whipple's triad:** Fasting hypoglycemia, blood sugar < 50 mg/dL during episodes, relief with glucose.
Gastrinoma	G cells/gastrin	Gastrinoma triangle, pancreatic head.	70% malignant; better prognosis if associated with multiple endocrine neoplasia type I (MEN-1).	Epigastric pain and ulcers refractory to medical treatment, diarrhea.
Glucagonoma	α cells/glucagon	Tail.	75% malignant with metastases.	**Migratory necrolytic erythema**, anemia, DM, protein malnutrition, hypercoagulability, stomatitis.
Somatostatinoma	δ cells/somatostatin	Head.	50% malignant with metastases.	DM, diarrhea, biliary tract disease.
VIPoma (Verner-Morrison syndrome; watery diarrhea, hypokalemia and achlorhydria [WDHA] syndrome)	D_2 cells/vasoactive intestinal peptide (VIP)	Body, tail.	50% malignant; 75% of these have metastatic disease.	**W**atery **d**iarrhea, **h**ypokalemia, **a**chlorhydria, ↑ Ca^{2+}.

Specific diagnostic and treatment options for these neoplasms include:

- **Insulinoma: Most common functional endocrine tumor of the pancreas**. Labs show ↓ **blood glucose, ↑ insulin, and ↑ C-peptide**. Preoperative localization with contrast-enhanced CT or MRI is successful in ~90%. Preoperative **diazoxide** is used to prevent hypoglycemia. Most tumors are small and amenable to **enucleation**; intraoperative ultrasound can be used. **Larger tumors (> 2 cm) require formal pancreatic resection.** Unresectable malignant tumors can be debulked followed by 5-FU and streptozocin. Octreotide can be used to control symptoms.
- **Gastrinoma:** Second most common functional endocrine tumor of the pancreas. More frequent in men and associated with **Zollinger-Ellison syndrome**. Confirm diagnosis with ↑ **serum gastrin levels** (> 1000 pg/mL versus 100 to150 pg/mL in normals) or ↑ **gastrin > 200 pg/mL in secretin stimulation test**. Somatostatin receptor scintigraphy (SRS) with radiolabeled octreotide can detect tumor location though might miss tumors < 1 cm and those found in the duodenal wall. Proton pump inhibitors may alleviate symptoms in symptomatic disease. Enucleation for small tumors; resection for larger (> 2 cm) tumors.
- **Glucagonoma: Fasting glucagon levels > 50 pg/mL are diagnostic.** Preoperative reversal of the catabolic state with octreotide, enteral nutrition, and amino acid supplementation (as patients commonly have protein malnutrition) are recommended. Surgery is curative; dacarbazine or streptozocin may be used if unresectable. Somatostatin, zinc, and amino acids may be effective in controlling associated stomatitis.
- **Somatostatinoma:** Usually unresectable at diagnosis. Chemotherapy includes streptozocin, dacarbazine, and doxorubicin. If resectable and at the pancreatic head, perform Whipple.
- **VIPoma:** Diagnosed by a combination of symptoms and ↑ serum VIP levels (> 200 pg/mL). Localize tumors with CT scan or SRS. Preoperative treatment with octreotide helps correct fluid and electrolyte imbalances. Resection is the recommended treatment.

Boundaries of the gastrinoma triangle–

(1) *Cystic duct*

(2) *Junction of the second and third portions of the duodenum*

(3) *Junction of the neck and body of the pancreas*

▶ SAMPLE QUESTIONS

What is the blood supply to the head of the pancreas?	SMA and the superior and inferior pancreaticoduodenal branches of the GDA.
What is the most common malignancy of the pancreas?	PDAC.
What are the classic ERCP findings in chronic pancreatitis? PDAC?	Chronic pancreatitis: Irregular main duct, ductal dilation, ductal strictures. PDAC: "Double duct" sign.
What are the CT findings of unresectable PDAC?	Extrapancreatic disease; encasement of SMA, HA, or celiac axis; occlusion of SMV-PV junction.
A 60-year-old male presents with an incidentally found cystic lesion of the pancreas. What is the classic ERCP finding for IPMN?	Mucin at the ampulla of Vater, as IPMNs communicate with the pancreatic duct.
A 50-year-old male with a history of chronic pancreatitis presents with bleeding gastric varices. What is the most likely cause? Curative treatment?	Most likely diagnosis is splenic vein thrombosis. As patient is bleeding, treat with splenectomy.
What is the most common location of an insulinoma? Gastrinoma? Glucagonoma?	Insulinoma: Evenly distributed throughout the pancreas. Gastrinoma: Gastrinoma triangle. Glucagonoma: Pancreatic tail.
A 45-year-old female presents with a cystic neoplasm of the pancreas. What is the most likely diagnosis? What histopathologic findings will be present?	Likely diagnosis is MCN. Treatment is resection, commonly a distal pancreatectomy. Pathology will reveal ovarian-like stroma and a mucinous epithelium.
A 65-year-old man presents with painless jaundice, and you suspect PDAC. What is the most sensitive radiographic modality to diagnosis PDAC?	Endoscopic ultrasound.
A patient with chronic pancreatitis presents with intractable pain. His evaluation reveals a pancreatic duct that is dilated to 1.2 cm. What surgery will you consider? What should be the length of your anastomosis?	Consider a Puestow procedure for pancreatic ducts dilated > 1 cm. To optimize outcomes, the anastomosis should extend over a distance of at least 6 cm.

CHAPTER 8

Hernias

Nicolas Melo, MD, MS
Reviewed by Charles M. Ferguson, MD

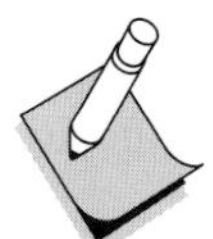

Abdominal wall fascial layers–
Camper's: Superficial and fatty.
Scarpa's: Deeper and fibrous.
Approximation of these layers reinforces closure.

Hernia Anatomy

Anatomy of the Abdominal Wall

Layers of the abdominal wall include skin, subcutaneous fat, fascia (Camper's and Scarpa's), external oblique (EO), internal oblique (IO), transversus abdominus, transversalis fascia, and peritoneum. The rectus abdominus is enveloped by the rectus sheath. Superior to the **arcuate line of Douglas**, the anterior sheath is composed of the EO and IO aponeuroses; the posterior sheath is composed of the IO aponeurosis and transversalis fascia. Inferior to the arcuate line, the posterior sheath is composed only of transversalis fascia.

Anatomy of the Inguinal Canal

There are number of ligaments and key structures that make up the inguinal canal (see Figure 8-1).

- **Deep (internal) ring**: Entrance to the inguinal canal, arising from transversalis fascia.
- **Superficial (external) ring**: Exit of inguinal canal, arising from the medial and lateral crura of the EO aponeurosis.

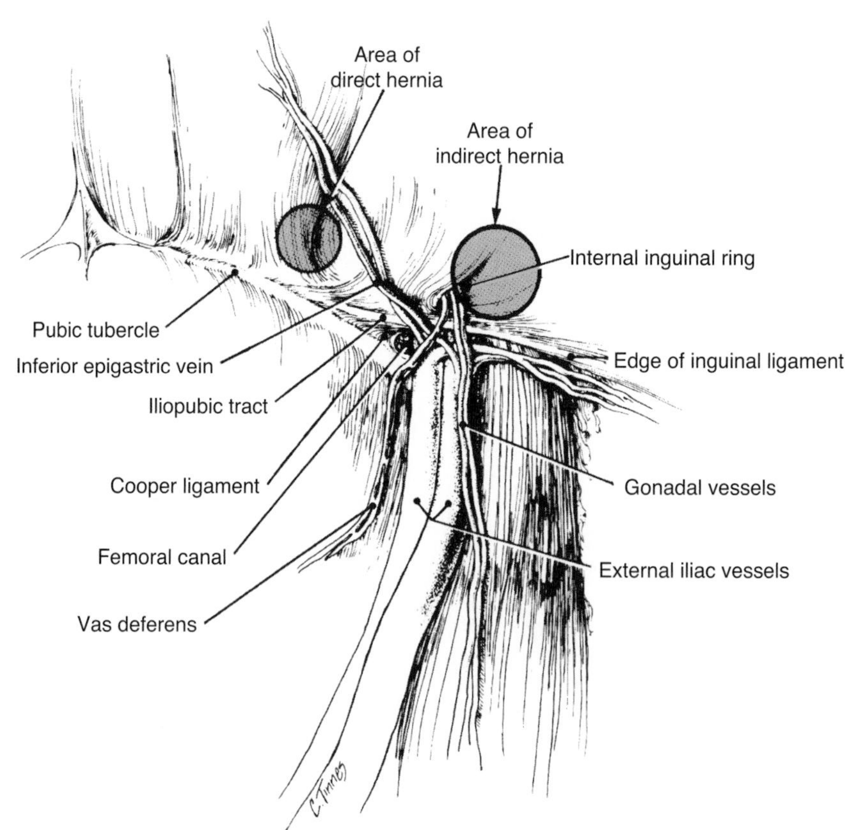

FIGURE 8-1. Ligaments of the inguinal canal.

(Reproduced, with permission, from Brunicardi FC, et al. *Schwartz's Principles of Surgery*. 8th ed. New York: McGraw-Hill, 2005:1363.)

- **Inguinal (Poupart's) ligament**: Arises from thickened portion of EO and connects the anterior superior iliac spine to the pubic tubercle.
- **Lacunar (Gimbernat's) ligament**: Medial, fan-shaped aspect of inguinal ligament that joins inguinal ligament at the pubic tubercle to the pectineal line of pubis.
- **Iliopubic tract**: Arises from the inferior aspect of transversalis fascia, parallel and deep to the inguinal ligament.
- **Cooper's (pectineal) ligament**: Arises from a thickening of the fascia at the pectineal line and appears to extend from the lacunar ligament.
- **Conjoint tendon (falx inguinalis)**: Arises from IO and transversus abdominus aponeuroses.

Boundaries of the inguinal canal–

Anterior: EO

Posterior: Transversalis fascia

Roof: IO, transversus abdominus

Floor: Inguinal ligament

Other important landmarks include:

- **Space of Retzius:** Preperitoneal space behind pubic symphysis. **Site of laparoscopic hernia repairs.**
- **Hesselbach's triangle**: Bordered by the inguinal ligament inferiorly, lateral border of the rectus sheath medially, and the inferior epigastric vessels superiolaterally.

Hernias affect 1–5% of the general population.

The **anatomic boundaries of inguinal canal** include:

- Anterior: **EO aponeurosis** with IO aponeurosis laterally
- Posterior: **Transversalis fascia** with conjoint tendon
- Roof: **IO** and **transversus abdominus**
- Floor: Superior aspect of the **inguinal ligament** with lacunar ligament medially.

The contents of the inguinal canal include the ilioinguinal nerve (superior to cord), spermatic cord (including the genital branch of genitofemoral nerve [posteromedial aspect], cremaster muscle, vas deferens, testicular artery, and pampiniform plexus) or round ligament, lymphatics, and vessels.

ANATOMY OF THE FEMORAL HERNIA

Femoral hernias occur at the medial aspect of the femoral canal. The anatomic boundaries associated with a femoral hernia include:

- Anterior: Inguinal ligament
- Posterior: Cooper's ligament with pubic ramus
- Medial: Lacunar ligament
- Lateral: Femoral vein

▶ CLINICAL SCIENCE

Inguinal Hernias

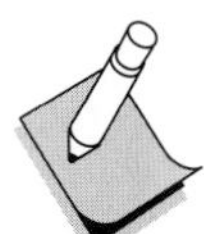

*Indirect inguinal hernias are caused by a congenital failure of the obliteration of the processus vaginalis and arise **lateral** to Hesselbach's triangle.*

*Direct inguinal hernias are acquired and arise **within** Hesselbach's triangle.*

DEMOGRAPHICS/RISK FACTORS

Most common type, comprising 75% of all hernias (50% indirect, 25% direct). Seven times more common in men. More common on the right, though bilateral inguinal hernias can occur. Risk factors include obesity, pregnancy, ascites, heavy exercise, and other conditions leading to ↑ intra-abdominal pressure (eg, straining, coughing).

TYPES

Indirect hernias are usually congenital (ie, **patent processus vaginalis**), arise **lateral to Hesselbach triangle**, and involve a protrusion of abdominal contents through the internal ring. The hernia sac is **anteromedial** to the cord and may descend into scrotum. **Acquired weaknesses** in the transversalis fascia allow direct hernias to protrude **through Hesselbach's triangle**.

SIGNS/SYMPTOMS

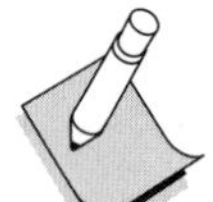

Ilioinguinal nerve: L1

Iliohypogastric nerve: T12, L1

Genitofemoral nerve: L1, L2

Usually presents as a painless, reducible protrusion near the scrotum or labia that is more evident with straining or Valsalva. If not reducible, may be **incarcerated** and can be associated with obstruction. If signs of ischemia are present (eg, skin changes, fever, ↑ white blood cell [WBC] count), suspect **strangulation**.

DIAGNOSIS

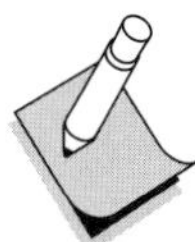

Early hernia recurrences are due to inadequate repairs. Late recurrences may be caused by loss of fascial strength.

Palpation of the inguinal canal with invagination of the finger through the external ring will facilitate diagnosis. However, distinguishing between indirect and direct forms can be difficult. Direct hernias tend to reduce with supine positioning; indirect hernias tend to extend into the scrotum. If a large hernia is not reducible, consider a **sliding hernia** involving the sigmoid colon (left), cecum (right), ovaries, fallopian tubes, or bladder. Radiologic studies are usually not indicated.

TREATMENT

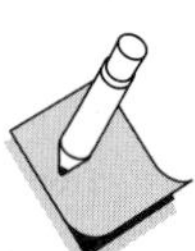

Consider laparoscopic inguinal hernia repair for bilateral or recurrent hernias. Avoid in the setting of incarcerated inguinal hernias.

*Avoid staples in the **trapezoid of doom** (lateral to femoral vessels and below iliopubic tract) where the lateral cutaneous, femoral branch of genitofemoral, and femoral nerves run.*

To minimize morbidity and mortality, emergent operative repair is indicated if strangulation is suspected. Repairs can include:

- Open, suture-based repairs.
  - **Bassini:** High ligation with repair of inguinal floor. Involves approximation of transversalis fascia, conjoint tendon, and shelving edge of inguinal ligament. Avoid sutures in the pubic tubercle to minimize incidence of **osteitis pubis**.
  - **Shouldice:** Similar to Bassini. Primary repair utilizing continuous running sutures in multiple layers.
  - **McVay:** Similar to Bassini. Closure involves **Cooper's ligament**. Used for both inguinal and femoral hernia repairs.
- Open, prosthetic-based repairs.
  - **Lichtenstein**: Tension-free repair that is used for direct and indirect hernias. Avoid a mesh repair if infection is present.
  - "Plug and Patch" or **Stoppa** repair.
- Laparoscopic repairs: Includes **transabdominal preperitoneal** or **totally extraperitoneal** approaches. Consider for **recurrent** (particularly after an anterior repair), **bilateral** (or suspected bilateral), or **femoral hernias**. Should not be used to treat strangulated hernias. Generally associated with less postoperative pain and earlier return to work. However, costs are greater than open repair, and recurrence rates are not yet clear.

In infants and children, high ligation of the hernia sac is sufficient to repair an indirect inguinal hernia. For children in whom bilateral inguinal hernias are suspected (age < 2 years particularly if left-sided hernia is present or females < 3 years), contralateral exploration may be performed.

COMPLICATIONS

Urinary retention (**most common early complication**), wound infection (2%), ischemic orchitis and testicular atrophy (caused by vessel disruption and thrombosis of spermatic vessels during dissection), nerve injury (pain, numbness), hernia recurrence (2–10%), seroma, hematoma, damage to the bladder or vas deferens. Signs of nerve injury include:

- Ilioinguinal injury: Loss of cremasteric reflex and sensation to ipsilateral penis, scrotum, and medial thigh.
- Iliohypogastric injury: Loss of sensation to the lower abdominal wall and inguinal region.
- Genitofemoral injury: Loss of sensation to the upper lateral thigh (femoral branch) or loss of scrotal sensation and cremasteric motor function (genital branch).

Most common early postoperative complication of hernia repair–
Urinary retention: Associated with ↑ IV fluids and type of anesthesia (spinal > general > local)

*Femoral hernias are **inferior** to the inguinal ligament. Repair requires re-approximation with Cooper's ligament.*

The ilioinguinal nerve is the most commonly injured nerve during hernia repair. Watch for it on top of the cord.

Femoral hernias are more common in women than in men. Most common hernia in women is inguinal hernia.

Femoral hernias are more likely than inguinal hernias to require emergent intervention for strangulation.

Femoral Hernias

DEMOGRAPHICS/RISK FACTORS

Comprise about 5% of hernias; bilateral in 15% of cases. **More common in women**, though **inguinal hernias are the most common hernias in women**. Risk factors are similar to inguinal hernias, except that femoral hernias are unlikely to be congenital in origin. Compared to inguinal hernias, greater incidence of incarceration and strangulation due to narrow neck.

SIGNS/SYMPTOMS

Usually presents as a protrusion at the **upper medial thigh, inferior to the inguinal ligament**. Look for signs of incarceration or strangulation.

DIAGNOSIS

Can be distinguished from inguinal hernia based on anatomy, as these most commonly lie **inferior** to inguinal ligament, along the upper medial thigh. Must distinguish from inguinal hernias, saphenous varix, lipomas, and lymphadenopathy.

TREATMENT

Bedside reduction is difficult. Due to high risk of strangulation (up to 45% by 2 years), **operative repair is always indicated**. Most common repair is **McVay** repair (see above). Emergent repair is indicated for strangulation. Recurrence rate is 5–10%.

Incisional (Ventral) Hernias

DEMOGRAPHICS/RISK FACTORS

Occurs in 10–20% of patients who undergo abdominal surgery, most commonly in the first postoperative year. Contributing factors include tissue ischemia, advanced age, presence of infection, malnutrition, obesity, ascites, tobacco use, corticosteroids, repair in an emergent setting, poor surgical technique, presence of aortic aneurysm, and immunosuppression.

SIGNS/SYMPTOMS

Symptoms vary from an asymptomatic bulge to an incarcerated or strangulated tender protrusion at the site of a previous operation. May be associated with overlying skin necrosis or bowel obstruction.

DIAGNOSIS

Clinical exam will support diagnosis, but radiographic studies can be used to confirm the presence of visceral contents and obstruction (if suspected). If protrusion is midline, distinguish from rectus diastasis (separation of rectus muscle vertically) as this does not require surgical treatment.

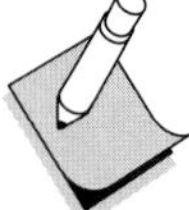

Primary repairs of incisional hernias are associated with a significantly greater recurrence rate compared to mesh repair.

TREATMENT

Like other hernias, the presence of incarceration or strangulation necessitates urgent or emergent surgical intervention. Surgical options include 1° repair, open repair with prosthetic device, and laparoscopic repair. Primary repair via an open approach is acceptable when the fascial edges are clean, the defect is small, and the repair can be performed without tension using nonabsorbable suture. If the fascia is not appropriate for 1° repair, if a tension-free repair is not possible, or if the defect is large, consider open repair with a nonabsorbable mesh (placed anteriorly or posteriorly), which has been found to have a **lower recurrence rate** compared to 1° repair (10% versus 50%). Laparoscopic repair is becoming increasingly utilized and relies on a posterior repair with nonabsorable mesh. Complications of incisional hernia repairs are similar to other hernia operations and include recurrence (greatest with 1° repair), wound infection, seroma, hematoma, and visceral damage (particularly with laparoscopic procedures).

A 47-year-old man with hepatitis C and Child-Pugh class B cirrhosis presents to the ER with an umbilical hernia. On exam, he has a temperature of 101.3°F, an HR of 110 bpm, and a BP of 90/64 mmHg. On exam, he is somnolent and has a distended abdomen with a palpable fluid wave and a nontender, reducible umbilical hernia that is slowly leaking ascites. What is the next step in management? Though the patient does not have a strangulated hernia, he is hemodynamically deteriorating and has an ascites leak at the site of his umbilical hernia. Stabilize the patient and obtain consent to perform an urgent hernia repair.

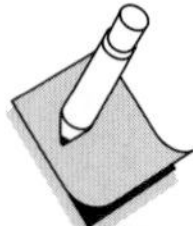

Repair of small, childhood umbilical hernias is usually delayed until 4 years of age due to a high rate of spontaneous closure.

Umbilical Hernias

DEMOGRAPHICS/RISK FACTORS

Arise from a fascial defect in linea alba at the level of umbilicus. Risk factors for congenital types (ie, persistent opening of the umbilical ring) include African American race and prematurity; risk factors for acquired forms include female gender and ↑ intra-abdominal pressure (eg, pregnancy, obesity, ascites, intra-abdominal mass). Whereas childhood umbilical hernias < 1 cm in size have a high rate of spontaneous closure by 4 years of age, **adult umbilical hernias rarely close spontaneously.**

SIGNS/SYMPTOMS

Congenital forms are usually associated with a small, asymptomatic bulge noted by the parents. Acquired forms vary from asymptomatic bulges to tender, erythematous bulges that may be associated with overlying skin necrosis, incarceration, or strangulation.

DIAGNOSIS

Confirm bulge at the umbilicus and try to define the associated fascial defect. Rule out additional etiologies including varices, metastatic tumors, or lymphadenopathy.

TREATMENT

Childhood umbilical hernias have a high rate of spontaneous closure, and repair is generally delayed until the child is 2–4 years old. These hernias rarely close spontaneously in adults and thus, require operative repair. Traditionally, an open approach with re-approximation of fascial edges with nonabsorbable suture is used. If the defect is large and cannot be primarily repaired without tension, a mesh repair (laparoscopic or open) might be necessary. Patients with cirrhosis have a particularly high incidence of morbidity and mortality associated with umbilical hernia repair. Medical optimization should occur prior to operative repair, but the presence of **incarceration, strangulation, or an ascites leak necessitate expeditious repair**.

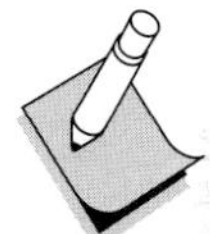

If ascites is present, optimize the patient's medical condition prior to repair unless an urgent or emergent indication exists.

> An 85-year-old woman presents to the ED with crampy, intermittent abdominal pain. She is hemodynamically stable and has a mildly distended abdomen. Though no hernia is palpated, she has medial thigh pain that is exacerbated with leg abduction, internal rotation, or extension. What is the most likely diagnosis? The patient likely has an obturator hernia based on the presence of the Howship-Romberg sign. A CT scan can confirm the diagnosis. Operative repair is indicated.

Miscellaneous Hernias

Additional hernias are summarized in Table 8-1.

TABLE 8-1. Miscellaneous Hernias

Type	Location
Spigelian	Hernia through the **linea semilunaris** (space extending lateral to the posterior rectus sheath to the medial aspect of the transversus abdominus), particularly where the line of Douglas intersects the linea semilunaris. High incidence (up to 20%) of incarceration. Operative repair is indicated.
Lumbar	
Petit's	Hernia through the **inferior lumbar triangle** (boundaries: posterior edge of the EO, latissimus dorsi, and iliac crest).
Grynfeltt's	Hernia through the **superior lumbar triangle** (boundaries: 12th rib, serratus, IO, quadratus lumborum, and erector spinae).
Epigastric	Midline hernia through muscular aponeuroses that form the linea alba, in an area extending from xiphoid to umbilicus.
Obturator	Hernia through the obturator foramen in pelvis. Hernias lie **anteromedial** to obturator nerve and vessels. Most common in **elderly women**. Associated signs include **Howship-Romberg sign**, bowel obstruction (acute or intermittent), and palpable **medial thigh mass**. Operative repair is indicated.
Richter's	Hernia involving one wall of bowel. Can cause ischemia and strangulation, leading to **perforation without associated obstruction**.
Littre's	Hernia involving a **Meckel's diverticulum**.
Pantaloon	Combination of indirect and direct inguinal hernias that straddle the inferior epigastric vessels.

▶ SAMPLE QUESTIONS

A 46-year-old man is unable to urinate 12 hours after an uncomplicated laparoscopic inguinal hernia repair under general anesthesia. What is the most common cause of his urinary retention?	General anesthesia and excessive IV fluid administration.
What are the 1° causes of early inguinal hernia recurrences? Late recurrences?	Early: Inadequate fascial repair, failure to identify and repair all hernias. Late: Loss of fascial strength.
A 63-year-old woman comes to your office with a protrusion at her upper inner thigh, inferior to the inguinal ligament. It is not reducible. What is the next step?	Rule out other diagnoses (assess for pulse or thrill). Prepare for urgent surgical repair of an incarcerated femoral hernia.
A 32-year-old male develops testicular atrophy after an indirect hernia repair. What is the most likely cause?	Ischemic orchitis due to venous congestion with venous thrombosis. Associated with indirect hernia repairs.
A 23-year-old male has an incarcerated inguinal hernia. What is the next step in management?	If strangulation is not suspected, attempt reduction with sedation and Trendelenburg position. After successful reduction, repair may be performed in 2–3 days. If unsuccessful, perform urgent operative repair.
What is the most common type of hernia in all-comers? In females?	All-comers: Indirect inguinal hernia. Women: Indirect inguinal hernia.
A 50-year-old female has a sliding indirect inguinal hernia. What organs are likely involved?	Ovary, fallopian tube, cecum (right), sigmoid colon (left), bladder.
What factors are associated with hernia recurrence? What type of hernia is most likely to recur?	Repair with tension, infection, tissue ischemia, preoperative size, emergent operation, tobacco use, presence of aortic aneurysm. Incisional hernias are most likely to recur.
How can a femoral hernia be differentiated from an inguinal hernia?	Femoral hernias typically lie inferior to the inguinal ligament, along the upper medial thigh.
During a McVay repair, bleeding is encountered. What is a possible source?	Aberrant obturator artery.

A 55-year-old man has pain radiating to his scrotum 2 months after an inguinal hernia repair. Sensation is intact. What are the possible causes? What is his prognosis? What is the first-line treatment?	Causes could include scar tissue, nerve compression/entrapment with sutures, reaction to foreign material. Postoperative herniorrhaphy pain usually resolves within 1 year. Nonsteroidal anti-inflammatory drugs (NSAIDs) are first-line therapy.
An 80-year-old female has medial thigh pain with leg abduction, internal rotation, or extension. What is the correct management?	Likely diagnosis is an obturator hernia. Surgical repair is always indicated due to high risk of incarceration and strangulation.
A 45-year-old man has a dull groin ache and painful ejaculation after an inguinal hernia repair. What therapy might cure his symptoms?	Vasectomy. Dysejaculation syndrome is likely caused by a partial obstruction of the vas deferens after an inguinal hernia repair.

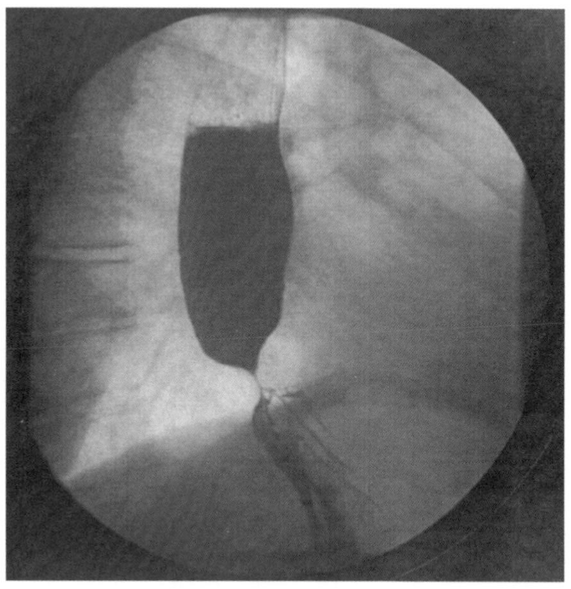

FIGURE 4-1. Esophageal achalasia.

(Reproduced, with permission, from Zinner MJ, Ashley SW. *Maingot's Abdominal Operations*, 11th ed. New York: McGraw-Hill, 2007.)

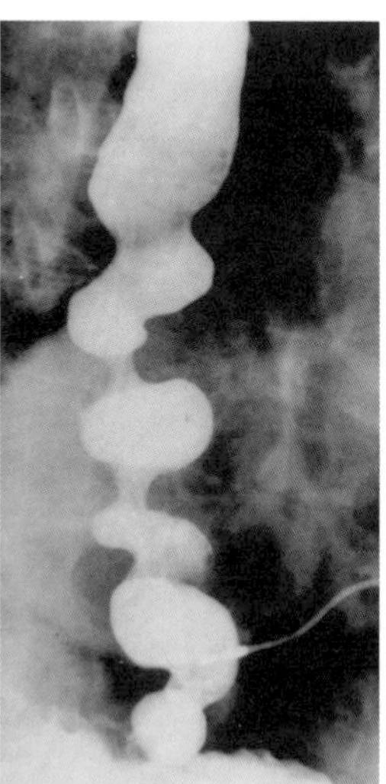

FIGURE 4-2. Diffuse esophageal spasm.

(Reproduced, with permission, from Brunicardi FC, et al. *Schwartz's Principles of Surgery*, 8th ed. New York: McGraw-Hill, 2005:88.)

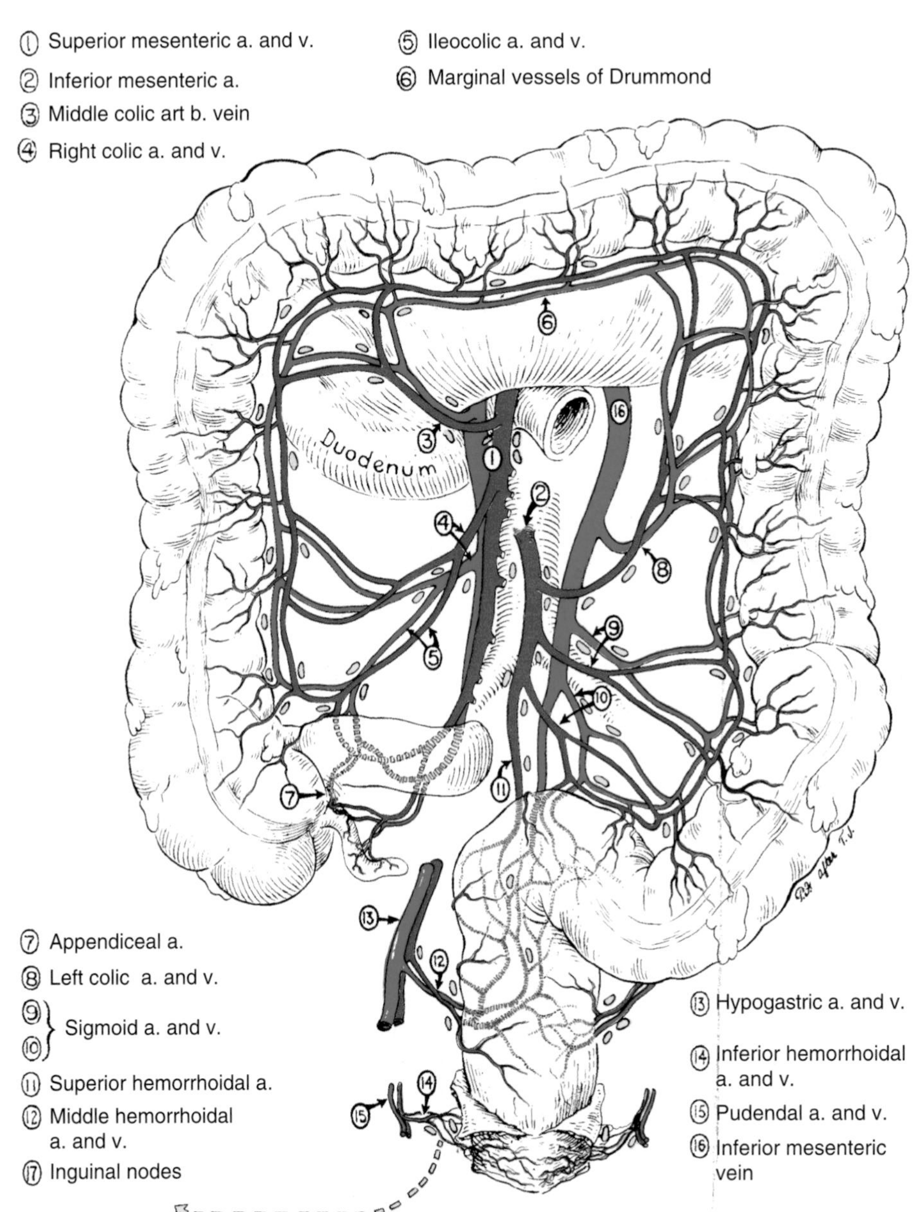

FIGURE 10-1. Arterial blood supply of the colon.

(Reproduced, with permission, from Zollinger RM Jr, Zollinger RM Sr. *Zollinger's Atlas of Surgical Operations*, 8th ed. New York: McGraw-Hill, 2003:17.)

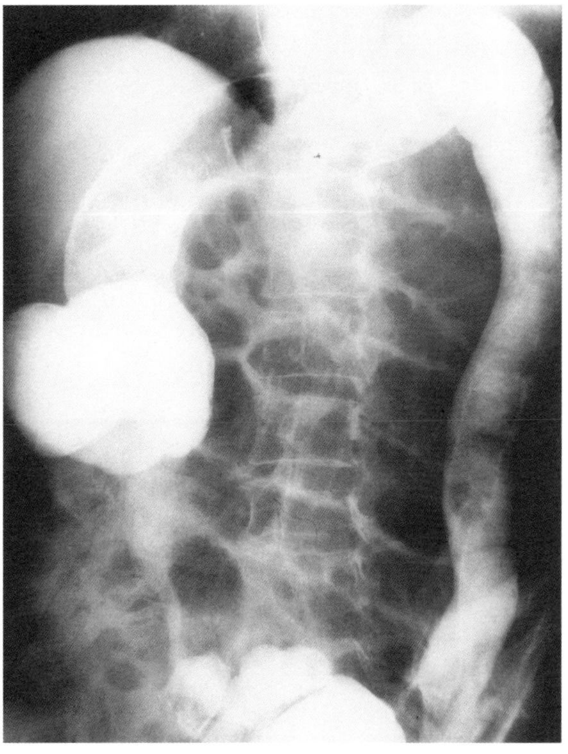

FIGURE 10-3. Large bowel obstruction.

(Reproduced, with permission, from Zinner MJ, Ashley SW. *Maingot's Abdominal Operations*, 11th ed. New York: McGraw-Hill, 2007:492.)

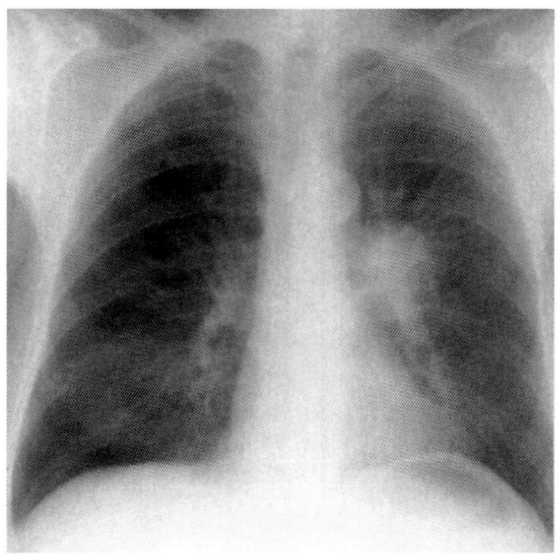

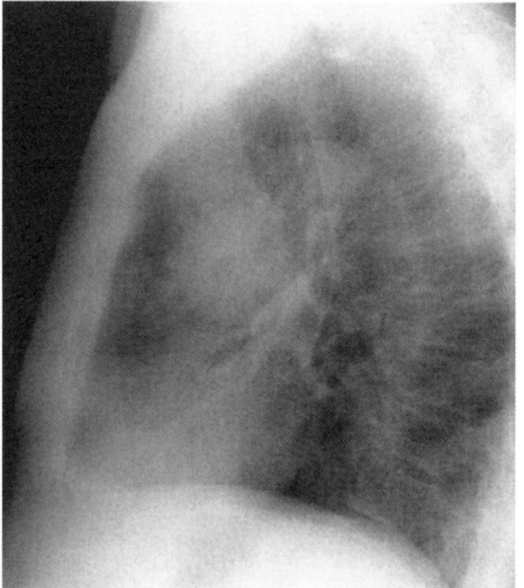

FIGURE 16-3. Radiographic appearance of lung cancer.

(Reproduced, with permission, from Chen MYM, et al. *Basic Radiology*. New York: McGraw-Hill, 2004:92.)

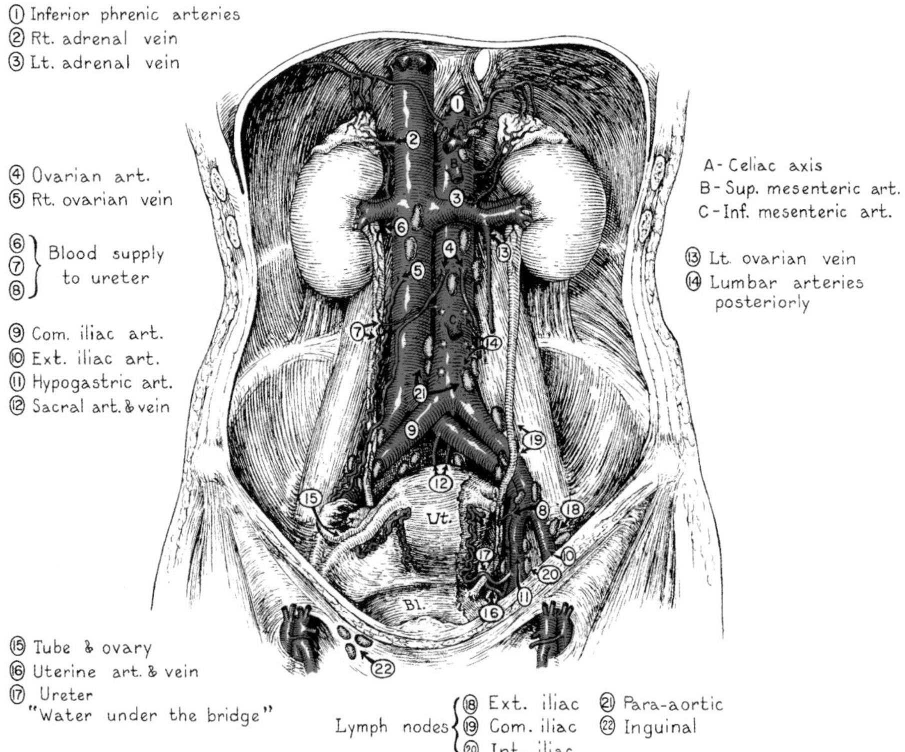

FIGURE 17-1. Anatomy of the abdominal arteries and veins.

(Reproduced, with permission, from Zollinger RM Jr, Zollinger RM Sr. *Zollinger's Atlas of Surgical Operations*, 8th ed. New York: McGraw-Hill, 2003:19.)

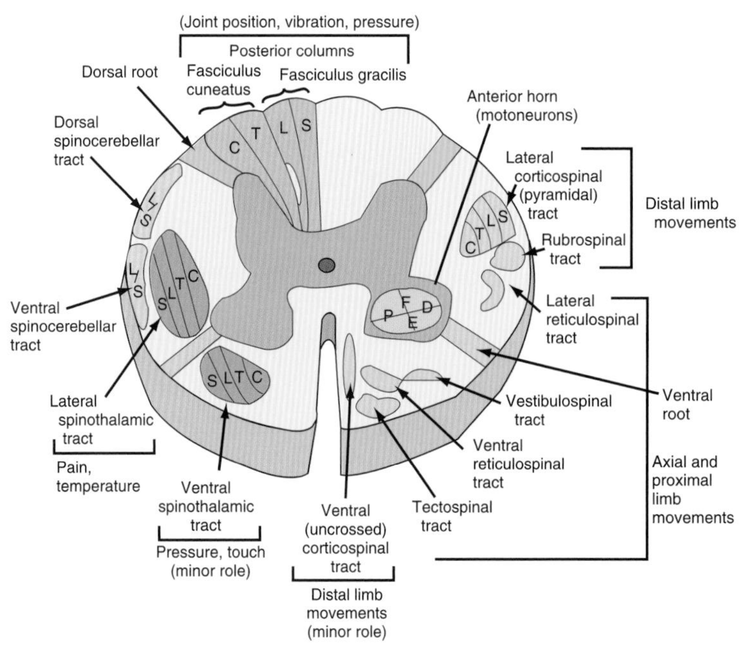

FIGURE 21-6. Spinal cord anatomy with pertinent sensory pathways.

(Reproduced, with permission, from Kasper DL, et al. *Harrison's Principles of Internal Medicine*, 16th ed. New York: McGraw-Hill, 2005:2440.)

CHAPTER 9

Small Intestine

Jennifer LaFemina, MD
Reviewed by Richard A. Hodin, MD

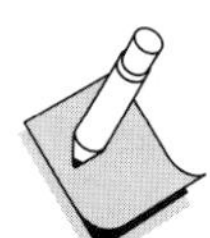

Meckel's diverticula are discussed in Chapter 19.

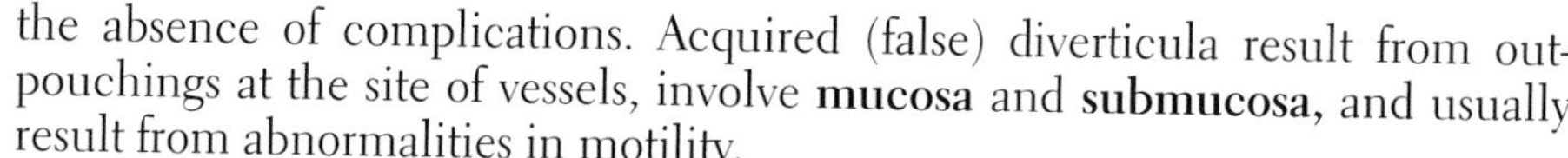

the absence of complications. Acquired (false) diverticula result from outpouchings at the site of vessels, involve **mucosa** and **submucosa,** and usually result from abnormalities in motility.

Although there is a low (~10%) risk of obstruction, recurrent pancreatitis, diverticulitis, hemorrhage, or perforation, **most SI diverticula are asymptomatic** and diagnosed incidentally. Asymptomatic lesions do not require resection. Surgical treatment for complications includes diverticulectomy (with patch or Roux-en-Y duodenojejunostomy for large defects), duodenal diverticularization, or resection of affected segment with anastomosis.

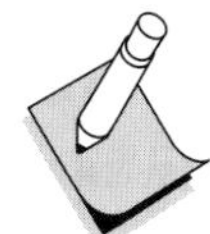

The majority of SI diverticula are found in the jejunum.

Post-ERCP Duodenal Perforations

Occur in 1% of endoscopic retrograde cholangiopancreatographies (ERCPs). Most commonly results in **retroperitoneal duodenal perforation** after sphincterotomy. Presentation varies from asymptomatic to peritonitis with shock. Diagnosis is confirmed with CT, which reveals retroperitoneal or free intraperitoneal air. Patients with mild illness may be managed with NPO status, NGT, serial abdominal exams, and IV antibiotics. Patients with peritonitis or who are hemodynamically unstable should undergo laparotomy.

Small Intestine Neoplasms

DEMOGRAPHICS

Comprise about 2% of GI malignancies and occur in the fifth to sixth decades.

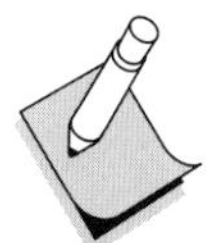

GISTs are discussed in Chapter 5. Carcinoids are discussed in Chapter 10.

TYPES

Benign tumors are most commonly **adenomas** and are found in the duodenum. May be associated with **familial adenomatous polyposis (FAP)**. Malignant tumors include:

- Adenocarcinoma: **Most common SI malignancy.** Most commonly found in the **duodenum**. Increased risk with Crohn's disease, FAP, and hereditary nonpolyposis colorectal cancer.
- Carcinoid: SI carcinoids are less frequent than appendiceal lesions and are found within 2 feet of the ileocecal valve.
- Lymphoma: May be 1° or disseminated disease. B cell lymphomas are the most common 1° type and affect the ileum. Risk factors include immunosuppression (eg, posttransplant lymphoproliferative disorder, acquired immune deficiency syndrome [AIDS]), celiac sprue, and Crohn's disease.
- Gastrointestinal stromal tumor (GIST): SI GISTs are less frequent than gastric lesions.
- Metastases: Primaries include **melanoma**, lung, renal cell, pancreatic, breast, and gastric.

> Most common 1° SI malignancies–**ACLS**:
> **A**denocarcinoma
> **C**arcinoid
> **L**ymphoma
> **S**tromal tumors (GIST)

SIGNS/SYMPTOMS

Benign lesions are most likely **asymptomatic** but may present with pain, bleeding, or obstruction. Malignancies are associated with symptoms late in the disease course, which can include **weight loss, abdominal pain**, obstruction, bleeding, palpable mass, or perforation. Carcinoids may be associated with carcinoid syndrome (eg, flushing, wheezing, tachycardia, right heart failure, hypotension). GISTs may be associated with **bleeding**.

Diagnosis

Labs may be unremarkable. Adenocarcinomas may be associated with anemia or guaiac + stool. Patients with carcinoid syndrome may have ↑ **5-HIAA** or **chromogranin A**. Evaluation includes esophagogastroduodenoscopy (EGD, proximal lesions), **enteroclysis** (for diagnosis), and CT scan (for staging).

About 80% of patients with SI adenocarcinoma will have metastases at the time of diagnosis.

Treatment

There is no clear role for chemoradiation. If resectable, surgical management varies by location. Periampullary adenocarcinomas and those in the second portion of duodenum require pancreaticoduodenectomy, distal duodenal lesions require duodenojejunostomy, and jejunoileal lesions require en bloc resections (six in margins) with lymphadenectomy. Disseminated or diffuse lymphomas are treated with chemotherapy. Localized 1° disease requires resection of SI and mesentery. Treatment of carcinoid and GISTs are addressed elsewhere.

Staging/Outcomes

Tumor, node status, metastasis (TNM) categories include

- T: T1 (extends into lamina propria or submucosa), T2 (extends into muscularis propria), T3 (extends into subserosa or into nonperitonealized adjacent tissue [< 2 cm]), T4 (extends > 2 cm into adjacent structures or into visceral peritoneum)
- N: N0 (– lymph nodes), N1 (+ lymph nodes)
- M: M0 (metastatic disease absent), M1 (metastatic disease present)

Staging includes

- Stage I: T1-2N0M0
- Stage II: T3-4N0M0
- Stage III: Any T, N1M0
- Stage IV: Any T, any N, M1

Five-year survival varies from 65% with stage I disease to 9% with stage IV disease.

Peutz-Jeghers Syndrome

Peutz-Jeghers syndrome (PJS) is caused by **autosomal dominant** inheritance of the *STK11* mutation (chromosome 19). Associated with **hamartomas** of the small and large bowel as well as **mucocutaneous hyperpigmentation**. Hamartomas may degenerate into malignancy and can be associated with ↑ risk of other malignancies (eg, gastric, esophageal, pancreatic, breast, endometrial, testicular, lung). Surveillance includes EGD and colonoscopy every other year beginning in adolescence as well as endoscopic ultrasound, mammography, and breast, gynecologic, and testicular exams. Surgery is indicated for hemorrhage, obstruction, or adenomatous lesions.

Short-Bowel Syndrome

Demographics/Risk Factors

Occurs in any age group and results from extensive resection of SI. Common indications for resection vary by age group. Pediatric disorders leading to short bowel syndrome (SBS) include **necrotizing enterocolitis**, midgut volvulus, intestinal

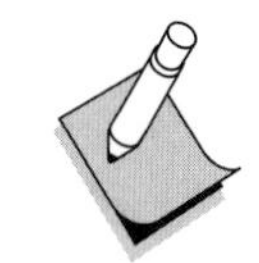

Mesenteric ischemia is discussed in Chapter 17.

atresia, and gastroschisis (see Chapter 19). Adult cases are often related to **Crohn disease**, mesenteric ischemia, trauma, malignancy, and radiation enteritis.

SIGNS/SYMPTOMS

Clinical syndrome occurs with < 200 cm of jejunoileal length (adults) or ≤ 30% of normal jejunoileal length for age (children). Malabsorption results in diarrhea, dehydration, steatorrhea, weakness, fatigue, depression, and possibly weight loss. Evaluation may reveal anemia (ie, iron and vitamin B_{12} deficiencies), edema, gallstones, nephrolithiasis, hypergastrinemia, dehydration, electrolyte abnormalities, and micro- and macronutrient deficiency.

DIAGNOSIS

Diagnosis is clinical. Look for history of extensive resection or intra-abdominal catastrophe in the setting of characteristic signs. Monitor albumin, liver function tests, electrolytes, hematocrit (HCT), vitamin levels, fecal fat (Sudan stain), and gastrin levels.

TREATMENT

Medical management includes fluid and electrolyte repletion, nutritional support with **TPN**, H_2-blockers or proton pump inhibitors (for hypergastrinemia), antidiarrheal agents (eg, diphenoxylate, loperamide), antibiotics (for bacterial overgrowth, when indicated), and advancement to enteral intake as adaptation proceeds. Surgical management may include a nontransplant procedure to ↑ bowel length, absorptive capacity, and transit time (ie, segment reversal). Small-bowel transplant with or without liver transplant is indicated for patients with SBS, long-term TPN dependence, and life-threatening complications (eg, recurrent dehydration, liver failure, recurrent sepsis).

OUTCOMES

Failure to wean from TPN is related to the remaining length of SI, presence of colon, and ileocecal valve competence. Preservation of the ileocecal valve allows for longer transit time, and prevents colonic bacteria from colonizing or infecting SI mucosa. With the colon present, a minimum of 70 cm of SI is needed; without the colon, the need is doubled due to further impairment of H_2O reabsorption. Complications include cholangitis and liver failure (due to prolonged TPN), infection, malnutrition, nephrolithiasis, and cholelithiasis. One- and 5-year survivals are 75% and 45%, respectively.

Intestinal Ostomies

Intestinal ostomies are summarized in Table 9-1. Generally placed through the rectus muscle, away from the belt line, and in an area easily visualized and accessed by the patient. Consultation with an enterostomal nurse improves functional outcome. Parastomal hernias associated with obstruction, pain, or appliance failure require relocation of ostomy with hernia repair.

TABLE 9-1. Ileostomies and Colostomies

TYPE OF OSTOMY	INDICATIONS	DURATION	COMPLICATIONS
Loop ileostomy, divided loop ileostomy	Protection of anastomosis.	Temporary.	**Diarrhea**, skin irritation, **dehydration/electrolyte imbalance**, **necrosis**, obstruction, stenosis, **retraction**, prolapse, parastomal hernia.
Brooke end ileostomy	Decompression of distal (eg, neoplasm), diversion after distal resection.	Permanent or temporary.	**Diarrhea**, skin irritation, **dehydration/electrolyte imbalance**, **necrosis**, obstruction, stenosis, **retraction**, prolapse, parastomal hernia.
Kock continent ileostomy	Decompression of distal (eg, neoplasm), diversion after distal resection.	Permanent or temporary.	**Valve dislodgement or incompetence, pouchitis,** diarrhea, dehydration/electrolyte imbalance, necrosis, retraction, parastomal hernia, prolapse.
Colostomy (end, double barrel, or loop; mucous fistula)	Decompression of distal protection of low anastomosis, treatment of perforation, diversion after resection.	Permanent or temporary.	**Necrosis**, **parastomal hernia**, prolapse, obstruction.

▶ SAMPLE QUESTIONS

Which GI organ has the quickest return of motility postoperatively? The slowest?	Small intestine (1 day) → stomach (2 days) → large intestine (3–5 days).
What is the 1° mode of transport of glucose and galactose? Fructose? Amino acids? Monoglycerides and free fatty acids?	Glucose/galactose: 2° Active transport. Fructose: Facilitated diffusion. Amino acids: 2° Active transport. Monoglycerides/free fatty acids: Passive diffusion.
What is the most likely SI malignancy in the duodenum? Ileum?	Adenocarcinoma (duodenum). Carcinoid (ileum).
A 20-year-old woman with hyperpigmented lips presents with intermittent abdominal pain and a palpable abdominal mass. Her mother has a history of "intestinal masses." What is the most likely diagnosis? Other associated cancers?	PJS. Associated with gastric, esophageal, pancreatic, breast, endometrial, testicular, lung cancers.
What determines mortality associated with enterocutaneous fistulas?	Site of origin, output, complications. Mortality is 15–20%.
What factors impair spontaneous closure of fistulas?	Foreign bodies, radiation, inflammatory bowel disease, infection, epithelialization, neoplasms, distal obstruction, sepsis.
What is the most common cause of SI hemorrhage in adults? In children?	Arteriovenous malformation (adults). Meckel's diverticulum (children).
A 55-year-old man undergoing cholecystectomy is found to have an incidental Meckel's diverticulum. Indications for resection?	Resection is not indicated for asymptomatic adults. Perform diverticulectomy for complications (bleeding, diverticulitis, obstruction).
What factors influence adaptation after SBS?	Luminal nutrients, hormones, growth factors, enteral feedings.
Exploration for appendicitis reveals a normal appendix, thickened and erythematous terminal ileum, and creeping fat. Most likely diagnosis? Intraoperative management?	Crohn's disease. If appendiceal stump is not involved, perform appendectomy but do not resect ileum.

What is the most common indication for surgery in Crohn's disease?	Obstruction.
After extensive SI resection (including ileocecal valve) for acute mesenteric ischemia with necrosis, a patient develops diarrhea and malnutrition. What is her initial medical management?	Patient has SBS. Fluid resuscitation, TPN for micro- and macro-nutrient repletion, H_2-blockers or proton pump inhibitors, antidiarrheal agents.

CHAPTER 10

Colorectal

Nicolas Melo, MD, MS
Reviewed by Paul C. Shellito, MD

▶ BASIC SCIENCE

Dentate line divides endoderm and ectoderm.

Embryology

Derived from **endoderm** (except the **ectoderm-derived** distal anal canal). Development begins during the fourth gestational week. Right colon and proximal two-thirds of the transverse colon are midgut-derived and superior mesenteric artery (SMA)-supplied; distal one-third of the transverse colon, left colon (descending), sigmoid, and proximal rectum are hindgut-derived and inferior mesenteric artery (IMA)-supplied. Between 6 and 10 weeks gestation, the midgut herniates and rotates counterclockwise 270° around the SMA. Hindgut development involves joining of endoderm and ectoderm at the dentate line and division of the urogenital sinus and rectum by the urorectal septum.

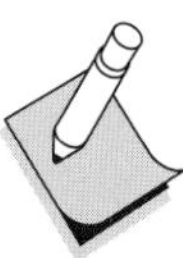

Colonic divisions are based on blood supply–
Midgut → right colon and proximal two-thirds transverse colon → SMA.
Hindgut → left, sigmoid, and distal one-third transverse colon and proximal rectum → IMA.

Anatomy

Macroscopic Anatomy

Right and left colon are retroperitoneal; transverse and sigmoid colon are intraperitoneal. Colon and rectum are composed of five layers

- Mucosa: Epithelium, lamina propria, muscularis mucosa.
- Submucosa: Resembles that of the small intestine (SI).
- Inner circular muscle: Coalesces in the anal canal to form the **internal sphincter (involuntary smooth muscle).**
- Outer longitudinal muscle: Comprises **tenia coli**, which extend from cecum to the distal sigmoid. In the rectum, the longitudinal muscle is circumferential.
- Serosa: Extends to mid-lower rectum at the peritoneal reflection.

Key colonic sites of pathology–
Cecum → largest diameter and thinnest wall → ↑ risk of perforation.
Sigmoid → most redundant → ↑ risk of volvulus.
Sigmoid → narrowest → ↑ risk of obstruction

The **external sphincter (voluntary striated muscle)** is contiguous and inferior to the pelvic floor muscles (eg, levator ani).

Fascial layers are important anatomic landmarks and include rectosacral (Waldeyer's) fascia (attaches to the presacral fascia posteriorly and the fascia propria of the mesorectum anteriorly). Denonvillier's fascia (separates the rectum from prostate and seminal vesicles or from vagina), and presacral fascia (covers the presacral venous plexus).

Colon can be differentiated from the SI by the presence of **appendices epiploicae** (intraperitoneal fat pads), noncircumferential **haustra** (circumferential plicae circulares in SI), and bands of outer longitudinal muscle in the form of **tenia coli**.

Microscopic Anatomy

Colonic and rectal mucosa contain a **simple columnar epithelium** with intestinal glands (ie, crypts of Lieberkühn) that secrete enzymes (eg, maltase, sucrase) and are deeper than those of the SI. Unlike the SI, the colon **lacks villi**. At the dentate line, about 2 cm proximal to the anal verge, the epithelium transitions to **stratified squamous**. Immediately proximal to the dentate line, the **anal transition zone** has a mix of columnar, cuboidal, and squamous epithelium.

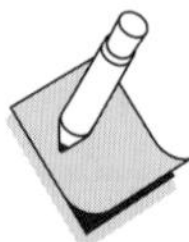

Difference between small bowel and colon–
Colon has Haustra
Appendices epiploicae
Tenia coli

Cell types include a population of undifferentiated cells as well as goblet and enteroendocrine cells similar to those in the SI (see Chapter 9).

Blood Supply

Arterial blood supply arises from the SMA and IMA (and their branches) as well as the middle and inferior rectal arteries (see Figure 10-1). The presence

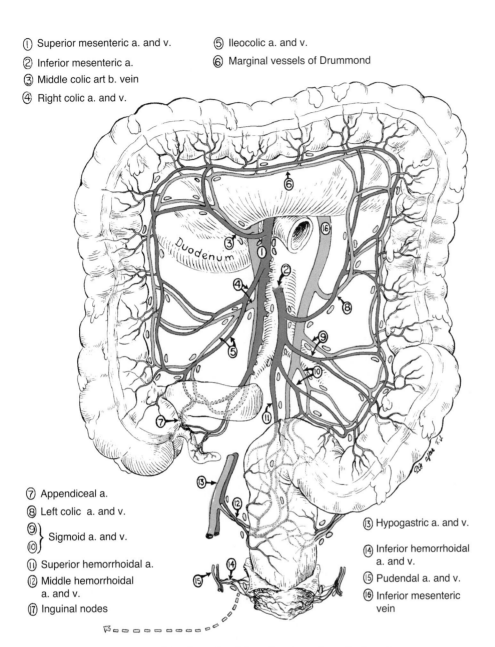

① Superior mesenteric a. and v.
② Inferior mesenteric a.
③ Middle colic art b. vein
④ Right colic a. and v.
⑤ Ileocolic a. and v.
⑥ Marginal vessels of Drummond
Duodenum
⑦ Appendiceal a.
⑧ Left colic a. and v.
⑨ ⑩ } Sigmoid a. and v.
⑪ Superior hemorrhoidal a.
⑫ Middle hemorrhoidal a. and v.
⑰ Inguinal nodes
⑬ Hypogastric a. and v.
⑭ Inferior hemorrhoidal a. and v.
⑮ Pudendal a. and v.
⑯ Inferior mesenteric vein

FIGURE 10-1. Arterial blood supply of the colon. See also color insert.

(Reproduced, with permission, from Zollinger RM Jr, Zollinger RM Sr. *Zollinger's Atlas of Surgical Operations*, 8th ed. New York: McGraw-Hill, 2003:17.)

of a middle rectal artery is variable and debatable. The **marginal artery of Drummond** connects the terminal branches of the arteries supplying the colon. Whereas the superior, middle, and inferior rectal arteries provide a rich arterial supply to the rectum making it resistant to ischemia, the **splenic flexure** is a **watershed area** (junction of SMA and IMA territories) and vulnerable to ischemia.

The splenic flexure is a watershed area and most prone to ischemia.

With the exception of the inferior mesenteric vein (IMV), colonic veins run parallel to arterial counterparts (the IMV drains into splenic vein). The rectal submucosal hemorrhoidal plexus drains into the superior, middle, and inferior rectal veins.

Anal sphincter innervation–

Internal anal sphincter: Sympathetic and parasympathetic.

External anal sphincter: Inferior rectal nerve (from pudendal)

INNERVATION

Innervation includes

- Sympathetic: Thoracic splanchnics (T10–T12) supply the right colon; L1–L3 supply the left colon and rectum.
- Parasympathetic: Vagus supplies the right colon; S2–S4 supply the left colon and rectum.
- Enteric nervous system: Includes Auerbach's and Meissner's plexuses. Regulate peristalsis and mucosal secretions, respectively.

Sensation to the anal canal and motor function to the external anal sphincter are supplied by the **inferior rectal nerve** (S2–S4, from the pudendal nerve). The internal sphincter has parasympathetic and sympathetic (via the pelvic plexus) innervation.

Total mesorectal excision (TME) is a key component of radical resection for rectal cancer.

LYMPHATIC DRAINAGE

Lymph drainage originates at the muscularis mucosa and includes the epicolic (bowel wall), paracolic (peripheral mesentery, adjacent to arcade), intermediate (around the mesenteric vessels), and main (origin of SMA or IMA) nodes. Rectum proximal to the anal canal drains to the IMA nodes (via the mesorectum). The mesorectum envelops the posterior and lateral aspects of the rectum. The proximal anal canal may drain to the IMA or inguinal nodes. Distal anus drains primarily to the inguinal nodes.

Physiology of the Colon

Short-chain fatty acids–

Most commonly derived from complex carbohydrates. Provide energy to colonocytes.

Primary function includes **passive H_20 absorption** (up to 5 L daily) and active absorption of Na^+, K^+, and Cl^-. Colonic bacteria produce short-chain fatty acids and ammonia.

Specialized Functions

Anal continence is maintained by adequate sensory innervation, compliance of the rectum, support from pelvic floor muscles, and tone from the internal and external sphincters. As feces reach the rectum, the pelvic floor and internal sphincter relax and the external sphincter contracts, allowing feces to approach the anus and anoderm (ie, **rectoanal reflex**). If contents are appropriate for release, defection occurs via ↑ intra-abdominal pressure, rectal contraction, and relaxation of the pelvic floor muscles. If contents are not released, they are stored in the rectum.

Internal and external anal sphincters maintain tonic contraction at rest.

Motility of the Colon

Unlike the stomach and SI, colon **lacks a migrating myoelectric complex**. However, vagal innervation regulates low-amplitude contractions (to ↑ H_2O and nutrient absorption) and high-amplitude contractions (to move contents distally).

Colorectal Tumor Progression Model

Colorectal tumor progression involves a number of mutations (eg, *APC*, *K-ras*, *DCC*, *p53*) involved in either tumor initiation or progression. The multistep process is summarized in Figure 10-2.

COLORECTAL

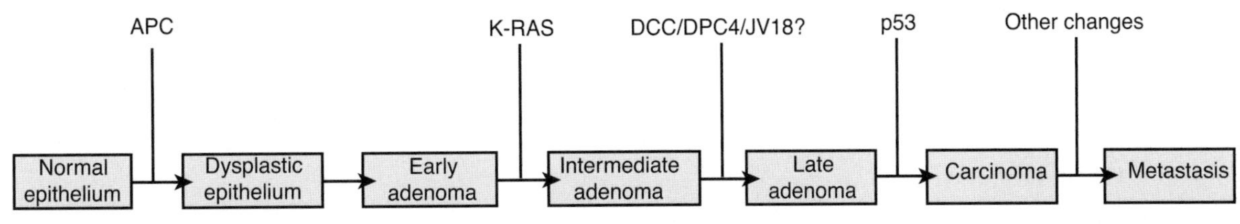

FIGURE 10-2. Colorectal tumor progression model and associated mutations.

(Reproduced, with permission, from Brunicardi FC, et al. *Schwartz's Principles of Surgery*, 8th ed. New York: McGraw-Hill, 2005:1085.)

COLORECTAL

▶ CLINICAL SCIENCE

A 19-year-old woman presents with right lower quadrant (RLQ) pain. She has a fever to 100.6°F but is hemodynamically stable. Her exam reveals RLQ rebound tenderness and guarding. Labs show WBC = 13 K/μL; human chorionic gonadotropin (hCG) is negative. CT confirms acute appendicitis without perforation. In the OR, an inflamed appendix is firmly attached to an inflamed, edematous ovary with purulence. What is the next step in management? Likely cause of her symptoms is pelvic inflammatory disease, leading to tubo-ovarian abscess and appendicitis. Attempt to salvage the ovary, but she will most likely require a right oophorectomy and appendectomy.

Acute Appendicitis

DEMOGRAPHICS

Most common surgical emergency of the abdomen. Affects 7% of the population, most commonly women in their second to fourth decades. Due to occlusion of the appendiceal lumen (eg, fecalith, lymphoid hyperplasia).

SIGNS/SYMPTOMS

Early disease is usually associated with nonspecific abdominal discomfort, anorexia, nausea, and low-grade fever. Later, pain usually shifts from the periumbilical region to the RLQ (**McBurney's point**) and becomes constant. Pain can be elicited with palpation of the left lower quadrant (LLQ; **Rovsing's sign**), hip flexion (**psoas sign**), or internal rotation of the right leg (**obturator sign**). If symptoms are present > 24 hours or if the patient presents with a high-grade fever or generalized peritonitis, suspect **perforation**.

Children < 5 years, pregnant women, and elderly patients usually present late with acute appendicitis, due to their atypical symptoms.

DIAGNOSIS

Labs demonstrate **mild leukocytosis** with or without left shift. Consider imaging if history and physical are not classic. Because of high sensitivity (95%), CT scans are the preferred in most populations and can demonstrate an **enlarged, enhancing appendix (> 6 mm) with or without a fecalith, periappendiceal fat stranding, and wallthickening**. Though associated with ↓ sensitivity, ultrasound is beneficial in pregnant women and children.

Open appendectomy techniques–
McBurney: Oblique incision
Rocky-Davis: Transverse incision.
Use tenia coli as a landmark to find the cecum and appendiceal base. Dissect the mesoappendix, divide the appendiceal artery, resect the appendix, and invert and oversew the base.

COLORECTAL

TREATMENT

Gold standard is open or laparoscopic appendectomy. If phlegmon is present, delay resection, start antibiotics, and perform **interval appendectomy**. There is a ~15% negative appendectomy rate in spite of advances in imaging and technology.

Carcinoid Tumor

DEMOGRAPHICS

Malignancy arising from neuroendocrine enterochromaffin cells. About 11,000 cases diagnosed annually. Up to 90% of cases arise in the appendix or distal ileum. **Most common malignancy of the appendix.**

SIGNS/SYMPTOMS

May be asymptomatic, discovered incidentally during appendectomy (as a **yellow** mass usually **< 2 cm at appendiceal tip**), or found in association with pain or obstruction. About 10% of cases are associated with **carcinoid syndrome** (eg, flushing, wheezing, edema, diarrhea, tricuspid insufficiency).

DIAGNOSIS

Carcinoids are most commonly found in the SI.

Usually a **clinical diagnosis**. If clinically suspected, confirm with ↑ **serum and urinary serotonin** or ↑ **chromogranin A**. Octreotide scan can localize the lesion. Pathology reveals a submucosal or intramural firm, yellow mass that stains positively for chromogranin A.

TREATMENT

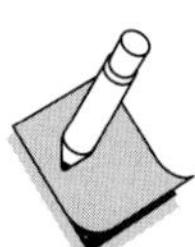

If tumor > 2 cm, involves the appendiceal base or terminal ileum, or is metastatic, perform a right hemicolectomy.

If < 2 cm, appendectomy is sufficient. If > 2 cm, associated with metastatic disease, or involving the terminal ileum or appendiceal base, perform a **right hemicolectomy**. Hepatic debulking is indicated for hepatic metastasis. **Octreotide** may alleviate symptoms; chemotherapy (eg, doxorubicin, streptozocin) may be used for palliation of unresectable metastatic disease.

Large-Bowel Obstruction

DEMOGRAPHICS/RISK FACTORS

Accounts for **15% intestinal obstructions**. Etiologies include **cancer (most common)**, diverticulitis, volvulus, fecal impaction, postoperative adhesions, hernias, or loss of peristalsis (ie, **pseudo-obstruction;** also called **Ogilvie's syndrome**). Pseudo-obstruction lacks mechanical obstruction and is usually associated with serious medical illness.

TYPES

Similar to small-bowel obstruction (SBO), may present as **partial or complete, simple or closed loop, gangrenous or nongangrenous** (see Chapter 9).

SIGNS/SYMPTOMS

Presentation can be acute or chronic with abdominal distension, vague abdominal pain, and failure to pass stool or flatus. Emesis is usually a late finding, as gastrointestinal (GI) contents move past the ileocecal valve and do not reflux.

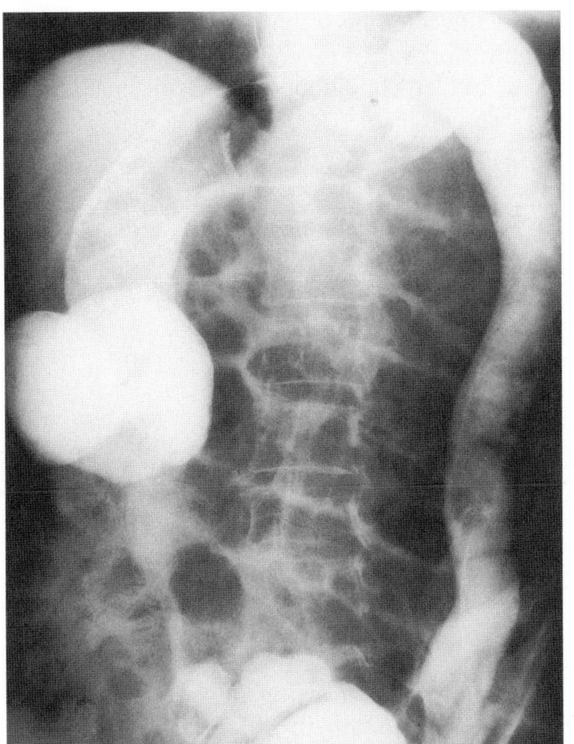

FIGURE 10-3. Large bowel obstruction. See also color insert.

(Reproduced, with permission, from Zinner MJ, Ashley SW. *Maingot's Abdominal Operations*, 11th ed. New York: McGraw-Hill, 2007:492.)

Diagnosis

Labs may be nonspecific, particularly if strangulation is not present. Imaging is helpful to differentiate etiologies. Abdominal radiographs may reveal colonic distention (see Figure 10-3); depending on ileocecal valve competency, SI air-fluid levels may be present. A dilated colon without air in the rectum suggests a mechanical obstruction; air in the rectum suggests pseudo-obstruction. CT confirms the diagnosis, though contrast enemas are an alternative.

Treatment

Initial treatment includes fluid resuscitation, correction of metabolic abnormalities, and placement of a nasogastric tube (NGT). Initiate antibiotics if ischemia is suspected. **In contrast to SBO, surgery is first-line treatment for large bowel obstruction (LBO)**. Depending on the condition of patient and viscera, can resect the pathologic area and perform a 1° anastomosis; however, it might be necessary to perform a resection with diverting ostomy and planned interval re-anastomosis. For pseudo-obstruction, NGT decompression and **neostigmine** (ie, reversible cholinesterase inhibitor to ↑ intestinal motility) may be necessary. Overall mortality rate for all patients with LBO approaches 20%.

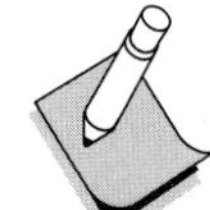

Unless an LBO is due to pseudo-obstruction, surgery is indicated.

Volvulus

Demographics/Risk Factors

Closed loop obstruction (ie, **obstruction in at least two locations**) caused by twisting of bowel ≥ 180° around its mesentery. Accounts for 5–7% of LBOs, occurring most frequently after the seventh decade of life. Most commonly seen in the sigmoid, cecum, and transverse colon. Risk factors include redundant segment, megacolon, bedridden condition, chronic constipation, and pregnancy.

Cecal bascule versus cecal volvulus–
Bascule → anteromedial folding of cecum on itself. Volvulus → axial rotation of the cecum around ileocolic vessels, resulting in twisting of the mesentery.

TYPES

Sigmoid volvulus involves rotation around the mesosigmoid. **Cecal volvulus** involves the rotation of the ileum, cecum, and ascending colon around the mesentery and ileocolic vessels. **Cecal bascule** presents similarly but involves anteromedial rotation of cecum onto itself.

SIGNS/SYMPTOMS

Similar to LBO, though volvulus may present with **sudden onset of abdominal distention and pain.** If ischemia is present, there may be peritonitis and hemodynamic instability.

Chilaiditi's syndrome–
Transverse colon loops that are interposed between the liver and diaphragm and are at risk for volvulus

DIAGNOSIS

Abdominal radiographs can confirm the diagnosis. Sigmoid volvulus may resemble a **bent inner tube,** narrowing into a **bird's beak**. Cecal volvulus may demonstrate a dilated cecum in a "**coffee bean**" shape that does not resolve with NGT placement.

TREATMENT

First-line therapy for nonstrangulated sigmoid volvulus involves gentle **endoscopic decompression** (eg, **sigmoidoscopy, colonoscopy**) and placement of a rectal tube. Passage of air and feces indicate reduction. Surgery is indicated to prevent recurrence but should be performed emergently if there is strangulation. Cecal volvulus necessitates emergent surgery (eg, cecopexy, right colectomy). Cecostomy is associated with a high rate of recurrence and should be reserved for select cases.

*Endoscopic decompression is first-line therapy for sigmoid volvulus but **not** cecal volvulus.*

A 43-year-old man presents with severe lower quadrant abdominal pain. He denies prior episodes, nausea, or vomiting. He has a temperature of 101.3°F but is hemodynamically stable. His abdomen is slightly distended and tender in the bilateral lower quadrants with guarding. His labs are significant only for leukocytosis. CT of the abdomen and pelvis demonstrates diverticulosis of the sigmoid colon with an adjacent diverticular abscess on the antimesenteric side of the sigmoid colon. There is no pneumoperitoneum. What is the next step in management? Admit the patient, make him NPO, and initiate IV antibiotics. Consider interventional radiology (IR) drainage if the abscess is in an amenable location.

Diverticular Disease

DEMOGRAPHICS/RISK FACTORS

Most common colonic pathology. Most commonly affects the **sigmoid colon** (95%) of elderly patients. Risk factors include low fiber diet, sedentary lifestyle, tobacco use, and chronic constipation. Lesions are typically **false**

diverticula involving herniation of mucosa and muscularis mucosa through the muscularis externa at an area of weakness (ie, near a vessel).

Right-sided diverticulum– *more common in young, Asian populations*

TYPES

Spectrum of disease includes

- **Diverticulosis**: Multiple, noninflamed lesions. Usually asymptomatic.
- **Diverticulitis**: Inflammation and infection of diverticulum (probably from a microperforation). May be **complicated** by abscess, gross perforation, or obstruction.

SIGNS/SYMPTOMS

Diverticulosis may be asymptomatic or cause the **sudden onset of painless bright red blood per rectum (BRBPR)**. Diverticulitis is associated with **LLQ pain, fever,** and **leukocytosis**. Perforation may present with peritonitis and hemodynamic instability.

DIAGNOSIS

Diverticulitis may be associated with leukocytosis with or without a left shift. Diagnosis is clinical but can be confirmed with CT scan. CT also identifies complications (eg, phlegmon, abscess, perforation, obstruction).

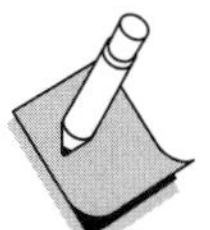

Indications for elective resection–

1. *Recurrent attacks of diverticulitis*
2. *Episode complicated by abscess or microperforation*
3. *Diverticulitis in young or immunosuppressed patient*

TREATMENT

Uncomplicated diverticulosis may be treated with a high fiber diet. Bleeding generally resolves spontaneously but may require surgery if continuous or recurrent. Treat uncomplicated diverticulitis with bowel rest and oral antibiotics. If complicated, admit patient and treat with IV antibiotics and IR drainage (if abscess is present). Emergent surgery is indicated for perforation (sigmoidectomy and Hartmann's procedure). **Delayed elective resection is indicated after an episode of complicated disease (eg, abscess), after an episode of diverticulitis in young or immunosuppressed patients, or after recurrent attacks.** For recurrent diverticulitis, the judgment concerning whether to proceed with elective surgery depends upon the frequency and severity of the attacks as well as the medical conditions and age of the patient.

Lower Gastrointestinal Bleeding

DEMOGRAPHICS/RISK FACTORS

Affects about 25/100,000 people. More common in men, particularly with ↑ age; mean age at diagnosis is 63–77 years. By definition, source of bleeding is distal to ligament of Treitz. Most commonly the result of **angiodysplasia, diverticulosis,** Meckel's diverticulum, ischemia, inflammatory bowel disease (IBD), infection (eg, *Escherichia coli, Clostridium difficile*), neoplasm, or hemorrhoids.

Most common causes of LGIB– *angiodysplasia and diverticulosis*

SIGNS/SYMPTOMS

Hematochezia and, possibly, melana, with or without hemodynamic instability. Additional signs and symptoms are related to etiology. Lower GI bleeding (LGIB) usually stops spontaneously.

A negative NGT aspirate **does not** rule out an upper GI (UGI) source for GI bleeding.

Diagnosis

History and exam may provide clues about the cause (eg, anticoagulation, chemotherapy, previous LGIB). Labs might show anemia, abnormal coagulation studies, thrombocytopenia, or leukocytosis. Perform digital rectal exam (DRE), anoscopy, and colonoscopy. The algorithm for evaluation is summarized in Figure 10-4. Capsule endoscopy can be employed to visualize the SI.

Treatment

All patients should be fluid resuscitated and have serial hematocrit (HCT) levels drawn. Treatment algorithms for life-threatening and non–life-threatening bleeds are summarized in Figure 10-4.

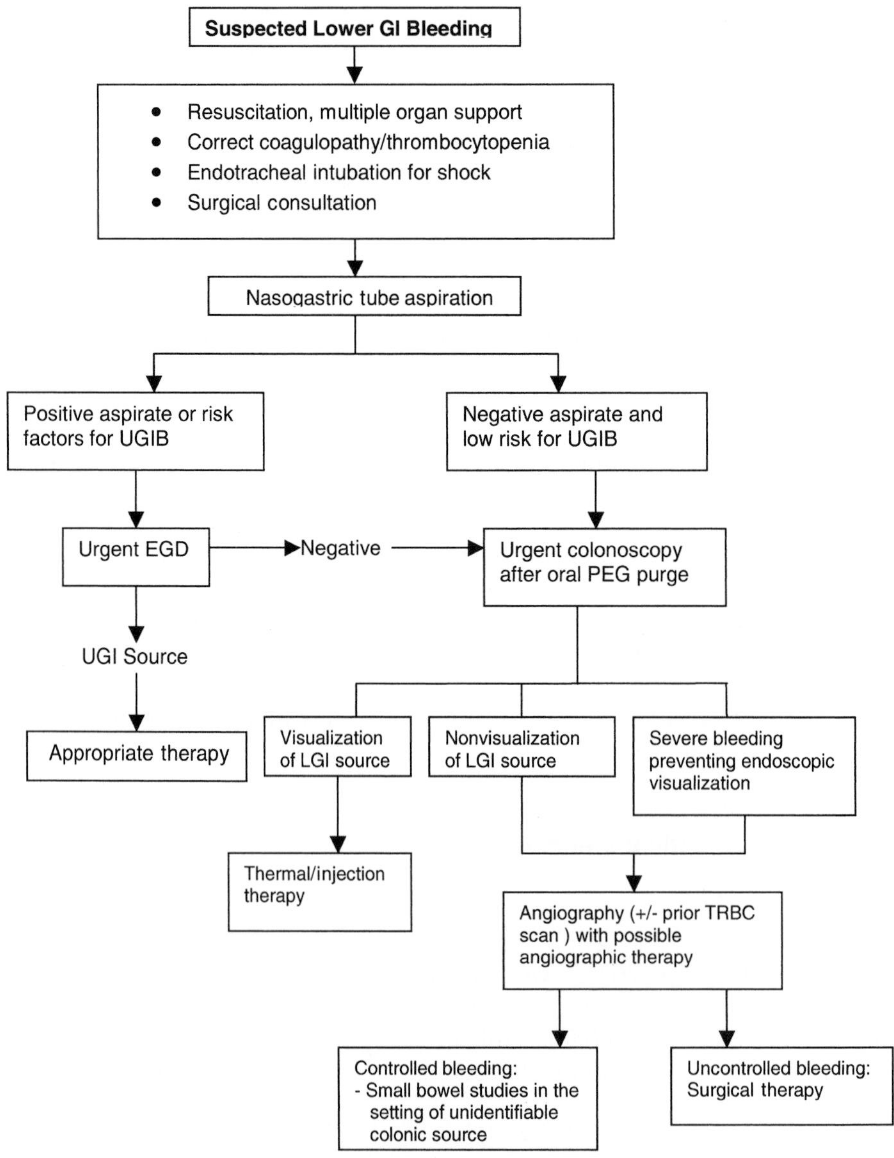

FIGURE 10-4. Workup and treatment of lower GI bleeding.

(Reproduced, with permission, from Hall JB, et al. *Principles of Critical Care*, 3rd ed. New York: McGraw-Hill, 2005:1273.)

Typhlitis

Necrotizing enterocolitis affecting the terminal ileum, cecum, and right colon. Risk factors include **leukemia** and immunosuppression (eg, acquired immune deficiency syndrome [AIDS], chemotherapy, immunosuppression due to transplantation). Patients typically present with diarrhea (bloody, watery), fever, emesis, and RLQ abdominal pain; signs and symptoms of sepsis or perforation may be present. **Because patients are generally immunocompromised, suspicion for typhlitis must be high.** CT can confirm diagnosis (eg, dilation of bowel, wall thickening, mesenteric stranding, pneumatosis intestinalis [if ischemia is present]) and differentiate from *C. difficile* colitis, radiation enteritis, and graft-versus-host disease. Management is primarily medical and should be immediately instituted: NPO status, NGT, fluid resuscitation, and broad-spectrum antibiotics. Consider resection for hemodynamic instability, perforation, hemorrhage, complete bowel obstruction, or sepsis.

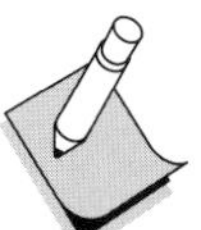

15% of IBD cases have an indeterminate cause.

5-ASA moiety is the active form of sulfasalazine.

Inflammatory Bowel Disease

Comprised of ulcerative colitis (UC) and Crohn's disease. Each disease has characteristic symptoms and pathologic features (see Table 10-1), though the underlying causes of IBD are not clear.

Extra-intestinal manifestations include **primary sclerosing cholangitis** (PSC, especially with UC), erythema nodosum, pyoderma gangrenosum, arthritis, sacroileitis, anemia, pancreatic insufficiency, pericarditis, ankylosing spondylitis, uveitis, and scleritis.

Due to risk of CRC, patients with IBD of the colon should have annual colonoscopies after disease has been present for 8–12 years.

Indications for emergent surgery for UC–
Toxic megacolon, fulminant/steroid-resistant disease, severe bleeding, perforation

Indications for elective surgery for UC–
Dysplasia or malignancy, stricture, intractable symptoms, inability to tolerate medical management, extra-intestinal disease, growth retardation

Colorectal Cancer

Demographics/Risk Factors

Second leading cause of cancer deaths in the United States. No gender predominance. Risk factors include age > 50 years, history of colon adenomas, IBD (especially UC), and family history of colorectal cancer (CRC) (see Hereditary Colon Cancer Syndromes).

Types

While hyperplastic, inflammatory, and hamartomatous polyps infrequently progress to cancer, adenomas are premalignant. Adenomas may be tubular (**most common**), tubulovillous, or villous (↑ **risk of cancer**) and pedunculated or sessile.

Specific syndromes associated with hamartomatous polyps are summarized in Table 10-2.

Indications for surgery for Crohn's disease–
Fistulas, abscesses, strictures/obstruction, failed medical management, perforation, hemorrhage, dysplasia/malignancy, growth retardation

Signs/Symptoms

Patients may be asymptomatic or present with **obstruction**, **rectal bleeding**, **changes in stool pattern or caliber,** tenesmus, or anemia. Exam might reveal guaiac + stool, palpable rectal mass, or signs of LBO.

Diagnosis

Labs might reveal anemia and ↑ **carcinoembryonic antigen (CEA)**. Screening tests for CRC include DRE, fecal occult blood testing (FOBT), flexible

Total proctocolectomy with IPAA is of the most common surgery for UC. Pouchitis is the most common complication. Surgery is curative for UC but not for Crohn's disease.

TABLE 10-1. Ulcerative Colitis and Crohn's Disease

	ULCERATIVE COLITIS	CROHN'S DISEASE
Demographics	Incidence: 10/100,000. Peak incidence: Third and seventh decades. ↑ Risk with Ashkenazi Jewish descent.	Incidence: 3/100,000. Peak incidence: Second and sixth decades. ↑ Risk with Ashkenazi Jewish descent.
Risk factors	↓ Risk with tobacco.	**↑ Risk with tobacco.**
Disease location	Colon (particularly left colon and **rectum**).	Anywhere in GI tract. **Most common in the terminal ileum**.
Signs/symptoms	**Diarrhea**, **hematochezia**, **abdominal pain** (crampy), fever.	Diarrhea, **obstruction**, abdominal pain, weight loss, hematochezia, fever.
Diagnosis	Colonoscopy, biopsy.	Colonoscopy with biopsy, small bowel follow-through CT scan.
Depth of involvement	**Mucosa and submucosa.**	**Transmural.**
Pathologic features	**Continuous**, friable mucosa, crypt abscesses, **pseudopolyps.**	**Skip lesions** (ulcerations with interspersed nl mucosa), **noncaseating granulomas**, **fistulas (perianal),** abscess, cobblestoning, strictures.
Complications	Fulminant UC, hemorrhage, **toxic megacolon, CRC,** extra-intestinal manifestations.	Fulminant colitis, toxic megacolon, extra-intestinal manifestations, colorectal and small bowel cancers.
Treatment	*For maintenance* → Sulfasalazine or 5-ASA; 6-mercaptopurine or azathioprine. *For acute attack* → Steroids, sulfasalazine or 5-ASA. **Infliximab** for severe disease. **Cyclosporine** if fulminant/steroid-refractory. *Emergent surgery* → Subtotal colectomy/proctocolectomy with end ileostomy. *Elective surgery* → Most commonly total proctocolectomy with ileal pouch-anal anastomosis (IPAA). Also total proctocolectomy and permanent ileostomy.	*Maintenance and management of acute attacks* → Similar to UC. Metronidazole for maintenance of perianal disease. *Elective surgery* → Resection of diseased portions (usually ileocolic resection, subtotal colectomy, total proctocolectomy, or small bowel resection). Consider **small bowel strictureplasty to minimize risk of short bowel syndrome.**

TABLE 10-2. Syndromes Associated with Hamartomatous Colorectal Polyps

SYNDROME	SYNDROME COMPLEX
Juvenile polyposis	Autosomal dominant. Hamartomatous polyps throughout GI tract. ↑ Risk of CRC.
Peutz-Jeghers syndrome	Autosomal dominant. Hamartomatous polyps most often located within the jejunum/ileum and possibly rectum. Concurrent hyperpigmentation of the buccal mucosa. **Slightly ↑ risk of adenomatous degeneration. ↑ Risk of extra-intestinal cancers** (eg, breast, gonads, pancreaticobiliary).
Cowden's syndrome	Autosomal dominant (*PTEN* mutation). GI polyps, mucocutaneous lesions, uterine leiomyomas, thyroid and breast tumors.
Cronkite-Canada syndrome	Sporadic. GI polyposis and epidermal changes including alopecia, nail plate dystrophy, and hyperpigmentation.

CRC screening guidelines for average risk patients starting at 50 years– *Annual FOBT and flexible sigmoidoscopy every 5 years or colonoscopy every 10 years or air-contrast barium enema every 5 years. Opinion is shifting to favor colonoscopy.*

sigmoidoscopy, air-contrast barium enema, **CT colonography** (ie, **virtual colonoscopy**), and **colonoscopy** (preferred method). Staging tools include **endoscopic ultrasound,** pelvic MRI (assess depth of local invasion), and CT (evaluate for distant metastases).

TREATMENT

Treatment for **colon cancer** includes

- Carcinoma in situ (or adenoma with high-grade dysplasia): Endoscopic resection.
- Invasive cancer in a polyp (ie, cancer invading through the muscularis mucosa): Segmental resection if lymphatic or vascular invasion, + margin, or poorly differentiated histology. Endoscopic resection if these criteria are absent.
- All other invasive colon cancers: Segmental resection. Add postoperative chemotherapy (usually 5-fluorouracil [5-FU], oxaliplatin, and leucovorin) if + lymph nodes.
- Lesions with associated metastatic disease: Hepatic or pulmonary resection is indicated for isolated, resectable metastases. If metastases are unresectable, consider palliative chemotherapy.

Resections should include at least 12 lymph nodes for optimal staging. If a tumor is perforated or obstructing, surgery is directed at the removal of malignancy, although intestinal bypass or colostomy may be all that is possible.

Unlike colon cancer, treatment for **rectal cancer** may include **radiation** with chemotherapy.

Outcomes for stage IV disease with hepatic metastases are improved if hepatic disease is resected.

- Carcinoma in situ: Endoscopic resection or transanal local excision.
- T1 disease: Radical resection or, for small accessible lesions, transanal, full thickness local excision.
- T2 or higher stage disease: Radical resection, including at least a 5 cm distal margin of rectum and mesorectum (for upper rectum and rectosigmoid) or TME with 1–2 cm distal margin of rectal wall (for mid- to low-rectal cancer).

Surgery for CRC involves segmental resection including the involved portion of the colon and lymphatic drainage to the root of the associated mesentery.

COLORECTAL

Perform abdominoperineal resections (APR) for very low-rectal cancers (near the anal canal or sphincters).

- T3 or node + disease: Add chemoradiation to radical surgery, preferably preoperatively (↓ morbidity compared to postoperative chemoradiation). Also add postoperative chemotherapy for any node + rectal cancer (as for colon cancer).
- Lesions with metastatic disease: Palliative surgery if possible.

STAGING/OUTCOMES

Tumor, node status, metastasis (TNM) categories include:

- T: T_{is} (does not invade submucosa), T1 (invades submucosa), T2 (invades muscularis propria), T3 (invades through muscularis propria into subserosa or nonperitonealized pericolic or perirectal tissue), T4 (invasion into adjacent organ or without invasion of the visceral peritoneum)
- N: N0 (- lymph nodes), N1 (1-3 + lymph nodes), N2 (≥ 4 + lymph nodes), N3 (+ lymph node adjacent to named major vessel)
- M: M0 (metastatic disease absent), M1 (metastatic disease present).

Staging includes

- Stage 0: T_{is}N0M0
- Stage I: T1-2N0M0
- Stage II: T3-4N0M0
- Stage III: Any T, N1-3M0
- Stage IV: Any T, any N, M1

Not as commonly used, the Duke's pathologic staging includes

- Stage A: Invasion of submucosa
- Stage B: Invasion of muscular propria with - lymph nodes
- Stage C: + Lymph nodes
- Stage D: Invasion into adjacent structures or the presence of metastatic disease

Five-year survival varies by stage.

- 95% for stage I (Duke's A)
- 85% for stage II (Duke's B)
- 30-60% for stage III (Duke's C)
- 5% for stage IV (Duke's D)

Routine surveillance includes colonoscopy, CEA levels, CT scans, and endoscopic ultrasound.

Amsterdam criteria for HNPCC (3,2,1 rule)–

≥ 3 relatives, 1 of whom is a first-degree relative, with an HNPCC-related cancer.

≥ 2 generations affected.

≥ 1 person affected < 50 years of age.

Confirmation that pathologic tumors are not FAP-related.

Hereditary Colon Cancer Syndromes

Approximately 20% of CRC patients have a family history of disease. Types include familial adenomatous polyposis (FAP) and hereditary nonpolyposis colon cancer (HNPCC); variants of FAP include Gardner's and Turcot's syndromes (see Table 10-3).

Presenting signs and symptoms are similar to CRC, though patients may be asymptomatic at time of screening and diagnosis. **FAP requires surgery**. Resections are based on age and presence of rectal disease: total proctocolectomy with ileostomy, total abdominal colectomy with ileorectal anastomosis, or total proctocolectomy with IPAA. For HNPCC with established CRC, **subtotal colectomy** (or sometimes segmental colectomy) is usually performed; consider total abdominal hysterectomy with bilateral salpingo-oophorectomy (TAH BSO) in

TABLE 10-3. Hereditary Colon Cancer Syndromes

Syndrome	Mutation	Diagnostic Criteria	Screening
FAP	*APC* mutation (chromosome 5q).	Colonic adenomas with **100% lifetime CRC risk.** **↑ Risk of periampullary,** thyroid, adrenocortical cancers.	If + *APC* mutation → flexible sigmoidoscopy annually starting at 10-15 years. Upper GI endoscopy every 1-3 years from 25 years.
Gardner's syndrome	*APC* mutation (chromosome 5q).	Colonic adenomas with ↑ risk of CRC; **desmoid tumors,** osteoid tumors, epidermoid skin cysts.	As for FAP.
Turcot's syndrome	*APC* mutation (chromosome 5q).	Colonic adenomas with ↑ risk of CRC, **brain tumors.**	As for FAP.
HNPCC (Lynch syndrome)	*hMLH1, hMSH2* mutations (DNA mismatch repair genes).	85% lifetime risk of CRC. **Lynch I:** Early-onset CRC. **Lynch II:** ↑ Risk of brain, stomach, SI, pancreaticobiliary, genitourinary, endometrial malignancies.	Screening colonoscopy annually starting at 20-25 years or 10 years earlier than the youngest CRC diagnosis. Endometrial biopsy or transvaginal ultrasound annually starting at 25-35 years.

affected women with Lynch II. **Outcomes are similar to sporadic CRC if early prophylactic resection is performed.**

Hemorrhoids

Demographics/Risk Factors

Engorged anal submucosal cushions (ie, connective tissue, arterioles, and venules; not varicose veins). Affect men and women of all ages. Major risk factors are related to increased **intra-abdominal pressure**: obesity, pregnancy, straining with defecation. Most common locations are right anterolateral, right posterolateral, and left lateral.

Types

Types include

- **Internal: Superior to the dentate line.** Transitional or columnar epithelium. **Relatively insensate.** Staged by degree of prolapse:
  - First degree: – Prolapse.
  - Second degree: + Spontaneously reducing prolapse.

- Third degree: + Prolapse requiring manual reduction.
- Fourth degree: + Nonreducible prolapse.
- **External:** Inferior to the dentate line. Squamous epithelium. **Innervated anoderm** → very sensitive to instrumentation or acute thrombosis.

Most common causes of acute anal pain—*thrombosis of an external hemorrhoid, perianal abscess, anal fissure*

SIGNS/SYMPTOMS

External hemorrhoids may cause **bothersome swelling and difficulties with hygiene**. Internal hemorrhoids cause **BRBPR** and occasionally, mucous discharge. Pain is an uncommon symptom of hemorrhoids unless there is acute thrombosis of an external hemorrhoid. In that case, exam reveals a firm, tender, blue-purple protrusion at the anal verge.

COLORECTAL

DIAGNOSIS

Anal inspection, DRE, anoscopy, and sigmoidoscopy. **If there is a family history of CRC, if the patient is > 40 years of age, or if there are any suspicious symptoms, perform flexible sigmoidoscopy or colonoscopy.**

TREATMENT

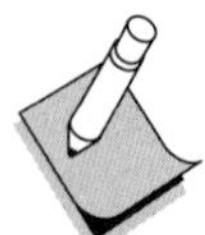

Complications of stapled and traditional hemorrhoidectomies—*pain, bleeding, urinary retention*

Increase H_2O and fiber intake, use stool softeners, and perform warm Sitz baths. Avoid sitting on the toilet for prolonged periods. Ointments, creams, and suppositories are neither harmful nor helpful. If medical management fails, consider rubber band ligation, sclerotherapy, infrared coagulation, or hemorrhoidectomy for internal hemorrhoids. Circular stapled hemorrhoidopexy can be employed for large, primarily internal, hemorrhoids. **Perform traditional formal hemorrhoidectomy if large hemorrhoids or a significant external component is present.** For a very painful, isolated, thrombosed external hemorrhoid < 4–5 days from onset, perform office excision under local anesthesia; if the patient presents later or is reluctant, treat with fiber and Sitz baths only as symptoms will eventually resolve spontaneously.

Anal Fissure

Tear or small ulcer in the anoderm **distal to the dentate line** usually at the midline (more commonly posterior). Likely caused by **hypertonic internal anal sphincter muscle**, perhaps from insufficient dietary fiber. Presents with pain and sometimes bleeding with and after defecation. Exam will reveal a small longitudinal ulcer in the anoderm perhaps with an associated **sentinel pile distally** or a **hypertrophic anal papilla proximally** (if chronic). Simple careful anal inspection shows the lesion and is the best way to diagnose fissures. DRE reveals **internal sphincter spasm and tenderness**. Anoscopy and sigmoidoscopy should be performed initially or at follow-up to rule out associated pathology, as for any anorectal condition. Treat with stool softeners, Sitz baths, **nifedipine ointment** (to relax the internal sphincter). If medical management fails, perform a **lateral internal sphincterotomy**. Injection of botulinum toxin in the internal anal sphincter is an alternative to lateral internal sphincterotomy but is less effective.

Minor incontinence is an occasional complication of lateral internal sphincterotomy.

Fistula In Ano

Fistula that develops between the anal canal and perineal skin. Classified as intersphincteric, trans-sphincteric, suprasphincteric, or extrasphincteric. Originates as an abscess in a crypt gland of the dentate line → intersphincteric abscess → perianal abscess. Most are idiopathic but may also be related to Crohn disease. Presents with bloody or purulent drainage from an external opening. Often there is a history of a perirectal abscess that was drained but never completely healed. Exam will demonstrate an external orifice. **Goodsall's rule** serves as a guide to location of tract: Anterior or anterolateral **external openings usually track directly radially** into the anal canal, while **posterior** or posterolateral openings track **curvilinearly to the posterior midline in the anal canal**. Treat with **fistulotomy. Fecal incontinence is a possible complication if sphincter is divided**. For fistulas that might encompass the external sphincter, use a staged fistulotomy with a noncutting **seton**. Fibrin glue instillation, collagen plug, endoanal flap closure, and sliding advancement flap of perianal skin are alternatives to fistulotomy. These are less likely to disrupt continence but also have a higher failure rate.

Always consider other Pathologies, such as Crohn's disease and malignancy, before treating fistula in ano or any other anorectal condition.

COLORECTAL

Pilonidal Cyst

Results from an infected hair-containing sinus in the gluteal cleft. Usually found in hirsute men aged 15–40 years. Commonly presents with pain superior to the gluteal cleft. Diagnosis is clinical and reveals an abscess or multiple pits or sinuses with hair. Treat with incision and marsupialization.

Proper evaluation for any anorectal complaint–

1. *Careful anal inspection*
2. *Rectal exam*
3. *Anoscopy*
4. *Sigmoidoscopy and sometimes colonoscopy*

Proctitis

Inflammation of the anorectum. Etiologies include syphilis, gonorrhea, herpes, human papilloma virus (HPV), cytomegalovirus (CMV), chlamydia, chancroid, UC, Crohn's disease, bacterial colitis, amebic colitis, *C. difficile*, or radiation. May present with rectal pain, urgency, BRBPR, and mucous discharge. Treatment is etiology-specific.

Rectal Prolapse

Protrusion of the entire rectal wall through the anus. Most often affects women > 60 years of age. The etiology is unknown but is usually associated with a weak pelvic floor. Typically presents as a mass protruding from the anus with associated incontinence, constipation, and possibly uterine or vaginal prolapse, cystocele, enterocele. True rectal prolapse can be differentiated from mucosal prolapse and hemorrhoids by the **circumferential mucosal folds** (versus **radial folds in mucosal prolapse**). Rarely the prolapsed rectum may become ischemic, causing tenderness. Evaluation includes **colonoscopy or contrast enema** (rule out other pathology). **Defecography** may be useful if occult rectal prolapse is suspected. Treatment depends on patient's health status. For poor operative candidates, less invasive procedures can provide relief (eg, Delorme's procedure, perineal rectosigmoidectomy). For good operative candidates, consider **laparotomy and rectopexy** with or without **rectosigmoid resection**.

Anal Cancer

Demographics/Risk Factors

Most commonly **squamous cell carcinoma (SCC)**, which is often caused by HPV infection. Adenocarcinoma makes up ~10% of cases and carries a worse prognosis. Treated the same as rectal cancer (see CRC). Anal SCC is most common in young men who engage in receptive anal intercourse. Other risk factors include **HIV**, Crohn's disease, Hodgkin's lymphoma, syphilis, herpes simplex virus 2, and tobacco use.

SIGNS/SYMPTOMS

Can be asymptomatic or associated with pain, pruritus, a sense of anal fullness, or **rectal bleeding**. Exam reveals an anal mass (above or below dentate line), occasionally with lymphadenopathy.

DIAGNOSIS

Biopsy will confirms diagnosis. Perform colonoscopy to rule out concomitant disease. Stage with CT of the abdomen and pelvis.

TREATMENT

Small lesions or those on the perianal skin are treated with wide local excision. Larger lesions or anal canal lesions are treated with **chemoradiation** (**Nigro protocol**—5-FU and mitomycin). Recurrent or persistent disease after chemoradiation is treated with an APR.

OUTCOME

Overall 5-year survival for all-comers is 60–70%.

▶ SAMPLE QUESTIONS

Which nerve(s) control the internal anal sphincter? External sphincter?	Internal: Sympathetic, parasympathetic. External: Inferior rectal nerve (Pudendal nerve).
What named artery connects the blood supply between the SMA and IMA?	Marginal artery of Drummond.
Which is the area of the colon most prone to ischemia and why?	Splenic flexure. Blood supply is lessrobust (watershed area).
During an appendectomy for suspected appendicitis, a 3 cm yellow mass is found at tip of a nonperforated appendix. Next step in management?	Because tumor is > 2 cm, right colectomy is indicated for likely carcinoid tumor.
What is the surgical procedure of choice for UC? Most common complication?	Total proctocolectomy with IPAA and sometimes total proctocolectomy with permanent ileostomy. Most common complication after IPAA is pouchitis.
What are the most common indications for surgery for Crohn's?	Failed medical management, fistulas, abscess, obstruction, perforation, hemorrhage, malignancy, growth retardation.
What is the first-line of treatment for nonstrangulated sigmoid volvulus? Cecal volvulus?	Sigmoid volvulus: Endoscopic decompression. Cecal volvulus: Exploratory laparotomy with cecopexy or right colectomy.
A 70-year-old man is diagnosed with colon cancer. What is the incidence of a synchronous lesion?	5–10% synchronous cancer. 20–50% synchronous adenoma.
What are the next steps in the evaluation of LGIB if UGI and LGI endoscopies are -, and the patient is hemodynamically stable?	Tagged red cell scan, angiography, capsule endoscopy.
What traits of a T1 colon cancer necessitate segmental resection rather than endoscopic resection?	Lymphovascular invasion, < 1 mm margin, poorly differentiated lesion.
A 25-year-old female is diagnosed with Lynch II syndrome. What are the screening recommendations?	Screening colonoscopy annually starting at 20–25 years of age or 10 years earlier than the youngest CRC diagnosis. Endometrial biopsy or transvaginal ultrasound annually starting at 25–35 years.

What is the adjuvant chemotherapy regimen for stage III colon cancer? What are the indications for adjuvant chemotherapy in stage II disease?	Stage III: FOLFOX. Stage II: Perforation, obstruction, high-grade lesion, lymphovascular invasion, < 12 lymph nodes in resected specimen.
On exam, how can one differentiate between rectal prolapse and mucosal prolapse?	True rectal prolapse: Circumferential mucosal folds. Mucosal prolapse: Radial folds.
For anal canal cancer, what therapy is usually indicated?	Chemoradiation with Nigro protocol (5-FU, mitomycin).

CHAPTER 11

Breast

Ugwuji Maduekwe, MD
Reviewed by Michelle C. Specht, MD

Embryology

Embryonic ectoderm forms the epithelium of the gland and ducts; supporting connective tissue is of mesenchymal origin. At 4–6 weeks of gestation, paired mammary ridges arise from the ectoderm on the ventral aspect of the embryo. A few days later, they regress except for a remnant, which is left at the fourth intercostal space on the thorax. Incomplete regression of this ridge may lead to **polythelia** (accessory nipples) or **polymastia** (accessory mammary glands).

Anatomic boundaries of the breast–

Superior: Second rib

Inferior: Sixth to seventh ribs

Medial: Sternal border

Lateral: Midaxillary line

Anatomy

Macroscopic Anatomy

Enveloped in superficial fascia of the anterior chest wall. Anatomic landmarks of the breast include

- Superior: Second rib
- Inferior: Sixth to seventh rib
- Medial: Sternal border
- Lateral: Midaxillary line

The nipple begins at the fourth intercostal space but may vary due to ptosis. The upper outer quadrant of breast tissue usually extends into the axilla forming the **tail of Spence**.

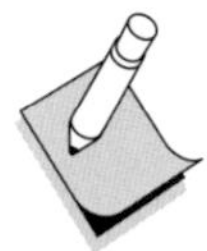

Mastectomy landmarks–

Superior: Clavicle

Inferior: Inframammary fold

Medial: Sternum

Lateral: Latissimus dorsi

Breast parenchyma is composed of a radial array of 15–20 glandular lobes supported by a connective tissue framework. Each lobe has a duct terminating at the nipple. These ducts widen underneath the areola to form lactiferous sinuses, which become the site of milk storage in the lactating breast. Suspensory ligaments of Cooper run between the lobes, forming the connective tissue framework of the breast by anchoring the dermis of the skin to the superficial fascia of the pectoralis major.

Microscopic Anatomy

Each glandular lobe consists of tubuloalveolar epithelium arranged in lobules. During lactation, milk is made in the branching alveoli of the breast lobules. Various alveoli drain into a single alveolar duct, which converge with others to form 15–20 lactiferous ducts. Each lactiferous duct drains a breast lobe.

Blood Supply

Arterial supply includes the internal thoracic, axillary, and third to fifth intercostal arteries. Venous system parallels the arterial supply (eg, internal thoracic, axillary, and third to fifth intercostal veins).

Innervation

Sensory innervation is supplied by the lateral and anterior cutaneous branches of the second to sixth intercostal nerves. Certain nerves must be identified during mastectomies to prevent injury:

- **Thoracodorsal nerve:** Innervates the latissimus dorsi. Damage causes weak internal rotation and abduction.
- **Long thoracic nerve:** Innervates the serratus anterior. Damage causes **"winged scapula."**

- **Medial and lateral anterior thoracic nerves:** Innervate portions of the pectoralis major (medial and lateral nerves) and minor (medial nerve only). Damage causes the atrophy of respective muscles.
- **Intercostobrachial nerve:** Arising from the lateral cutaneous branch of the second intercostal nerve. Provides sensation to the **upper, inner aspect of the arm** including axilla. Damage causes numbness in this distribution.

LYMPHATIC DRAINAGE

Superficial areas of the breast drain into the subareolar lymphatic plexus, which then drains into the deeper lymphatic plexus. Deep tissues drain via axillary and internal thoracic routes. Ultimately, drainage is primarily to the axillary nodes followed by the internal mammary nodes.

Classification of the three lymph nodes levels includes:

- Level I: Lateral to pectoralis minor
- Level II: Deep to pectoralis minor
- Level III: Medial to pectoralis minor

Rotter's nodes are a group of nodes between the pectoralis major and the pectoralis minor.

Relevant lymph node levels in breast cancer–

Level I: Lateral to pectoralis minor

Level II: Deep to pectoralis minor

Level III: Medial to pectoralis minor

Mastectomy Resection Margins

Mastectomy resection margins include

- **Simple mastectomy:** Removal of all breast tissue.
- **Modified radical mastectomy (MRM):** Removal of all breast tissue and pectoralis fascia with an axillary lymph node dissection (ie, resection of level I and II nodes).
- **Radical mastectomy:** Removal of all breast tissue and pectoralis major and minor with an axillary lymph node dissection.

Physiology of the Breast

A number of physiologic conditions impact the breast.

PUBERTY

In females, estrogen acts on the primordial breast bud to induce ductal development. In men, androgen acts on a similar location to destroy the ductal epithelium.

MENSTRUATION

During the follicular phase, follicle stimulating hormone and luteinizing hormone cause an ↑ in estrogen, resulting in ductal epithelial proliferation. Later, the progesterone surge results in ductal dilation and epithelial differentiation into secretory cells. Ductal epithelial regression occurs with the onset of menstruation.

PREGNANCY

Estrogen, progesterone, prolactin, growth hormone (GH), placental lactogen, and chorionic gonadotropin induce growth of the ductal, alveolar, and lobular compartments. As pregnancy progresses, there is a shift of the breast

Important breast cancer risks–

BRCA1*: 80% risk of breast cancer*

BRCA2*: 60% risk of breast cancer*

↑ Risk with Ashkenazi Jewish descent

↑ Risk of male breast cancer with BRCA2

↑ Risk of ovarian cancer with BRCA1

Indications for genetic testing for hereditary breast/ovarian cancer syndrome–

1. *Member of family with known* BRCA *mutation*
2. *Personal history of breast cancer*
   - *Personal history of ovarian cancer,*
   - *Diagnosis of breast cancer ≤ 40 years of age (+/- family history of disease),*
   - *Diagnosis of breast cancer ≤ 50 years of age* or *two 1° breast cancers (bilateral disease or ≤ 2 ipsilateral 1° tumors)* and *≤ 1 first, second, or third degree relative with breast cancer ≤ 50 years* and/or *≤ 1 first, second, or third degree relative with ovarian cancer, or*
   - *First, second, or third degree male relative with breast cancer*
3. *Personal history of ovarian cancer*
4. *Personal history of male breast cancer especially in the setting of ≥ 1 of the following criteria:*
   - *≥ 1 first, second, or third degree male relative with breast cancer*
   - *≥ 1 first, second, or third degree female relative with breast* or *ovarian cancer*

toward a secretory organ as the epithelium develops into cells capable of synthesizing and secreting milk. Under the influence of **oxytocin**, the myoepithelium proliferates and differentiates so that lactation might occur in the postpartum period.

Lactation

Postpartum declines in estrogen, progesterone, and placental lactogen lead to lactation. Prolactin, GH, and insulin induce the production of milk. Secretion of milk is regulated by the action of oxytocin, which is released from the pituitary gland in response to suckling. After weaning, the secretory cells and myoepithelium regress. The change in the breast lobules toward a more glandular and less stromal architecture persists.

Menopause

Ovarian decline causes regression of the glandular and ductal aspects of the breast. Adipose is preserved.

Obesity and Cirrhosis

Obesity and cirrhosis are associated with hyperestrogenemia, resulting in stimulation of breast tissue.

Genetics of Breast Cancer

Five to 10 percent of breast cancers are hereditary in nature. Various genes and hereditary syndromes ↑ breast cancer susceptibility.

BRCA1

Located on **chromosome 17q** and transmitted in autosomal dominant fashion. Increased risk of **breast** (80%) and **ovarian** (40%) **cancers**. Associated with early disease onset and bilaterality. **Prophylactic mastectomies with bilateral salpingo-oophorectomy** may be considered.

BRCA2

Located on **chromosome 13q** and normally involved in DNA repair. Results in ↑ risk of **breast cancer** (60%, including **male breast cancer**) and an ↑ **risk of ovarian cancer** (15–25%).

Syndromes Associated with Breast Cancer

Include **Li–Fraumeni syndrome** (p53 mutation leads to soft tissue sarcoma, osteosarcoma, breast cancer, brain tumors, leukemia), **Cowden's syndrome** (*PTEN* mutation leads to breast, gastrointestinal [GI], central nervous system, skin, eye, thyroid, genitourinary, bone cancers), **Peutz–Jeghers syndrome** (*STK11* mutation results in GI hamartomas, pigmented lesions, breast cancer), **ataxia-telangiectasia** (DNA repair defect results in telangiectasias, cerebellar ataxia, ↑ risk of breast cancer), **hereditary nonpolyposis colon cancer** (HNPCC; mismatch repair gene defect results in ↑ risk of colon, endometrial, ovarian, urinary, breast cancers). See Chapters 2 and 10 for additional details.

Evaluation of a Breast Mass

The goal of the evaluation of breast abnormalities is early diagnosis of breast cancer. The algorithm for breast mass evaluation is summarized in Figure 11-1.

Certain features are suggestive of breast cancer:

- **Nipple discharge**: Unilateral, spontaneous, bloody (rather than serous or green), and clear (rather than milky) discharge is associated with cancer.
- **Mass characterization: Fixed, firm** masses, particularly if they are associated with **nipple retraction** and **skin changes** (ie, **peau d'orange**), are more likely to be cancer.

Clinical breast exam is indicated for women 20–39 years of age every 2–3 years and for women ≥ 40 years of age annually. Annual mammography is recommended in asymptomatic, average-risk women ≤ 40 years of age. Breast self-exams are encouraged but are not associated with improved survival.

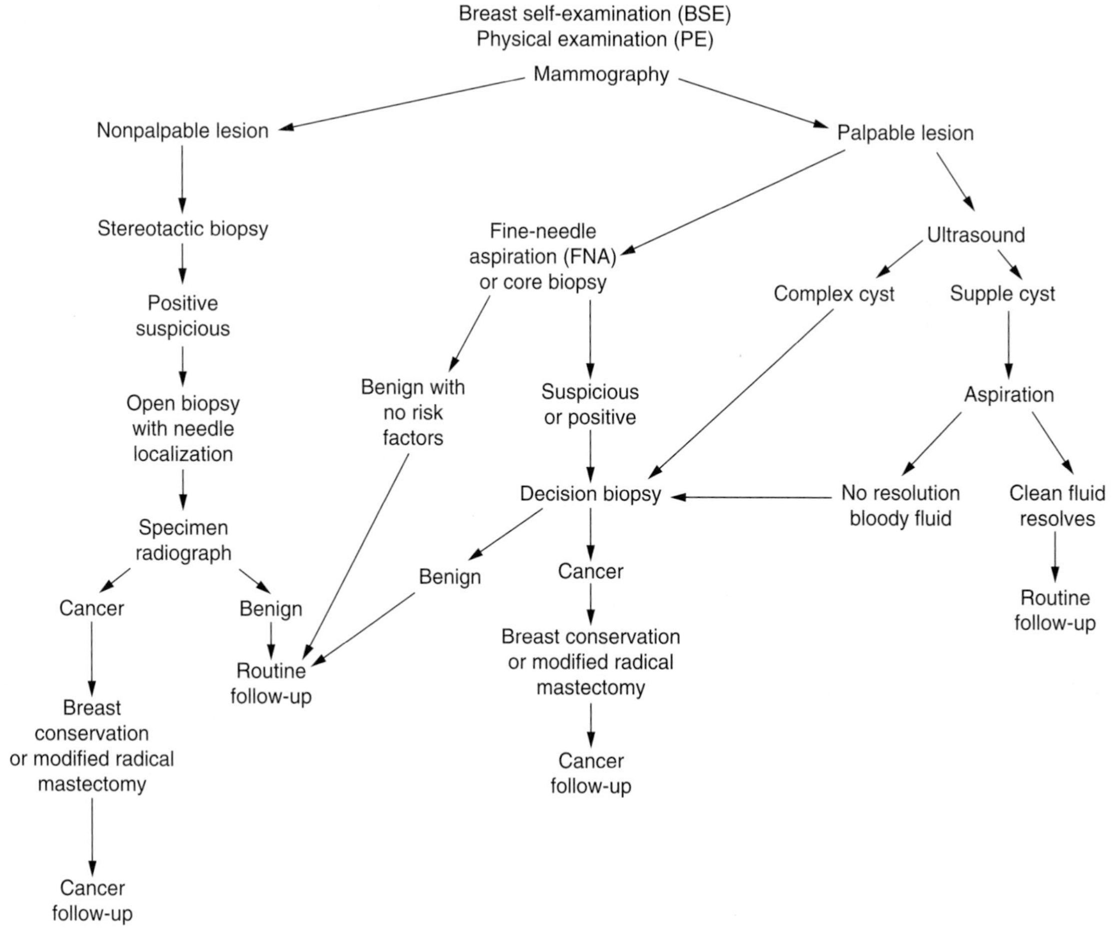

FIGURE 11-1. Approach to a patient with a breast abnormality.

(Reproduced, with permission, from Bland KI, et al. *Surgical Oncology—Contemporary Principles and Practice*. New York: McGraw-Hill, 2001:956.)

BREAST

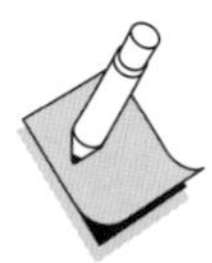

Breast cancer screening–

Clinical breast exam: Every 2-3 years from age 20-39 years; annually ≤ 40 years

Mammography: Annually ≤ 40 years

MRI: Consider for patients with known BRCA *mutations, women who have not undergone genetic testing but who have a first degree relative with* BRCA *mutation or premenopausal breast cancer, women with > 20–25% lifetime risk of breast cancer, women exposed to chest irradiation between 10 and 30 years of age.*

Radiologic options include

- **Ultrasound:** Useful in distinguishing between solid and cystic masses, particularly in women < 35 years of age in whom mammography is more difficult to interpret.
- **Mammography:** Of limited value in women < 35 years of age because of ↑ density of breast tissue. Views in screening mammography include **craniocaudal** and **mediolateral oblique**. Additional views to better characterize lesions are employed in diagnostic mammography. Findings suggestive of malignancy include **solid mass with or without stellate characteristics, asymmetric thickening, and clustered microcalcifications.** Sensitivity and specificity are > 90% but can be lower in younger women. BI-RADS classification includes 0 (additional evaluation needed), 1 (- test), 2 (benign finding), 3 (probably benign; follow-up in 6 months), 4 (lesion suspicious for cancer; biopsy indicated), 5 (highly suggestive of malignancy; biopsy indicated), and 6 (known malignancy).
- **MRI:** Not a replacement for mammography or ultrasound. Useful as a supplemental tool for detecting and staging breast cancer. **Screening MRI is recommended for women with a known *BRCA* mutation, those who have not undergone genetic testing but who have a first degree relative with a known mutation or premenopausal breast cancer, women with > 20–25% lifetime risk for breast cancer, and women who have a history of chest irradiation between 10 and 30 years of age.** Diagnostic breast MRIs are indicated for new diagnoses of breast cancer, particularly in the presence of lobular cancer or dense breast tissue.

Pathologic diagnoses can be made via a number of modalities:

- **Fine needle aspiration (FNA):** May be done in the office and yields rapid results. Cannot differentiate carcinoma in situ from invasive cancer.
- **Core biopsy:** Indicated for palpable lesions and for screening of lesions detected by mammography, ultrasound, or MRI. Tissue architecture is maintained, allowing for determination of invasive versus noninvasive.
- **Excisional biopsy:** Operative biopsy with or without preoperative needle localization. Indicated for **nonpalpable lesions**. Needle localization reduces false-biopsy results.

If core biopsy reveals lobular carcinoma in situ (LCIS), radial scar, atypical lobular or ductal hyperplasia, inadequate tissue, or results that are discordant with radiologic findings, proceed with excisional biopsy.

Mastodynia

Breast pain that may be benign (ie, cyclic) or pathologic. Cyclic mastodynia is associated with the menstrual cycle and is most intense before menstruation. Pain is usually at the bilateral upper, outer quadrants. Treatment includes evening primrose oil, **supportive bra, nonsteroidal anti-inflammatory drugs (NSAIDs), and ↓ caffeine intake.**

Gynecomastia

Male breast buds due to abnormal hormonal stimulation. Causes include relative androgen deficiency, chronic disease (eg, hepatic, renal), and medications (eg, antipsychotics, cimetidine, omeprazole, spironolactone). Diagnosis is clinical, but if not caused by physiologic changes, correctable etiologies should be sought.

A 33-year-old female recently gave birth and is lactating. She presents with a diffusely erythematous and tender breast. Her exam reveals a temperature of 101°F, a tender breast without masses, and leukocytosis. What is the differential diagnosis and treatment? Differential includes puerperal mastitis, breast abscess, and inflammatory breast cancer. Puerperal mastitis is the most likely diagnosis given fever, leukocytosis, and lack of a fluctuant lesion. Continue breast feeding and treat for *Staphylococcus aureus*.

Mastitis and Breast Abscess

DEMOGRAPHICS/RISK FACTORS

Inflammation of the breast that may be associated with an infected fluid collection (ie, abscess). Includes puerperal (peripartum) and nonpuerperal (periductal) forms. Puerperal mastitis and abscesses occur in lactating mothers. Usually caused by ***S. aureus*** that enters at sites of skin breakdown or at the nipples during breastfeeding. Periductal mastitis and abscesses are commonly found in young female smokers or in older diabetic women with ductal ectasia. Associated with growth of polymicrobial, anaerobic flora in the setting of ductal obstruction or fibrosis.

Mastitis and breast abscesses–

Lactating women: S. aureus

Nonlactating women:

Polymicrobial, anaerobic flora

SIGNS/SYMPTOMS

Mastitis is associated with erythema, warmth, induration, and tenderness of the breast skin. Abscesses present similarly and may be associated with a palpable, tender, and fluctuant mass; nipple discharge and fever may be present.

DIAGNOSIS

Mastitis is a clinical diagnosis and may be associated with leukocytosis. Abscesses will also be associated with leukocytosis and may be confirmed with ultrasound or needle aspiration of purulent fluid.

TREATMENT

- **Puerperal**: Gram+ cocci antibiotic coverage (eg, dicloxacillin, cephalosporin), warm packs, continuation of breastfeeding. If abscess is present, consider needle aspiration or incision and drainage.
- **Nonpuereral**: Antibiotics to cover mixed flora (eg, dicloxacillin and metronidazole). If abscess is present, consider needle aspiration or incision and drainage. If abscess is recurrent, consider subareolar duct excision.

A diagnostic mammogram should be considered for women with breast mastitis or abscess once the infection has resolved in order to rule out malignancy.

Sclerosing Adenosis

Involves the overgrowth of lobular tissue due to ductal proliferation and stromal fibrosis. Occurs in women in their reproductive and perimenopausal years.

Patients may report pain and a breast mass. May be confused with cancer on exam and mammography. Though the lesion is not associated with cancer, excisional biopsy is sometimes considered to rule out cancer.

Radial scars of sclerosing adenosis may be confused with cancer. Biopsy is always warranted.

Intraductal Papilloma

Lesion associated with **bloody discharge** from a single duct; may present as a lesion detected on mammographic screening. Occurs in premenopausal women. Workup may include ductal lavage, ductography, or mammography and generally reveals an epithelial-derived polyp. Though the malignant potential is low, treatment includes **excision of the affected ductal system**.

Fibroadenoma

DEMOGRAPHICS

Benign mass of stromal and glandular elements. **Most common solid breast lesion in women < 30 years**.

SIGNS/SYMPTOMS

Firm, mobile masses that may be painful, bilateral, or multiple. Pain and size may vary with hormonal stimulation (eg, phase of menstrual cycle, postmenopausal state).

DIAGNOSIS

Triple test of clinical exam (rubbery, mobile mass), ultrasound (lack of cyst cavity), and biopsy (proliferation of stroma and epithelium) confirms the diagnosis.

TREATMENT

For lesions that are small and biopsy-confirmed fibroadenomas, observation is sufficient. However, if lesions are symptomatic or if lesion size ↑ (particularly in postmenopausal women), consider resection.

Fibrocystic Disease

DEMOGRAPHICS

Benign breast disease associated with proliferation of fibrous tissue, resulting in cysts and nodularity. Due to **estrogen stimulation** of breast tissue. **Most common breast lesion.** Usually found in women 30 to 50 years of age.

SIGNS/SYMPTOMS

Firm, mobile breast masses that may be asymptomatic but are often tender to palpation. May be multiple and bilateral. Size and pain vary with menstrual cycle phase: **premenstrual cycle is associated with ↑ lesion size and ↑ pain.**

DIAGNOSIS

FNA can confirm histopathologic diagnosis and can also serve as a means to drain cyst fluid.

TREATMENT

Control pain by minimizing caffeine intake or taking vitamin E or danazol. As estrogen levels ↓ (ie, postmenopausal women), tumors regress and symptoms usually improve. **If the lesion fails to regress after aspiration, has bloody cyst fluid, or if the lesion is suspicious for cancer, excise tumor.**

Phyllodes Tumor

Most common nonepithelial breast tumor. Associated with large, painless, mobile, and rapidly growing lesion that histologically, has a **leaf-like appearance**. Classified as benign and malignant (ie, **cystosarcoma phyllodes**). Wide local excision (WLE) is indicated with a **minimum of 1 cm margins. In large or recurrent tumors, perform mastectomy. Lymph node dissection is not indicated** as metastatic spread rarely occurs via lymphatics.

Syndromes of the Breast

MONDOR'S SYNDROME

Sclerosing thrombophlebitis of anterior chest wall following radical mastectomy. Presents as a cord-like mass. Treat with NSAIDs.

POLAND'S SYNDROME

Hypoplasia or absence of pectoralis major with lack of breast development and ipsilateral hand development anomaly.

Ductal Carcinoma In Situ

DEMOGRAPHICS

Breast cancer without invasion of the basement membrane. Involves proliferation of ductal epithelium, resulting in a papillary, cribriform, or comedo growth pattern. Considered a ductal **adenocarcinoma precursor** and associated with a **5-fold ↑ in ipsilateral breast cancer**. Affects women in their fifth to sixth decades. Comprises 15–20% of female and 5% of male breast cancer cases.

Always suspect DCIS or IDC when Paget's disease of the breast is present.

SIGNS/SYMPTOMS

May be asymptomatic or may present as a palpable breast mass. **Paget's disease of the breast** is an eczematoid lesion of the nipple, which is usually associated with underlying ductal carcinoma in situ (DCIS) or invasive ductal carcinoma (IDC).

DIAGNOSIS

Mammography reveals a mass with associated **microcalcifications.** Biopsy confirms diagnosis. Grade is determined by the **presence of necrosis** (comedo-type) and **nuclear atypia**: High-grade nuclear atypia and necrosis indicate high-grade DCIS → ↑ risk of microinvasion and lymph node metastasis. Paget's disease must be differentiated from melanoma, and an underlying lesion should always be sought.

TREATMENT

The Van Nuys prognostic index helps guide treatment with WLE, with or without radiation, versus simple mastectomy. Tamoxifen ↓ risk of contralateral breast cancer and recurrence.

> A 45-year-old woman has a breast biopsy that reveals LCIS. Postoperatively, she seeks advice on her risk of breast cancer and her prevention options. How do you counsel her? LCIS is associated with an increased risk of malignancy in either breast. Tamoxifen can decrease the risk of cancer. Management can include observation or bilateral prophylactic mastectomies.

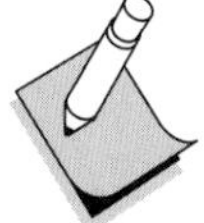

DCIS is indicative of ↑ risk of cancer in ipsilateral breast. LCIS is indicative of ↑ risk of cancer in either breast at multiple sites.

Lobular Carcinoma In Situ

Proliferation of terminal duct lobules. Though not a preinvasive lesion to ductal adenocarcinoma, LCIS is associated with **~30% risk of ductal adenocarcinoma in either breast**. Most commonly found in premenopausal Caucasian women in the fifth decade and may be bilateral or multicentric. Commonly asymptomatic. Workup might be normal or might reveal adjacent calcifications on mammography. Treatment can include observation or bilateral prophylactic mastectomies and tamoxifen.

ABCs of breast cancer risks:
Advanced age
***B**RCA1/**B**RCA2*
Caucasian race
Delayed menopause or first pregnancy
Early menarche
Family history of breast cancer
Genetic syndromes
History of breast cancer/atypical ductal hyperplasia

Ductal Adenocarcinoma of the Female Breast

DEMOGRAPHICS/RISK FACTORS

Most **common cancer in females**. Commonly presents in postmenopausal woman. Lifetime incidence is one in every 8–9 women. Risk factors include female gender, Caucasian race, age > 50 years, early menarche, nulliparity, late first pregnancy, late menopause, history of breast cancer in first-degree relatives, prior breast cancer or atypical ductal hyperplasia, and presence of genetic syndromes (eg, *BRCA1*, *BRCA2*).

SIGNS/SYMPTOMS

Classically presents as painless, firm, and fixed mass. As disease progresses, skin retraction, nipple inversion, skin changes (ie, peau d'orange), bleeding, and ulceration may occur. Can be associated with Paget's disease of the breast. Additionally, may present with a clinically suspicious axillary lymph node.

Diagnosis

All patients with a clinically suspicious breast lesion should undergo a diagnostic workup with bilateral mammography and targeted ultrasound, followed by a biopsy (ie, FNA, core biopsy, excisional biopsy).

Treatment

Therapy is determined by stage of lesion and includes surgery, chemotherapy, and radiation therapy.

- **Surgery**: Goals of surgery include **control of local disease** (ie, **lumpectomy or mastectomy) and evaluation of nodal disease. Contraindications to breast-conserving surgery include** Previous radiation to the affected breast, multicentric disease, large tumor relative to breast size that would result in an unacceptable cosmetic result, and high risk of local recurrence. Studies show **no difference in overall or disease-free survival** comparing lumpectomy with radiation to MRM. Evaluation of nodal disease can be via sentinel lymph node biopsy (SLNBx) with pathologic evaluation or via axillary lymph node dissection. The latter is indicated for + SLNBx, known lymph node + disease based on preoperative FNA or clinical exam, or the presence of inflammatory breast cancer.

SLNBx is performed with preoperative isosulfan blue or methylene blue and ^{99m}Tc sulfur colloid. Sensitivity is 85–100% based on center.

- **Radiation therapy**: Used to ↓ rate of local recurrence, particularly when used in combination with breast-conserving surgery. **Contraindicated in first and second trimesters** of pregnancy or in patients with a prior history of chest wall irradiation. Radiation may be forgone in elderly patients with small hormone receptor + tumors who are treated with adjuvant hormonal therapy.
- **Chemotherapy**: Beneficial to all patients with high risk of relapse **regardless of nodal status**. Can generally be withheld in patients with tumors < 1 cm and - lymph nodes. Decreases recurrence rate by 30%. Combinations vary, but those containing **anthracyclines** (eg, doxorubicin-cyclophosphamide, 5-fluorouracil [5-FU]-doxorubicin-cyclophosphamide) are most effective. Anthracyclines in combination with taxanes (eg, paclitazel) may also be effective.

Contraindications to tamoxifen use–
Uterine cancer, allergy, history of venous thrombosis

- **Hormonal therapy**: Reduces recurrence and mortality in patients with estrogen receptor + (ER+) tumors. Also helps prevent contralateral breast cancer and cancer in high-risk patients. ***HER2/neu*** is located on chromosome 17q and is a member of the **epidermal growth factor receptor** family. Overexpression is associated with ↓ **disease-free breast cancer survival**.
  - Tamoxifen: **Selective estrogen receptor modulator**. Standard regimen recommended is 20 mg/d for 5 years. **Reduces risk of recurrent and contralateral breast cancer and improves overall and disease-free survival.** Also used for 1° prevention in high-risk groups (risk ↓ up to 50%). **Increased risk of endometrial cancer, stroke, and thromboembolic events.** Benefits also include ↑ **bone density** and ↓ low-density lipoprotein (LDL) cholesterol.
  - Anastrozole: Aromatase inhibitor that **can be used in postmenopausal women, particularly in those with contraindication to tamoxifen.** May improve disease-free survival and risk of contralateral cancer compared to tamoxifen alone.
  - Trastuzumab: Monoclonal antibody to HER2 that may be used with *HER2/neu* + breast cancer patients in both the adjuvant and metastatic setting. Side effects include cardiomyopathy.

Response to hormonal therapy–
ER+/PR+ > ER–/PR+ > ER+/PR– > ER–/PR–

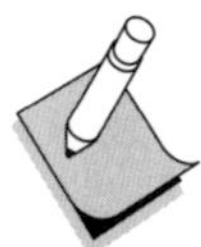

High-yield breast cancer staging–

Inflammatory breast cancer, – nodes: Stage IIIB

Paget's disease without mass: Stage 0

Cancer > 5 cm: Stage II if – lymph nodes; stage III if + lymph nodes

Any size cancer, + ipsilateral, internal mammary lymph nodes: Stage IIIA

Any size cancer, + ipsilateral, supraclavicular lymph nodes: Stage IIIB

Distant metastasis: Stage IV

Site of breast cancer metastases–

Bone, lung, brain

STAGING

The tumor, node status, metastasis (TNM) categories for pathologic and clinical staging include

- T: T0 (no evidence of 1° tumor), T_{is} (DCIS, LCIS, Paget's disease without tumor), T1 (mass ≤ 2 cm), T2 (mass > 2 cm and ≤ 5 cm), T3 (mass > 5 cm), T4 (tumor of any size with chest wall extension, edema, or ulceration of the skin, or satellite skin nodules; inflammatory breast cancer)
- N (pathological; pN): pN0 (histologically - lymph nodes), pN1 (1-3 histologically + axillary and/or internal mammary lymph nodes that are not clinically apparent), pN2 (4-9 histologically + axillary lymph nodes *or* clinically apparent + internal mammary lymph nodes without + axillary lymph nodes), pN3 (≥ 10 histologically + axillary lymph nodes *or* + infraclavicular lymph nodes *or* clinically apparent ipsilateral internal mammary lymph nodes *with* ≥ 1 + axillary lymph node *or* ≥ 3 + axillary lymph nodes with histologically + but not clinically apparent internal mammary lymph nodes *or* + ipsilateral supraclavicular lymph nodes)
- N (clinical): N0 (- lymph nodes), N1 (+ **mobile,** ipsilateral axillary nodes), N2 (+ **fixed**, ipsilateral axillary nodes or clinically apparent, ipsilateral internal mammary nodes without clinically evident axillary node disease), N3 (+ ipsilateral infraclavicular lymph nodes with or without axillary node disease *or* clinically apparent, ipsilateral internal mammary nodes with clinically apparent axillary node disease *or* ipsilateral supraclavicular lymph nodes with or without internal mammary or axillary node disease)
- M: M0 (metastatic disease absent), M1 (metastatic disease present).

  Staging includes

- Stage 0: T_{is}N0M0
- Stage I: T1N0M0
- Stage II: T0N1M0 *or* T1N1M0 *or* T2N0M0 *or* T2N1M0 *or* T3N0M0
- Stage III: T0N2M0 *or* T1N2M0 *or* T2N2M0 *or* T3N1M0 *or* T3N2M0 *or* T4, any N, M0 *or* Any T, N3M0
- Stage IV: Any T, any N, M1

COMPLICATIONS

Skin changes from radiation, brachial plexus damage due to axillary irradiation, chronic lymphedema after axillary dissection, **Stewart-Treves' syndrome** (lymphangiosarcoma in the setting of chronic lymphedema following MRM).

Lobular Carcinoma of the Breast

Comprises about 10% of breast cancer cases. Compared to ductal adenocarcinoma, often associated with an ill-defined fibrotic mass. More likely to be ER+/progesterone receptor positive (PR+), multicentric, and bilateral. Histology reveals characteristic "**indian-filing**" of tumor cells.

Inflammatory Breast Cancer

Comprises about 5% of breast cancer cases. Commonly affects **younger women**. Characterized by a **rapid onset of breast erythema, edema, warmth, and pain.** Must be differentiated from mastitis, which is associated with leukocytosis, fever, and response to antibiotics. Generally a clinical diagnosis, but workup can include a skin biopsy that reveals **tumor invasion into the lymphatics.** Treatment includes induction chemotherapy, MRM, radiation, and hormonal therapy if ER+. Portends **worst prognosis of all breast cancer types**.

Male Breast Cancer

Rare entity, ↑ prevalence in men > 60 years of age. Risks include ***BRCA2* mutation**, family history of breast cancer, gynecomastia, Ashkenazi Jewish descent, **Klinefelter' syndrome** (ie, 47,XXY), and radiation exposure. Presents as **painless, retroareolar mass with nipple changes** (eg, erythema, discharge). Must differentiate from gynecomastia, which is mobile, painful, and rubbery. Resect with MRM and consider tamoxifen, as **most tumors are ER+.** Metastatic disease may also be treated with tamoxifen or orchiectomy.

Breast Cancer in the Pregnant Woman

Diagnosed during pregnancy or within 1 year of delivery. During the **first and second trimesters, breast irradiation is contraindicated, and treatment includes MRM.** If cancer warrants chemotherapy or radiation in the first trimester, consider pregnancy termination. If diagnosed during the **third trimester**, options include lumpectomy with radiation or lumpectomy with axillary node dissection if radiation is deferred. Chemotherapy should be delayed until after delivery. For postpartum cases, breast-conservation surgery or MRM may be used. Lactation should be suppressed, and patient should be advised to avoid pregnancy for at least 1 year.

SLNBx in pregnancy remains controversial. Previously contraindicated due to the theoretical risk of radioisotope and dye exposure. Newer studies have shown that effective doses of these agents are unlikely to affect mother or fetus. Nevertheless, the question of whether pregnancy affects lymphatic flow is still unanswered and thus, SLNBx may be unreliable. The current approach to decision-making in this instance should involve discussion of the risks and benefits with the pregnant patient who has clinically - nodes.

▶ SAMPLE QUESTIONS

A 55-year-old woman has numbness of the inner arm after axillary lymph node dissection. What nerve is likely affected?	Intercostobrachial nerve.
What is the difference between simple mastectomy and MRM?	Simple mastectomy removes breast tissue. MRM additionally removes pectoralis fascia and axillary lymph nodes.
A postpartum woman is unable to lactate. What hormone might be implicated?	Oxytocin.
What prophylaxis is indicated for patients with a *BRCA1* mutation?	Bilateral salpingo-oophorectomy after childbearing, possible bilateral risk-reducing mastectomies. Patients have a 30% ↓ breast cancer risk after bilateral oophorectomy. Can follow with screening MRI and mammography.
What mutation is associated with male breast cancer? Li-Fraumeni?	Male breast cancer: *BRCA2*. Li-Fraumeni: p53.
Overexpression of which oncogene is associated with ↓ disease-free survival from breast cancer?	*HER2/neu*.
What is the recommended screening for breast cancer?	Mammography annually ≤ 40 years. Clinical breast exam every 2–3 years from age 20 to 39 and annually ≤ 40 years.
What treatment options are indicated for axillary metastases without a known 1° tumor?	1. Ipsilateral MRM and chemotherapy. 2. Axillary lymph node dissection, whole breast radiation therapy, systemic chemotherapy.
A 20-year-old female presents with a rubbery 1 cm mass of the left breast. What is the likely diagnosis?	Fibroadenoma.
A 40-year-old female presents with bilateral cyclical painful breast masses. What is the most likely diagnosis?	Fibrocystic disease.
A 35-year-old female presents with an 8-cm mass. Histology reveals leaf-like appearance. What is the most likely diagnosis? Treatment?	Phyllodes tumor. Because of large size, perform mastectomy or wide excision with 1-cm margins.

A 39-year-old female with a family history of breast cancer is diagnosed with LCIS of the right breast. What are her options? What if she was diagnosed with DCIS?	LCIS: Careful observation versus bilateral prophylactic mastectomy. DCIS: Lumpectomy with radiation or simple mastectomy (and possibly prophylactic contralateral mastectomy).
A 54-year-old female with a history of Hodgkin's lymphoma s/p mantle radiation therapy presents with a 1 cm breast carcinoma. What is the appropriate management?	Simple mastectomy with SLNBx or MRM.
Ten years s/p mastectomy, a woman presents with Stewart-Treves' syndrome. What is the appropriate treatment?	Amputation of the affected limb.

CHAPTER 12

Endocrine

Gregory R. Veillette, MD
Reviewed by Antonia E. Stephen, MD

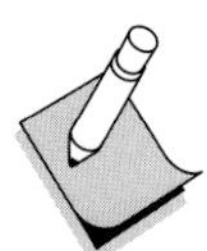

Failure to obliterate the thyroglossal duct results in a thyroglossal duct cyst. See Chapter 19 for details.

▶ BASIC SCIENCE

Embryology

Embryology of the Thyroid

Derived from endoderm during the third gestational week, thyroid descends from **foramen cecum** to just below the cricoid. Thyroglossal duct is an epithelial-lined structure serving as the attachment for thyroid passage. These epithelial cells ultimately become thyroid follicular cells with colloid production beginning at 11 weeks. **Neuroectodermal ultimobranchial bodies** (from the **fourth branchial pouch**) give rise to **calcitonin-producing C cells**. Ectopic thyroid is present when thyroid migration arrests at another anatomic location.

Embryology of the Parathyroid

Superior glands are derived from the **fourth branchial pouch; inferior glands** and **thymus** arise from the **third branchial pouch**.

Embryology of the Adrenal

Adrenal cortex is derived from mesoderm. Adrenal medulla is derived from ectodermal **neural crest**. Neural crest cells migrate to the cortical mesoderm and become surrounded by it.

Embryology of the Pituitary

The anterior pituitary is derived from a pouch of ectoderm (**Rathke's pouch**) from the roof of the mouth. The posterior pituitary is derived from a neuroectodermal pouch from the hypothalamus. The two join to form the pituitary gland.

Anatomy

Macroscopic Anatomy of the Thyroid

Composed of two lobes joined by an isthmus and occasionally including a pyramidal lobe. Anatomic boundaries include:

- Anterior: Sternohyoid and sternothyroid muscles
- Superior: Midaspect of thyroid cartilage
- Lateral: Sternocleidomastoid, carotid sheath
- Inferior: Sternal notch and clavicles.

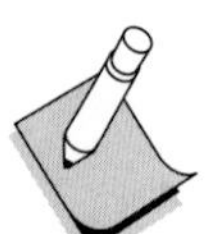

Ectopic parathyroid locations–
Superior glands: Tracheoesophageal groove, tracheal bifurcation, retroesophageal space, retropharyngeal space, carotid sheath
Inferior glands: Thymus, intrathyroidal, carotid sheath

Microscopic Anatomy of the Thyroid

Lobules are divided into functional units called **follicles**. Follicles are lined by a cuboidal epithelium and store colloid, the storage form of thyroid hormone. C cells secrete **calcitonin** and are found in the interfollicular spaces.

Macroscopic Anatomy of the Parathyroid

Two **superior glands** are usually located **posterolateral to the recurrent laryngeal nerve (RLN)**; two **inferior glands** are usually located **anteromedially**. Supernumerary glands or glands in ectopic positions may be present.

Microscopic Anatomy of the Parathyroid

Composed of two main cells types: chief cells and oxyphil cells. **Chief cells** secrete parathyroid hormone (PTH). **Oxyphil cells** also secrete PTH but may have additional roles.

Macroscopic Anatomy of the Adrenal

Small, bilateral glands that rest on the superomedial aspect of each kidney. Dark, tan-to-orange color makes them easily distinguishable.

Organ of Zuckerkandl– *Extra-adrenal neuroectodermal tissue located at the aortic bifurcation*

Microscopic Anatomy of the Adrenal

Divided into cortex and medulla. Cortex is divided into **zona glomerulosa** (produces mineralocorticoids), **zona fasciculata** (produces glucocorticoids), and **zona reticularis** (produces sex steroids). Medulla is composed of **chromaffin cells** that secrete epinephrine and norepinephrine.

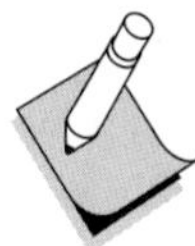

Isthmus is usually located inferior to the cricothyroid membrane.

Macroscopic Anatomy of the Pituitary

Small, teardrop-shaped gland in the **sella turcica**. Divided into anterior (adenohypophysis) and posterior (neurohypophysis) sections. Posterior pituitary is largely made of axons (ie, pituitary stalk) from the hypothalamus.

Microscopic Anatomy of the Pituitary

Anterior pituitary contains acidophils, basophils, and chromophils that secrete luteinizing hormone (LH), follicle-stimulating hormone (FSH), thyroid-stimulating hormone (TSH), growth hormone (GH), prolactin, and adrenocorticotropic hormone (ACTH). Posterior pituitary contains neurosecretory granules of hormones delivered from the hypothalamus (ie, antidiuretic hormone [ADH], oxytocin).

Pituitary stalk is vulnerable to injury and is easily damaged by head trauma.

Blood Supply

Blood supply varies by organ.

- **Thyroid:** Arterial supply arises from the **inferior thyroid artery** (from the thyrocervical trunk) and **superior thyroid artery** (from the external carotid). Venous drainage occurs via the superior, middle, and inferior thyroid veins. The inferior drains into the innominate vein, while the superior and middle drain into the internal jugular.
- **Parathyroid:** Supplied by the **inferior thyroid artery.**
- **Adrenal:** Supplied by the aorta (middle adrenal artery) as well as inferior phrenic (superior adrenal artery) and renal (inferior adrenal artery) arteries. A single adrenal vein drains to the inferior vena cava (**IVC**) **on the right** and **renal vein on the left.** Most blood to the adrenal cortex filters through the medulla.
- **Pituitary: Hypothalamic-hypophyseal portal system** (HHPS) provides blood to the anterior pituitary. Allows for direct transport of hypothalamic hormones to the anterior pituitary, bypassing systemic circulation.

HHPS, with two capillary beds in series, causes ↓ perfusion pressure to the pituitary. Consequently, it is at high risk for infarction during hypotensive episodes (ie, Sheehan's syndrome after peripartum bleeding).

INNERVATION

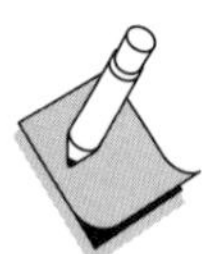

Inferior thyroid artery is associated with the RLN. Identify the nerve before ligating the artery. Middle thyroid vein travels with inferior thyroid artery, with the vein being more anterior and superficial.

Surgically relevant innervation includes:

- **Thyroid: RLNs** arise from the vagus and **innervate all intrinsic laryngeal muscles except the cricothyroid.** The left branch loops around the aorta (at the ligamentum arteriosum) to ultimately lie in the tracheoesophageal groove; the right RLN loops around the right subclavian artery. In 1% of people, the nerve is not recurrent. **Superior laryngeal nerve** also arises from the vagus and gives rise to internal and external branches. **Internal branch** provides sensation to the larynx, while the **external branch** provides motor function to cricothyroid muscle.
- **Parathyroid:** Innervated by branches of the vagus and cervical sympathetic ganglia.
- **Adrenal**: Cortex receives stimulation via the hypophyseal-pituitary-adrenal (HPA) axis. Medulla receives **preganglionic sympathetic fibers**.
- **Pituitary:** Anterior pituitary is stimulated by hypothalamic releasing factors. Posterior pituitary is composed of hypothalamic axons.

LYMPHATIC DRAINAGE OF THE THYROID

Central and lateral neck lymph nodes drain the thyroid. Look for lymph node metastases, particularly in thyroid cancers prone to lymph node spread (eg, medullary, papillary). **Thyroid cells located within a lymph node almost always represent a metastatic focus of papillary thyroid cancer.**

Physiology of the Endocrine System

PHYSIOLOGY OF THE THYROID

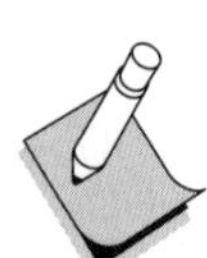

Superior thyroid artery and vein are associated with the superior laryngeal nerve. Identify the nerve during mobilization of the superior pole.

Na^+/I^- symporter is inhibited by ***perchlorate****.*

Hypothalamic thyroid releasing hormone (TRH) stimulates pituitary TSH, which then drives production of thyroid hormone. The follicle contains tyrosine-rich thyroglobulin (Tg), which is involved in the production and storage of thyroid hormone. Production involves a number of steps (see Figure 12-1):

- Transport of I^-: Basal Na^+/I^- symporter drives I^- intracellularly via active transport.
- Oxidation of I^- to I_2: Involves thyroperoxidase.
- Tg iodination: Results in mono-iodotyrosines (MITs) and di-iodotyrosines (DITs).
- DIT and MIT coupling: DIT + DIT → T_4 (thyroxine); MIT + DIT → T_3.
- Hydrolysis of Tg: Releases free MIT, DIT, T_3, and T_4.
- Hematogenous release of T_3 and T_4: After TSH stimulation.

T_4 is the 1° hormone produced in the thyroid (80–85%). T_3 (from thyroid and peripheral conversion of T_4) is more active and has a shorter half-life ($t_{1/2}$).

Functions of thyroid hormone include stimulation of catabolism, gastrointestinal motility, β-adrenergic activity (ie, inotropic, chronotropic), brain and skeletal maturation, bone growth, and basal metabolic rate.

PHYSIOLOGY OF THE PARATHYROID

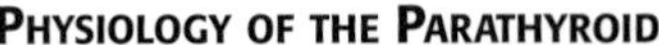

PTH is secreted by the chief cells in response to ↓ Ca^{2+}. PTH regulates total and ionized Ca^{2+} levels via renal, bone, and intestinal effects (see Figure 12-2):

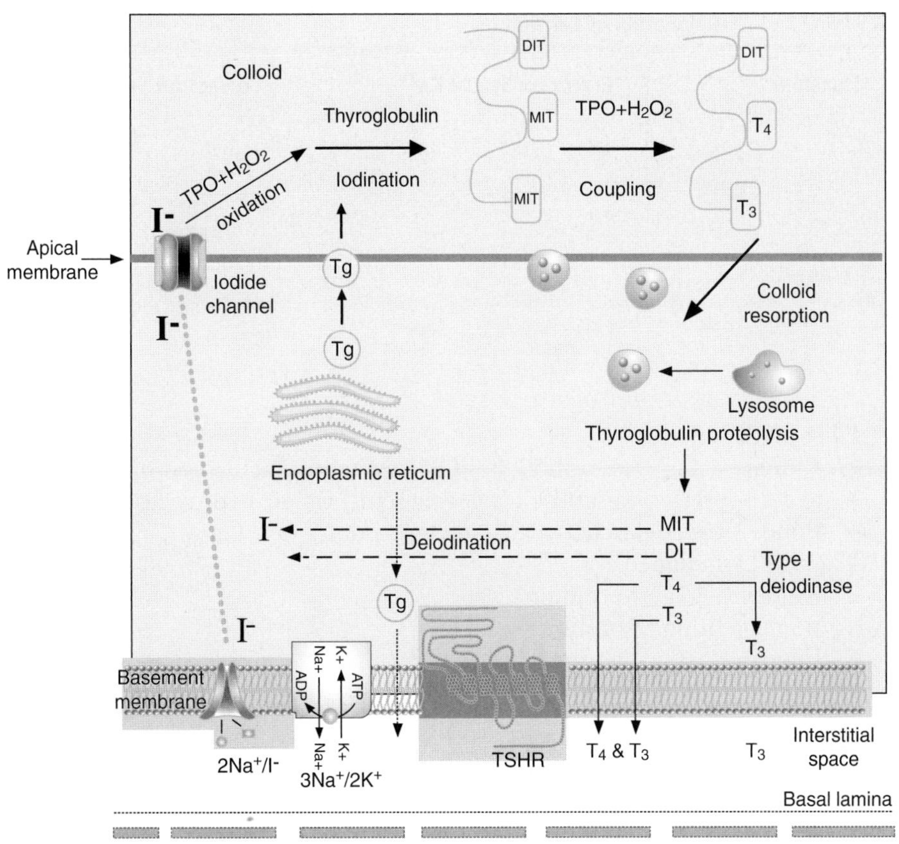

FIGURE 12-1. Thyroid hormone production.

(Reproduced, with permission, from Molina PE. *Endocrine Physiology*, 2nd ed. New York: McGraw-Hill, 2006:78.)

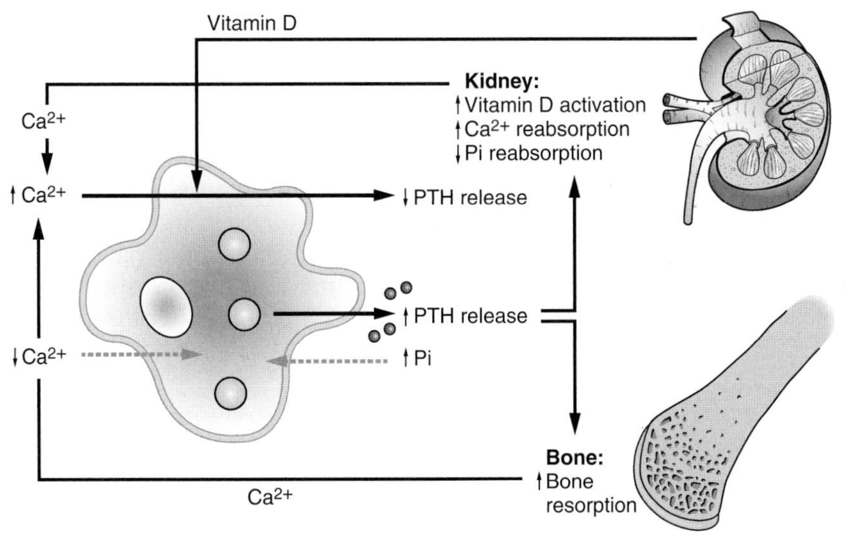

FIGURE 12-2. Calcium regulation.

(Reproduced, with permission, from Molina PE. *Endocrine Physiology*, 2nd ed. New York: McGraw-Hill, 2006:96.)

Corrected total Ca^{2+} formula–
Corrected total Ca^{2+} = Measured total Ca^{2+} + (0.8 × [4.0 – serum albumin])

TABLE 12-1. Regulation of Calcium

HORMONE	EFFECT ON SERUM Ca^{2+}	EFFECT ON SERUM PO_4^{3-}
PTH	↑	↓
Vitamin D	↑	↑
Calcitonin	↓	↓

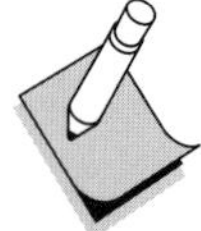

Signs of hypercalcemia–
Kidney stones, diabetes insipidus, mental status changes, abdominal pain, constipation, bone pain.

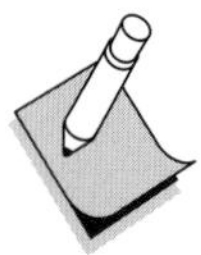

Signs of hypocalcemia–
Trousseau's sign, Chvostek's sign, tetany.

- PTH-mediated
  - Kidney: ↑ Ca^{2+} resorption, ↑ PO_4^{3-} excretion, activation of vitamin D to 1,25-$(OH)_2$ vitamin D (cholecalciferol) via 1α-hydroxylase
  - Bone: ↑ Osteoclast activity (bone resorption) → ↑ Ca^{2+}.
- Vitamin D-mediated
  - Kidney: ↑ Ca^{2+} resorption
  - Bone: ↑ Bone resorption → ↑ Ca^{2+}
  - Intestine: ↑ Ca^{2+} absorption.

Calcitonin is secreted by the thyroidal C cells and acts as a **PTH antagonist**.

PTH, calcitonin, and vitamin D regulate Ca^{2+}-PO_4^{3-} homeostasis (see Table 12-1).

Total Ca^{2+} depends on protein levels (↓ albumin → ↓ **total** Ca^{2+}). Acid-base status impacts ionized Ca^{2+} (↓ pH → Ca^{2+} displacement → ↑ ionized Ca^{2+}).

Mg^{2+} is involved in Ca^{2+} homeostasis. Similar to ↑ Ca^{2+}, ↓ Mg^{2+} inhibits PTH, leading to hypocalcemia. Correct Mg^{2+} before correcting Ca^{2+}.

PHYSIOLOGY OF THE ADRENAL

Releases mineralocorticoids (eg, aldosterone), glucocorticoids (eg, cortisol), androgens (eg, dehydroepiandrosterone [DHEA]), and catecholamines. Adrenal cortical steroid production is summarized in Figure 12-3. Initial reaction (**cholesterol → pregnenolone**) is the **rate-limiting step**.

- Aldosterone: Released in response to renin-angiotensin system and ↓ circulating blood volume. Results in ↑ Na^+ resorption (in the distal nephron) as well as ↑ K^+ and H^+ secretion. Causes HTN, hypokalemia, and metabolic alkalosis.
- Cortisol: ACTH stimulates production from pregnenolone via serial enzymatic conversions (**21-hydroxylase, 11β-hydroxylase,** and **17α-hydroxylase**). Acts synergistically with catecholamines in response to stress to cause HTN. Also causes hyperglycemia, insulin resistance, protein and fat catabolism, easy bruising, and muscle weakness.
- Androgens: Androstenedione (and ultimately, testosterone) is produced by way of DHEA or 17α-hydroxyprogesterone in response to ACTH. Involved in sexual maturation and reproductive biology.
- Catecholamines: Produced from **tyrosine**, which is converted to L-DOPA → dopamine → norepinephrine → epinephrine. Production is mediated by preganglionic sympathetic fibers and cortisol concentrations. Enzyme phenylethanolamine N-methyltransferase (PNMT) converts norepinephrine to epinephrine. Metabolized to by-products, including **vanillylmandelic acid** and **homovanillic acid.**

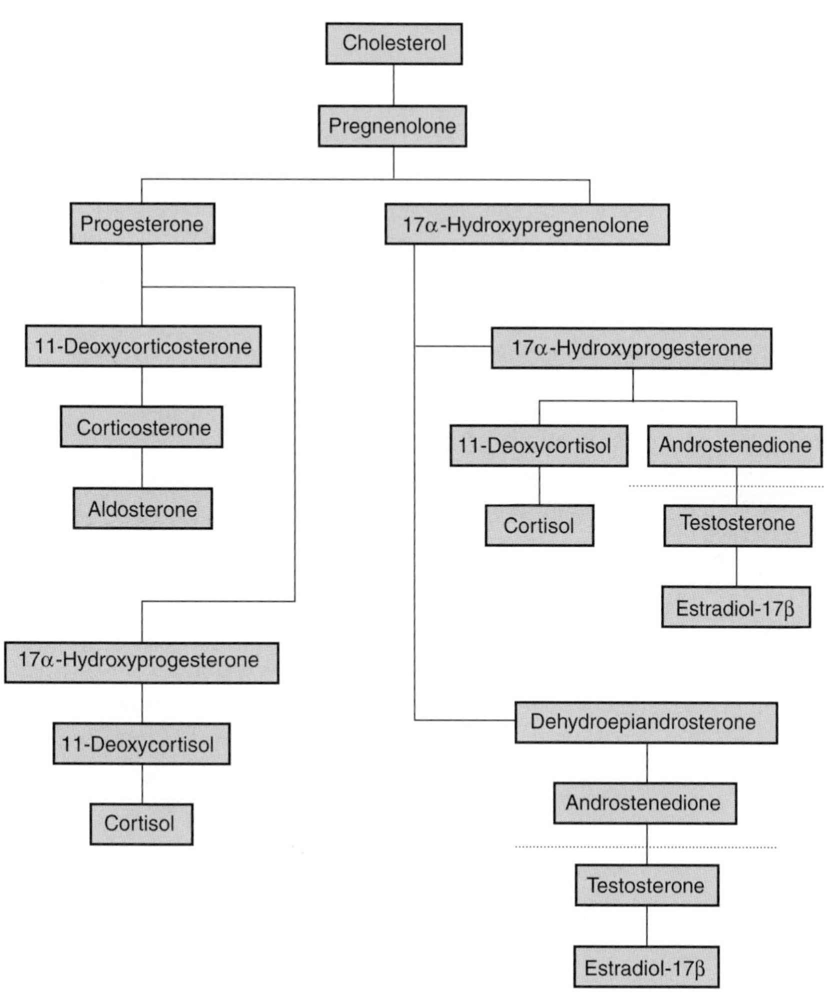

FIGURE 12-3. Adrenal cortical steroid production.

(Reproduced, with permission, from Molina PE. *Endocrine Physiology*, 2nd ed. New York: McGraw-Hill, 2006:128.)

*Secretory granules in the anterior pituitary are **made in** and **released from the anterior pituitary** under the influence of hypothalamic releasing factors. Secretory granules in the posterior pituitary are **made in the hypothalamus** and **released from the posterior pituitary.***

Physiology of the Pituitary

Anterior and posterior pituitary hormones are summarized in Table 12-2.

▶ CLINICAL SCIENCE

Asymptomatic Thyroid Nodules

Thyroid cancer comprises about 5% of thyroid nodules. Ask about the duration of symptoms, history of head and neck radiation exposure, and family history of thyroid cancer, endocrine tumors, and multiple endocrine neoplasia (MEN) syndromes. Assess for nodule size, tenderness, and fluctuance as well as airway obstruction and constitutional symptoms. Diagnostic workup to rule out malignancy includes (see Figure 12-4):

- Thyroid function tests (TFTs): Free T_4 (FT_4; **preferred test** as not affected by thyroid-binding globulin), total T_4 (varies with amount of thyroid-binding globulin, liver disease, pregnancy), TSH, and T_3 resin uptake (T_3RU; allows for calculation of free thyroxine index to normalize thyroid-binding globulin differences).

TABLE 12-2. Pituitary Hormones

LOCATION	HORMONE	STIMULATING FACTOR	FUNCTION
Anterior pituitary	TSH	TRH.	Stimulates thyroid hormone release.
	ACTH	Corticotropin-releasing hormone (CRH).	Stimulates adrenal cortical steroid production.
	Prolactin	↓ Dopamine.	Stimulates breast development and milk production.
	GH	Growth hormone-releasing hormone (GHRH).	Stimulates insulin-like growth factor-I production.
	FSH	Gonadotropin-releasing hormone (GnRH).	Acts on gonads.
	LH	GnRH.	Acts on gonads.
Posterior pituitary	Oxytocin	Childbirth, breastfeeding → stimulation from paraventricular nuclei and supraoptic nuclei.	Uterine contractions, milk let-down.
	ADH (vasopressin)	↓ Blood volume, ↑ serum osmolarity.	Acts on renal collecting duct. Inserts aquaporin channels to allow free H_2O resorption and maximal urine concentration. Causes vasoconstriction of splanchnic and peripheral vessels.

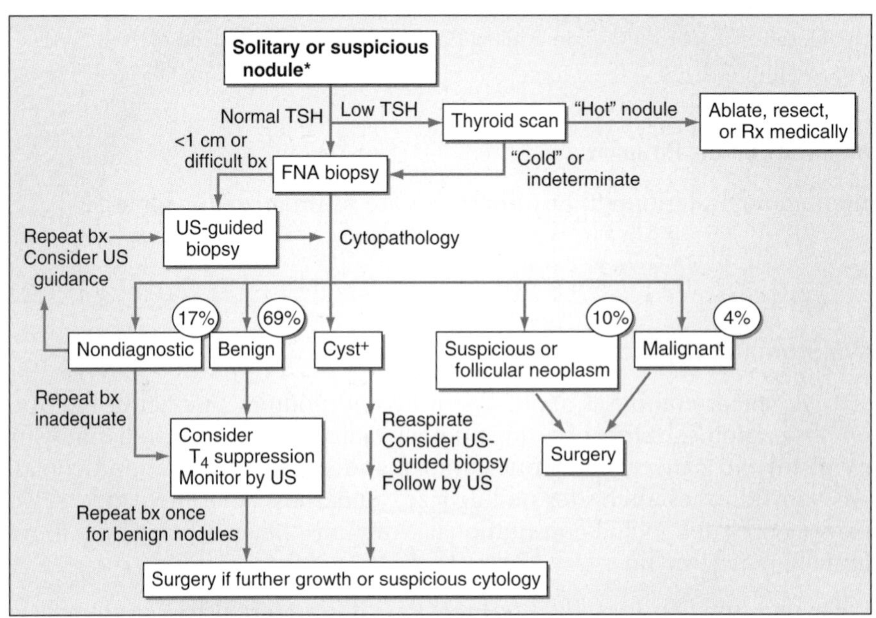

FIGURE 12-4. Evaluation of a thyroid nodule.

(Reproduced, with permission, from Kasper DL, et al. *Harrison's Principles of Internal Medicine*, 16th ed. New York: McGraw-Hill, 2005:212.)

- Thyroid ultrasound: Noninvasive means to screen for nonpalpable nodules and to assess for nodule size, solid and cystic components, and adjacent lymphadenopathy.
- Fine needle aspiration (FNA): Indicated for most thyroid nodules > 1 cm in size. Provides diagnosis in up to 90% of cases. Associated with ~3% false-rate.
- Radionuclide scan: Evaluates I_2 uptake. Useful in differentiating hyperthyroid states and should only be done when the TSH is suppressed. **Not to be used for routine workup of nodule.**

Quick review of TFTs–

↓ TSH → hyperthyroidism.

↑ TSH → hypothyroidism.

↑ Total T_4, ↑ free T_4 → ↑ T_3RU.

↑ Total T_4, ↑ thyroid-binding globulin → ↓ T_3RU.

Hyperthyroidism

Demographics

Excess circulating FT_3 or FT_4. Most commonly affects females 20–40 years of age.

Types

Due to abnormal gland stimulation (eg, **Grave's disease**, molar pregnancy, choriocarcinoma, TSH-secreting tumor), **thyroid gland autonomy** (eg, toxic adenoma, toxic multinodular goiter, I_2-induced, amiodarone toxicity), or **inflammation** (eg, thyroiditis).

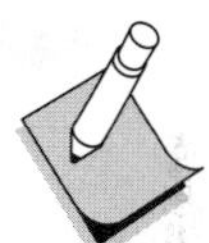

Hot nodules (functioning) = benign.

Cold nodules (nonfunctioning) = possibly malignant.

- **Grave's disease: Most common cause of hyperthyroidism**, particularly in women aged 20–40 years. Symptoms include anxiety, weakness, diarrhea, and weight loss. Exam reveals warm, moist skin, tachycardia (possibly **atrial fibrillation**), tremor, hyperactive reflexes, **goiter, pretibial myxedema, and ophthalmopathy**. Workup will reveal ↓ TSH, ↑ FT_4, ↑ total T_4, ↑ FT_4 index, ↑ ^{123}I uptake, and **anti-TSH receptor antibodies**. Initial treatment includes control of hyperthyroidism with antithyroid medication (eg, methimazole, propylthiouracil [PTU], and β-blockers). If the patient cannot be controlled medically or does not sustain a euthyroid state with medication discontinuation, then definitive therapy is indicated. Definitive treatment options include radioactive iodine or thyroidectomy. **Surgery is preferred for pregnant women or large goiters**.
- **Thyroiditis:** Inflammation of the thyroid with acute (eg, suppurative), subacute (eg, de Quervain's, postpartum), and chronic (eg, Hashimoto's, amiodarone-induced) forms (see Table 12-3). Can see initial hyperthyroidism from gland inflammation and release of preformed hormone, followed by a hypothyroid phase from gland impairment.

Human leukocytic antigens (HLA) B8 and DR3 are associated with Grave's disease.

Hypothyroidism

Demographics/Risk Factors

Affects ~1% of population. Most common causes include **thyroid resection**, irradiation, ^{131}I ablation, cretinism, thyroiditis, and medication (eg, lithium, amiodarone).

Signs/Symptoms

May be asymptomatic or associated with fatigue, depression, constipation, weight gain, brittle or thinning hair, or cold intolerance. Exam may reveal hypothermia, myxedema, ileus, ↓ BP, ↓ HR, or heart failure. **Cretinism** is

TABLE 12-3. Types of Thyroiditis

TYPE/SUBTYPE	ETIOLOGY	SIGNS/SYMPTOMS	DIAGNOSIS	TREATMENT
Acute				
Suppurative	Bacterial	Painful, enlarged thyroid with fluctuance, erythema, fever.	↑ WBC, ↑ ESR.	Antibiotics, incision and drainage of abscesses.
Subacute				
De Quervain's	Viral	Painful, enlarged thyroid with neck pain, viral-like symptoms, dysphagia, preceding URI.	↑ FT_4, ↓ TSH (initial hyperthyroidism), ↑ **ESR.** ↓ I_2 uptake on radionuclide scan.	Acetylsalicylic acid (ASA) or nonsteroidal anti-inflammatory drugs (NSAIDs), steroids. Usually resolves in 4-6 months.
Postpartum	Autoimmune	Typically asymptomatic. Occurs in postpartum period.	Similar to de Quervain's, except **ESR is normal.**	Treat hyperthyroidism symptoms.
Chronic				
Hashimoto's	Autoimmune	**Painless, firm, rubbery**, enlarged thyroid. Subclinical or symptomatic hypothyroidism in later stages.	↑ FT_4, ↓ TSH (initial hyperthyroidism) → ↓ TSH, ↓ FT_4 ↑ ESR. ↓ I_2 uptake on radionuclide scan. ↑ **Anti-Tg antibody,** ↑ **antithyroperoxidase antibody**.	Treat hypothyroidism.
Riedel's	Likely autoimmune	Painless, "woody," enlarged thyroid. Can compress airway or esophagus.	Lymphocytic infiltration of thyroid.	Surgery to ↓ compressive symptoms. Tamoxifen or steroids.

congenital hypothyroidism caused by I_2 deficiency, genetic causes, or unknown causes. Associated with characteristic facies, mental retardation, and stunted growth.

Patients with Hashimoto's thyroiditis can develop thyroid cancers including thyroid lymphoma. Continue to monitor for thyroid nodules.

DIAGNOSIS

Characteristic labs findings including ↓ FT_4, ↑ TSH, and ↓ radioactive iodine uptake. Anemia, hyponatremia, and hyperlipidemia may also be present.

TREATMENT

Treat with **levothyroxine**. Stabilize any patient with **myxedema coma**: secure airway, correct hypothermia, and administer IV levothyroxine. Associated with high mortality rate.

A 40-year-old male presents for his annual physical exam. He has a 3-cm right-sided thyroid nodule. He denies symptoms of thyroid dysfunction or compression, family history of thyroid cancer, or history of radiation exposure. FNA reveals a microfollicular neoplasm. What is the correct surgical management? Choices include a right thyroidectomy with isthmusectomy to confirm follicular adenoma without follicular carcinoma. If carcinoma is present, patient requires a completion (ie, left) thyroidectomy. May also opt to perform 1° total thyroidectomy in order to avoid a second procedure.

Thyroid Cancer

DEMOGRAPHICS/RISK FACTORS

Most commonly affects women 25–65 years of age. Increased risk associated with family history of thyroid cancer, history of neck irradiation, history of goiter, and genetic mutations (eg, *PTEN*, *p53*, *p16*, *RET*).

TYPES

Summarized in Table 12-4.

5 H's of myxedema coma:
Hypothermia
Hypotension
Hypoventilation
Hyponatremia
Hypoglycemia

AMES scoring system:
↑ Risk of death (46%) associated with–
Age: > 51 years (women), > 41 years (men)
Metastasis: Present
Extent of disease: Extrathyroidal papillary carcinoma or follicular carcinoma with capsular involvement
Size (diameter) of tumor: ≥ 5 cm

Hyperparathyroidism

Causes and impact on PTH, Ca^{2+}, and PO_4^{3-} vary by type (see Table 12-5). Hypercalcemia results in nephrolithiasis, abdominal cramps, nausea, constipation, and depression. Nephrogenic diabetes insipidus, short QT interval, and mental status changes are induced by extremely high Ca^{2+} levels. In addition to checking PTH, Ca^{2+}, and PO_4^{3-} levels, check a parathyroid hormone-related protein (PTHrP) level if malignancies or paraneoplastic syndromes are suspected. Rule out other causes of hypercalcemia (eg, multiple myeloma, thiazide diuretics, bone metastases, sarcoidosis, vitamin D intoxication, Paget's disease). Localize abnormal gland(s) with sestamibi scan (~85% accurate for adenomas).

Hypoparathyroidism

Caused by ↓ **PTH** with subsequent ↓ Ca^{2+} and ↑ PO_4^{3-}. **Most common cause is parathyroid resection.** Hypocalcemia results in neuromuscular excitability, **Trousseau's** (ie, carpopedal spasm) and **Chvostek's** (ie, facial muscle contraction with tapping of facial nerve) signs, and tetany. Treat with Ca^{2+} and vitamin D supplements. If Mg^{2+} is low, replete this first.

Differentiate 1° disease from **pseudohypoparathyroidism**, which is caused by **abnormal activity of PTH**. Labs reveal ↓ **Ca^{2+} and ↑ PO_4^{3-} with ↑ PTH.**

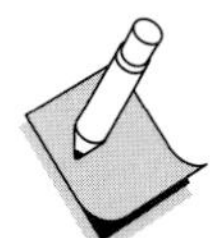

If FNA pathology reveals follicular neoplasm, perform lobectomy to demonstrate capsular or vascular invasion. If + invasive disease, perform a completion thyroidectomy. Another option is a total thyroidectomy during the first procedure.

Parathyroid Carcinoma

Rare condition affecting people > 30 years of age. Compared to benign hyperparathyroidism, presents with significantly ↑ **Ca^{2+} (> 14 mg/dL)** and PTH. Signs and symptoms are consistent with **severe hypercalcemia**; a firm, palpable neck mass may be present. If resectable, treatment includes en bloc resection of parathyroid, thyroid, and any involved structures. Chemoradiation can be used for palliation. Five-year survival is 50–75%.

TABLE 12-4. Thyroid Cancers

Type	Demographics	Pathologic Findings	Treatment	Prognosis
Papillary	80% **(most common).** Most common in **women** 20-40 years. Associated with radiation exposure.	**Psammona bodies, Orphan Annie cells** (intranuclear cytoplasmic inclusions). **Lymphatic spread. Lateral aberrant thyroid** = metastatic papillary carcinoma.	If < 1 cm → lobectomy with isthmusectomy. If > 1 cm, bilateral, or high-risk tumor, total thyroidectomy. Central neck dissection for + central node disease; modified radical neck dissection (MRND) for + lateral node disease. Postoperative ^{131}**I** for lesions > 1.5 cm or high-risk tumors. Follow postoperative Tg levels.	95% 10-year survival. TNM and AMES are two systems that determine mortality risk.
Follicular	10%. Most common in women > 50 years. **Hürthle cell-variant** is more likely to be bilateral/multifocal.	Unlike adenoma, + **capsular or vascular invasion. Hematogenous spread.** Hürthle cell = eosinophilic cells and ↑ rate of lymphatic spread.	**FNA shows microfollicles.** Perform lobectomy or total thyroidectomy. If + cancer after a lobectomy, perform completion thyroidectomy with postoperative ^{131}**I.** Follow postoperative Tg levels.	85% 10-year survival. Hürthle cell has ↑ mortality rate.
Anaplastic	3%. Most common in women > 65 years.	**Undifferentiated.** Local invasion with metastatic disease at diagnosis.	**Resection indicated only for airway control.** Palliative chemoradiation.	**10% 2-year survival.** Median survival = 4 months.
Medullary	5%. Women = men. 25% have MEN-2 (↑ multicentric, bilateral disease).	↑ Calcitonin (hyperplastic C cells), ↑ CEA, + *RET* mutation. Look for other MEN-2 signs/symptoms.	If present, resect pheochromocytoma first. Total thyroidectomy, central node dissection. Parathyroidectomy if hyperparathyroidism. **No role for** ^{131}**I.**	80% 10-year survival if - nodal disease; 40% if + nodal disease.
Lymphoma	1%. More common in women. ↑ Risk with **Hashimoto's thyroiditis.**	**Non-Hodgkin's** type.	Secure airway if rapidly expanding with impending airway compromise. Chemotherapy.	50% 5-year survival; 35% if + extrathyroidal disease.

TABLE 12-5. **Types of Hyperparathyoidism and Laboratory Findings**

Type	Etiology	PTH	Serum Ca^{2+}	Serum PO_4^{3-}	Treatment
1°	Single adenoma (85%), 4-gland hyperplasia, carcinoma.	↑	**↑ Serum Ca^{2+}; ↑ urine Ca^{2+}**	↓	Parathyroidectomy for complications from hypercalcemia. For adenoma → resect adenoma. For hyperplasia → resect $3^1/_2$ glands or four glands with autotransplantation. Intraoperative PTH level should fall by 50%.
2°	Chronic renal failure.	↑	Nl/↓	↑	Parathyroidectomy for complications. PO_4^{3-} binders. Renal transplant. Watch for **calciphylaxis**.
3°	Autonomous PTH release after renal transplant.	↑	↑	↓	Parathyroidectomy if symptomatic or persistent disease 1 year after transplant.
Familial hypocalciuric hypercalcemia	Ca^{2+}-sensing gene mutation.	Nl/↑	**↑ Serum Ca^{2+}; ↓ urine Ca^{2+}**	↓	Usually no treatment required as patients are asymptomatic.

Endocrine-specific nerve injuries—

Damage to 1 RLN → abduction of vocal cord with voice hoarseness.

Damage to both RLNs → airway obstruction.

Damage to the external branch of the superior laryngeal nerve → inability to tense vocal cord and sing high notes.

A 40-year-old man presents to the ED with moderate left lower quadrant (LLQ) pain. On exam, his BP is mildly elevated. Labs are significant for a K^+ = 3.0 mEq/L. CT scan reveals uncomplicated diverticulitis and a 4-cm right adrenal mass. He is treated with antibiotics for his diverticulitis. On followup, his BP remains elevated and K^+ = 3.1 mEq/L. What additional steps should be taken? Check his serum aldosterone and aldosterone-to-renin ratio. If labs suggest a functional adrenal tumor (eg, aldosteronoma), perform adrenalectomy.

Adrenal Incidentaloma

Inadvertently discovered adrenal lesion during workup of nonadrenal condition. Present in about 3% of people > 50 years old. Tumors may be functioning or nonfunctioning and benign or malignant. Specific causes include adrenal adenoma or cyst, pheochromocytoma, aldosteronoma, cortisol-secreting lesion, **metastatic disease (eg, breast, lung, renal, melanoma)**, or adrenocortical carcinoma. Workup includes:

- Hormonal evaluation (functional versus nonfunctional): Urine and plasma metanephrines (for pheochromocytoma), K^+, aldosterone (> 20 ng/dL), aldosterone-to-renin ratio (> 30 with aldosteronomas), overnight dexamethasone suppression test (for cortisol-secreting tumors).
- Radiologic evaluation: CT and magnetic resonance imaging (MRI) are equivalent in differentiating benign and malignant lesions. Lesions < 4 cm, smooth, and homogenous with < 10 Hounsfield units (HU) are likely to be benign. Lesions that are heterogeneous, > 6 cm, or have high HU are likely to be malignant.
- Pathologic evaluation: **After excluding pheochromocytoma, FNA may be used to confirm metastatic disease or adrenocortical carcinoma**.

Malignancy in a nonfunctional adrenal incidentaloma–

< 4 cm → 2%

4–6 cm → 6%

> 6 cm → 25%

Adrenalectomy (open or laparoscopic) is indicated for all functional tumors. For nonfunctional tumors, resect lesions that are suspicious for malignancy. For indeterminate size lesions (4–6 cm), repeat CT in 6 months. Avoid laparoscopic adrenalectomy for resection of adrenocortical carcinomas or for cases not amenable to laparoscopic resection (eg, large size).

Functional Adrenal Tumors

Multiple types, including aldosteronomas, cortisol-secreting tumors, pheochromocytomas, and adrenocortical carcinomas.

- Aldosteronoma: Most commonly caused by single adenoma (70–80%) or bilateral hyperplasia (20–30%). Patients present with **HTN, ↓ K^+, and nonanion gap metabolic acidosis.** Serum aldosterone and serum aldosterone-to-renin ratio are ↑. If serum aldosterone-to-renin ratio is ↑ with a discrete unilateral mass, perform adrenalectomy. If ratio is ↑ without a discrete mass or with bilateral adrenal lesions, consider adrenal vein sampling. If sampling localizes lesion to one side, perform adrenalectomy. Administer spironolactone if tumor does not localize.
- Cortisol-secreting tumors: Can be caused by adrenal oversecretion of cortisol (ie, due to cortisol-secreting tumors), pituitary oversecretion of ACTH (ie, Cushing's disease, resulting in bilateral adrenal hyperplasia), or ectopic ACTH source (ie, malignancy). Patients present with HTN, ↑ glucose, striae, amenorrhea, hirsutism, buffalo hump, easy bruising, muscle weakness, and depression. Evaluation includes 24-hour urinary cortisol level or a low-dose (ie, 1 mg), overnight dexamethasone suppression test. If cortisol is not suppressed, Cushing's syndrome is confirmed. Next, if ACTH is ↓, there is an **ACTH-independent** source; order a abdominal CT to look for a cortisol-secreting adrenal tumor, which should be resected. If ACTH is ↑, there is an **ACTH-dependent** source, which might include an ectopic ACTH-secreting tumor or Cushing's disease (resulting in bilateral adrenal hyperplasia). For ACTH-dependent sources, a high-dose dexamethasone suppression test suppresses cortisol if the source is pituitary in origin. If no suppression occurs, ectopic ACTH production is the source. Confirm pituitary source with MRI. Consider CT of the chest and abdomen to look for malignancy causing ectopic ACTH production.
- Pheochromocytoma: Lesions of the adrenal or the organ of Zuckerkandl; contain PNMT and produce epinephrine. Ten percent of lesions are extra-adrenal, malignant, familial, or bilateral. Patients present with

episodic headaches, palpitations, diaphoresis, chest pain, anxiety, abdominal pain, panic attacks, and syncope. Workup includes serum and urinary metanephrines. Perform a CT or MRI to localize the lesion. On CT, lesion will be large, round, vascular and have > 10 HU; MRI shows a **T2-bright lesion**. Metaiodobenzylguanidine (**MIBG**) is selectively taken up by chromaffin tissue and can be used to further localize the lesion. Lesions should be resected. Start **phenoxybenzamine** preoperatively. When α-blocked (to prevent unopposed vasoconstriction), administer β-blockers.

- **Adrenocortical carcinoma:** Rare, aggressive lesion that is usually large and locally invasive at time of presentation. About 60% are functional. Complete resection is curative. With complete resection, 5-year survival is about 40%; without complete resection, survival is < 1 year. **IVC and renal vein thrombus are considered regional involvement and are not contraindications to surgery.**

CT characteristics of adrenal tumors–

- *Adenoma: Small, homogeneous, < 10 HU, no necrosis, slow-growing, solitary, rapid washout of contrast*
- *Adrenocortical carcinoma: Large, irregular, heterogeneous, > 10 HU, vascular, rapid growth, necrosis, unilateral, < 50% washout at 10 minutes*
- *Pheochromocytoma: Large, round, vascular, slow-growing, > 10 HU, < 50% washout at 10 minutes*
- *Metastasis: Bilateral, irregular, vascular, < 50% washout at 10 minutes*

Congenital Adrenal Hyperplasia

Most commonly caused by a deficiency or lack of **21-hydroxylase**, resulting in ↓ aldosterone and ↓ cortisol. Patients have **virilization with hypotension, ↓ Na^+, ↑ K^+, ↑ 17α-progesterone, ↑ androstenedione,** and **↑ testosterone**. 11β-hydroxylase deficiency is also associated with **virilization but not with hypotension and salt-wasting.**

Adrenal Insufficiency

Found in up to 30% of critically ill patients. Primary adrenal insufficiency results from failure of the gland due to stress, atrophy, **hemorrhage (ie, Waterhouse–Friedrichsen syndrome)**, infection, or infarct. Secondary adrenal insufficiency results from suppression of the hypothalamic-pituitary-adrenal axis, most commonly caused by **exogenous steroid administration**. Presentation varies from subtle (eg, weight loss, weakness, hyperpigmentation, abdominal pain, constipation, orthostatic hypotension) to severe (eg, persistent hypotension, tachycardia). Labs reveal **↓ Na^+, ↑ K^+, nonanion gap metabolic acidosis,** and **↓ random cortisol level.** If ↓ random cortisol level, perform a cortisol stimulation test. Nonresponders have adrenal insufficiency. Secure airway and treat with fluid resuscitation, electrolyte and glucose correction, and IV hydrocortisone (glucocorticoid) and fludrocortisone (mineralocorticoid) administration.

*Suspect metastasis in patients with **bilateral** adrenal masses.*

Prolactinoma

Most common pituitary adenoma. Differentiated into microadenomas (< 1 cm) or macroadenomas (> 1 cm). Tumors secrete prolactin and cause amenorrhea, infertility, galactorrhea, headache, and **bitemporal hemianopsia** (ie, optic chiasm compression). Rule out other causes of hyperprolactinemia: pregnancy, breastfeeding, estrogen use, dopamine antagonists (eg, haloperidol, metoclopramide), and other medical conditions (eg, chronic renal insufficiency, hypothyroidism, sarcoidosis). Confirm diagnosis with MRI. Medical therapy with dopamine agonists (eg, bromocriptine) is effective. Transsphenoidal resection is reserved for patients who cannot tolerate medical therapy or who fail medical therapy.

Multiple Endocrine Neoplasia Syndromes

Summarized in Table 12-6.

TABLE 12-6. MEN Syndromes

TYPE	MUTATION	FEATURES	TREATMENT
MEN-1 (Wermer syndrome)	Autosomal dominant mutation of *MENIN* (chromosome 11).	**Pituitary tumors** (prolactinoma), **hyperparathyroidism** (four gland hyperplasia), **pancreatic/neuroendocrine tumors** (most common—**gastrinoma**).	First—parathyroidectomy ($3^1/_2$ gland) to correct hypercalcemia. Second—resect additional tumors.
MEN-2A (Sipple syndrome)	Autosomal dominant mutation of *RET* (chromosome 10).	Hyperparathyroidism, **medullary thyroid cancer, pheochromocytoma.**	*RET* testing. Prophylactic thyroidectomy with node dissection by 5 years.
MEN-2B (Gorlin syndrome)	Autosomal dominant mutation of *RET* (chromosome 10).	**Medullary thyroid cancer, pheochromocytoma,** mucosal neuromas, marfanoid body habitus.	*RET* testing. Prophylactic thyroidectomy and node dissection in infancy.

▶ SAMPLE QUESTIONS

A 50-year-old female with kidney stones, diabetes insipidus, and mental status changes has a serum Ca^{2+} = 14 mg/dL and a painless, firm neck mass. What is the most likely diagnosis?	Parathyroid carcinoma.
A 30-year-old female undergoes a right thyroid lobectomy with isthmusectomy for a 2-cm thyroid nodule. One week later the pathology returns as follicular carcinoma. What do you do next?	Take her back to the operating room and perform a completion thyroidectomy.
A 40-year-old male has sporadic medullary thyroid cancer. What is the correct management?	Check for *RET* mutation and rule out pheochromocytoma. If -, perform total thyroidectomy with central node dissection.
A 60-year-old female with a history of Hashimoto's thyroiditis presents with a thyroid nodule. What is the most likely malignant diagnosis?	Papillary or follicular carcinomas are the most likely diagnoses for thyroid nodules in patients with Hashimoto's. However, do think about lymphoma.
A 50-year-old female with a family history of hypercalcemia presents with a mildly ↑ serum Ca^{2+}, ↓ urinary Ca^{2+}, and a PTH level that is at the upper limit of normal. What is the most likely cause of her hyperparathyroidism? How should she be treated if she is asymptomatic?	Familial hypocalciuric hypercalcemia. No treatment is indicated if she is asymptomatic.
A patient has bilateral adrenal masses on CT. What is the most likely diagnosis? What 1° lesions are likely to be the cause?	Nonfunctional adrenal adenomas are most common. Rule out metastatic 1° disease from breast, lung, renal, or melanoma.
A 35-year-old male has HTN, hypokalemia, and muscle cramps. What is the most likely diagnosis? Test to confirm this diagnosis?	Hyperaldosteronism (Conn's syndrome). Perform a serum aldosterone-to-renin ratio. If ↑ in the setting of ↑ aldosterone and ↓ renin, diagnosis is confirmed.
A 60-year-old male in the ICU has persistent hypotension in spite of vasoactive medications. Labs show hyperkalemia with a nonanion gap metabolic acidosis. What is the most likely diagnosis? Workup? Treatment?	Adrenal insufficiency. Confirm with random cortisol test (which will be low) and a cortisol stimulation test (to which he will not appropriately respond). Treat with IV hydrocortisone and IV fludrocortisone.

A 30-year-old male has episodic palpitations, chest tightness, anxiety, panic attacks, headaches, and diaphoresis. What mutation is associated with this lesion? What syndrome?	Pheochromocytomas are associated with *RET* mutations and MEN-2A and MEN-2B. Confirm with serum and/or urinary metanephrines. CT and/or MRI will demonstrate lesion. Treat with phenoxybenzamine (preoperatively) and adrenalectomy.

CHAPTER 13

Skin and Soft Tissue

Mark M. Melendez, MD, MBA
Reviewed by Marc J. Shapiro, MS, MD, FACS, FCCM

▶ BASIC SCIENCE

Anatomy of the Skin

Layers include (see Figure 13-1)

- Epidermis: Superficial cellular layer composed of **stratified squamous epithelium**. Sublayers (ie, horny, granular, spinous, basal) include cells that progressively differentiate as they migrate from deep to superficial levels.
- Basal membrane: Dermal-epidermal junction. Anchors dermis to epidermis.
- Dermis: Composed of papillary and deeper, reticular layers. In comparison to the papillary layer, reticular dermis has a thick layer of dense connective tissue, larger blood vessels, and nerve endings. Collagen (primarily **type I**) comprises 70% of this layer and provides **tensile strength.** Also contains dermal appendages and hair follicles (which house pluripotential cells that are critical in wound healing).

Specialized functions of dermal nerves–

Meissner's corpuscles: Light touch.

Pacinian corpuscles: Pressure.

Specialized cell types and appendages differ by skin level. Melanocytes (produce pigment), Langerhan's cells (function as immune cells), and Merkel cells (function is unclear) are found in the epidermis. Hair follicles, sebaceous glands, apocrine glands, and specialized nerve cells (ie, Meissner's and Pacinian corpuscles) are found in the dermis.

Skin and Soft Tissue Syndromes

Multiple skin and soft tissue syndromes are associated with characteristic signs and genetic mutations (see Table 13-1).

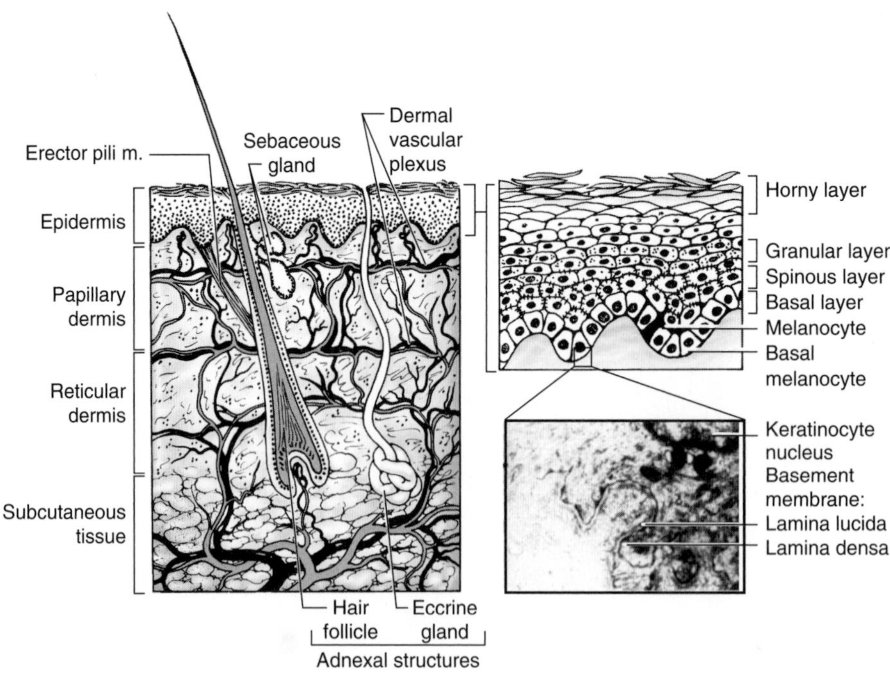

FIGURE 13-1. Anatomy of the skin.

(Reproduced, with permission, from Brunicardi FC, et al. *Schwartz's Principles of Surgery*, 8th ed. New York: McGraw-Hill, 2005:430.)

TABLE 13-1. Presentations and Mutations of Skin and Soft Tissue Syndromes

SYNDROME	CHARACTERISTIC SIGNS/SYMPTOMS	GENETIC MUTATIONS
Neurofibromatosis, type I (NF1; von Recklinghausen's disease)	Hyperpigmented macules (**café au lait spots**), **neurofibromas**, iris hamartomas (**Lisch nodules**), optic gliomas, **freckling** of non–sun exposed areas (eg, axilla). ↑ Risk of astrocytomas, **pheochromocytomas,** and neurofibrosarcomas.	*NF1* gene (chromosome 17). **Autosomal dominant**. Involved in *Ras* pathway. More common than *NF2*.
Neurofibromatosis, type II (NF2)	**Bilateral vestibular (CN VIII) schwannomas**, intracranial or intraspinal tumors (eg, gliomas, meningioma).	*NF2* gene (chromosome 22). **Autosomal dominant**. Involved in cytoskeleton.
Tuberous sclerosis	**Adenoma sebaceum**, **shagreen patches, ash leaf macules**, hamartomas (of brain, lung, kidney), epilepsy, mental retardation.	*TSC1* and *TSC2* genes (chromosomes 9 and 16, respectively). **Autosomal dominant** or sporadic. Involved in GTPase activity.
Gardner's syndrome	**Gastrointestinal (GI) polyps** (ampullary, small intestine [SI], large intestine [LI]), **desmoid tumors**, sebaceous cysts, osteomas. Variant of **familial adenomatous polyposis (FAP)**.	*Adenomatous polyposis coli (APC)* gene (chromosome 5). **Autosomal dominant.** Involved in cell adhesion, interaction, cytoskeleton.
Familial atypical multiple mole melanoma syndrome (FAMMM)	Inclusion criteria: 1. ≤ 1 first- or second-degree relative(s) with melanoma; 2. multiple atypical moles; and 3. moles with specific microscopic features. Associated with ↑ risk of pancreatic cancer.	*CDKN2A (p16)* and *CDK4* genes (chromosomes 9 and 12, respectively). **Autosomal dominant**. Involved in cell-cycle progression through G1-S transition.

Key genetic mutations in skin and soft tissue syndromes–

NF1*: Chromosome 17*

NF2*: Chromosome 22*

APC *(Gardner's syndrome, FAP): Chromosome 5.*

TSC1, TSC2 *(Tuberous sclerosis): Chromosomes 9 and 16.*

CDKN2A *and* CDK4 *(FAMMM): Chromosomes 9 and 12.*

A 45-year-old woman presents to your office with a painful 5 mm subungual, bluish nodule on her right index finger. Her symptoms are exacerbated with cold weather and cold water. What is the most likely diagnosis? Treatment? Lesion is likely a glomus tumor. Excise lesion. Use a lateral approach if the lesion is present at a nail margin.

▶ CLINICAL SCIENCE

Glomus Tumor

Benign digital tumors composed of blood vessels and nerves arising from the dermal glomus body, which normally **regulates distal digital perfusion**. Most common location is the **subungual area**. Often affects women aged 30–50 years. Presents as a painful, **subungual, bluish nodule**; symptoms are

exacerbated by cold exposure. Exam reveals a blanching blue to purple nodule, usually < 1 cm. May be mistaken for hemangioma or venous malformation. Excise via nail bed or via a lateral approach if at the nail margin.

Actinic and Seborrheic Keratoses

Demographics/Risk Factors

Actinic keratoses (AK) are commonly found in fair-skinned Caucasian males with sun exposure. Lesions are considered **premalignant** and can lead to **squamous cell carcinoma** (SCC). Seborrheic keratoses (SK) are **benign** and appear with an equal prevalence in males and females. May ↑ in size with pregnancy, hormone therapy, or malignancy but are unrelated to sun exposure.

Signs/Symptoms

Differentiating signs and symptoms are summarized in Table 13-2.

Diagnosis

Clinical diagnosis based on lesion appearance.

Treatment

Excise lesion or apply topical 5-fluorouracil (5-FU) ointment to AKs. SKs rarely require intervention.

Hemangioma

Most common benign head and neck tumor in adults. Frequently demonstrate accelerated growth during the first 2 years of age but **usually involute** and do not require therapy. Approximately 50% spontaneously resolve by 5 years of age; 70% resolve by 7 years of age. Types include capillary hemangioma (typically involute), cavernous hemangioma (may not involute), and port wine stain (does not involute). Typically asymptomatic but can cause a cosmetic defect. Nonsurgical treatments include intralesional steroid injections, steroids, and IFNα-2a; invasive therapies involve surgical excision, laser or cryotherapy, and embolization. Early therapy or surgical excision should be considered for patients with visual or airway impairment, bleeding or ulceration, infection, **Kasabach-Merritt syndrome** (ie, consumptive coagulopathy due to

TABLE 13-2. Signs and Symptoms of Keratoses

Actinic Keratosis	Seborrheic Keratosis
▪ ↑ With sun exposure	▪ ↑ With pregnancy, hormone therapy, malignancy
▪ Tender	▪ Not affected by sun exposure
▪ Face, backs of hands, forearms (sun-exposed regions)	▪ Nontender, pruritic
	▪ Chest, back, abdomen
▪ Elevated, scaly, warty	▪ Elevated, scaly, waxy/oily plaques
▪ Red-yellow, brown, or black lesions	▪ Yellowish, brown, or brownish-black **"stuck-on"** macules
▪ **Hyperkeratotic scale**	

a hemangioma, resulting in thrombocytopenia and possibly, disseminated intravascular coagulation [DIC]), congestive heart failure, or persistence into adolescence (as rate of spontaneous involution ↓).

Pyoderma Gangrenosum

Inflammatory nodule associated with underlying systemic disease (eg, **ulcerative colitis**, regional ileitis, rheumatoid arthritis, dysproteinemia, leukemia, lymphoma). Most commonly presents with rapidly enlarging, **erythematous, necrotic ulcers with purple edematous borders** involving the **lower extremities**. Generally a clinical diagnosis. Treatment includes identification and treatment of underlying systemic disease. For skin lesions, treat with systemic **steroids** and **cyclosporine**; skin grafts are sometimes needed. For underlying bowel disease, some patients respond to **resection of the affected bowel**.

Think pyoderma gangrenosum if—
Necrotic ulcer with violet border and surrounding erythematous halo

Benign Nevus

Demographics

Benign overgrowth of melanocytes. May be **congenital or acquired**. Congenital nevi develop in approximately 1% of children; acquired nevi appear after the first few months of life. Acquired nevi can include junctional, compound, intradermal, Spitz, or blue types.

Signs/Symptoms

Congenital lesions may be flat, elevated, verrucous, or nodular with a brown, black, or blue appearance. **Junctional nevi** are typically flat, nonpalpable, brown lesions, presenting on the palms and soles of infants. **Compound nevi** are elevated, dome-shaped, pigmented lesions. **Intradermal** nevi are elevated, skin-colored lesions that may contain hair. **Spitz nevi** are solitary brown or pink, dome-shaped nodules on the face or upper extremities. **Blue nevi** are blue to black dome-shaped nodules.

Diagnosis

Usually a clinical diagnosis that may be confirmed with skin biopsy. Junctional nevi have a characteristic melanocyte proliferation at the epidermal-dermal junction. Intradermal and blue nevi have melanocyte proliferation only in the dermis. Compound nevi demonstrate melanocyte proliferation both in the dermis and the epidermal-dermal junction. Spitz nevi demonstrate a large number of mitoses.

Treatment

Excise lesions to treat and confirm the absence of malignancy.

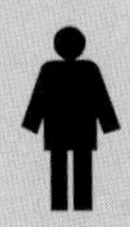

A 65-year-old woman presents with a forehead lesion. Exam is notable for an 8-mm lesion with a rolled border and underlying telangiectasias. What is the next step in the management of this patient? Surgical excision with 4-mm margins for a likely basal cell carcinoma (BCC).

Basal Cell Carcinoma

Demographics/Risk Factors

Most common cancer. Risk factors include **exposure to UV radiation**; p53 mutations are common. Presents most commonly in fair-skinned men (eg, Celtic ancestry) on sun-exposed areas (eg, face). Can occur at any age but typically after the fifth decade.

Signs/Symptoms

Typically presents as a small, slow-growing, translucent or shiny ("**pearly**"), elevated nodule. Central ulceration with **rolled pearly edges**, scab, or **telangiectasias** may be present.

Diagnosis

Shave or punch biopsy confirms malignancy arising from the basal layer of epidermis.

Treatment

Electrodissection and curettage for small lesions < 2 mm. Excision (via Moh's micrographic surgery) for larger lesions. For patients unable or unwilling to undergo surgery, consider radiation, topical 5-FU, imiquimod, or intralesional interferon.

Staging/Outcome

The tumor, node status, metastasis (TNM) categories include

- T: T1 (≥ 2 cm in greatest dimension), T2 (> 2 cm and ≥ 5 cm in greatest dimension), T3 (> 5 cm in greatest dimension), T4 (invasion into extradermal structures)
- N: N0 (- regional lymph nodes), N1 (+ regional lymph nodes)
- M: M0 (metastatic disease absent), M1 (metastatic disease present).

Staging includes

- Stage I: T1N0M0
- Stage II: T2-3N0M0
- Stage III: T4N0M0 *or* Any T, N1M0
- Stage IV: Any T, any N, M1

Though recurrences occur, up to 95% of cases are cured with treatment. Metastases are rare.

Squamous Cell Carcinoma

Demographics/Risk Factors

Second most common cancer in fair-skinned populations. Most commonly occurs in sun-exposed areas (eg, lower lip, ears, backs of hands). Risk factors include UV or ionizing radiation exposure, presence of AK, hydrocarbon exposure, tobacco use, chronic infection (eg, human papilloma virus infection), immunosuppression, burns (**Marjolin's ulcer**), and chronic, nonhealing wounds.

SIGNS/SYMPTOMS

Erythematous plaque or nodule that may be associated with **central ulceration** or indistinct margins. Advanced disease may be associated with **pain, bleeding, or pruritus**.

DIAGNOSIS

Usually a clinical diagnosis that can be confirmed with biopsy (ie, shave, punch, incisional, excisional). Pathology will show atypical keratinocytes invading into the dermis with associated **keratin pearls**. **Bowen's disease** is squamous cell carcinoma in situ.

TREATMENT

Excise lesions with **1 cm margins**. Regional lymph node excision is indicated for clinically palpable nodes.

STAGING/OUTCOME

Staging is similar to BCC. As SCC has a greater propensity to metastasize, prognosis is worse than BCC: 3-year survival for all-comers is ~85% and is dramatically ↓ if metastatic disease is present.

Melanoma

DEMOGRAPHICS/RISK FACTORS

Diagnosed in about 160,000 patients annually in the United States; **leading cause of skin cancer-related deaths**. Risk factors include UV exposure, family history (eg, FAMMM), or congenital nevi. Most commonly affects fair skinned males, particularly those who have a significant history of sun exposure during their teenage years.

TYPES

Table 13-3 summarizes the four histologic types of melanoma.

TABLE 13-3. Types of Melanoma

Type	Location	Features
Lentigo maligna	Sun-exposed areas (eg, neck, face, back of hands).	Patients are typically older. **Best prognosis.**
Superficial spreading	Anywhere, but palms and soles are spared.	**Most common**. Exhibits primarily radial growth.
Acral lentiginous	Palms, soles, subungual.	**Least common**. More commonly affects dark-skinned populations.
Nodular	Palms, soles, subungual.	**Most aggressive** type. **Lacks radial growth.**

> **ABCDE**s of melanoma:
> **A**symmetry
> **B**orders (irregular, ill-defined)
> **C**olor (pigmented)
> **D**iameter (> 6 mm)
> **E**volution of lesion

SIGNS/SYMPTOMS

Lesions are typically pigmented, asymmetric, and have irregular borders. Lesions > 6 mm that have recently changed or that are **associated with pruritis (suggesting neural invasion)** are particularly concerning.

DIAGNOSIS

Excisional biopsy confirms diagnosis. Orient incision so that it can be incorporated into subsequent wide local excision (WLE), if necessary.

TREATMENT

WLE is standard of care; margins are based on thickness:

- < 1 cm for lesion < 1 mm
- 1–2 cm for lesions 1–2 mm
- 2 cm for lesions 2–4 mm
- 2–3 cm for lesions > 4 mm.

Perform **sentinel lymph node biopsy** (SLNBx) for melanomas > 1 mm without clinically + nodes or for lesions > 0.75 mm with high-risk signs (ie, ulceration). Lymph node dissection is indicated for clinically + nodes. Though chemotherapy has not been shown to be particularly effective, **IFNα-2b** improves disease–free and overall survival in patients with stage IIB or III disease.

STAGING/OUTCOME

Staging is based on **tumor thickness** (see Figure 13-2). The tumor, node status, metastasis (TNM) categories include:

- T: T1 (0.1-1.0 mm thick), T2 (1.01-2.0 mm thick), T3 (2.01-4.0 thick), T4

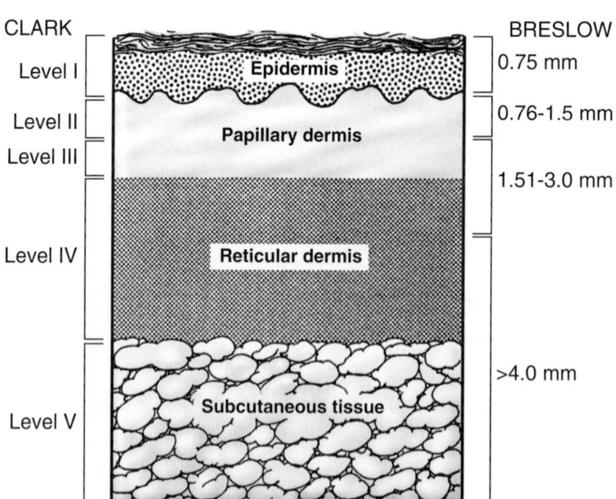

FIGURE 13-2. Melanoma staging.

(Reproduced, with permission, from Brunicardi FC, et al. *Schwartz's Principles of Surgery*, 8th ed. New York: McGraw-Hill, 2005:442.)

(> 4.0 mm thick; T status is further designated as "a" or "b" for without or with ulceration, respectively)

- N: N0 (- regional lymph nodes), N1 (1 + lymph node), N2 (2-3 + lymph nodes *or* in-transit lesion with - lymph nodes), N3 (≥ 4 + regional lymph nodes, matted nodes, *or* in-transit lesions with + lymph nodes)
- M: M0 (metastatic disease absent), M1 (metastatic disease present)

Staging includes

- Stage I: T1N0M0 *or* T2aN0M0
- Stage II: T2bN0M0 *or* T3N0M0 *or* T4N0M0
- Stage III: Any T, N3, M0 *or* Any T, N1, M0 *or* Any T, N2, M0
- Stage IV: Any T, any N, M1

Five-year survival varies from 90% with stage I disease to 25% with stage IV disease.

Soft Tissue Neoplasms

Specific neoplasms are summarized in Table 13-4.

Merkel Cell Carcinoma

Neuroendocrine lesion of the dermis, usually affecting elderly patients. May have **synchronous or metachronous SCC** (25% of cases). Presents as a red to purple painless nodule of the head or neck. Confirm diagnosis with + immunohistochemical staining for **neuron specific enolase (NSE)** and **neurofilament protein**. Treatment includes **WLE with 3-cm margins**; perform lymph node dissection for palpable lymph nodes. Five-year survival is 30–40%; rate of lymph node metastases is high.

Desmoid Tumor

Benign tumor that arises from muscular fascial planes. Presents during the third to fourth decade of life. Etiology is not clear, but these tumors are associated with **Gardner's syndrome**, prior surgery, and pregnancy. May be asymptomatic or present with signs and symptoms related to compression or invasion of adjacent structures (eg, pain, obstruction). Confirm diagnosis with biopsy, which shows spindle cells surrounded by collagen. Immunohistochemical stains are + for smooth muscle actin, vimentin, and desmin. Have a high level of suspicion for this diagnosis in patients with FAP or Gardner's syndrome. Large size and extensive involvement of adjacent structures makes management difficult. If possible, perform **WLE with 2- to 4-cm margins**.

Rectus Sheath Hematoma

Injury to the **superior or inferior epigastric vessels** or to collaterals of the rectus sheath. May be related to ↑ pressure on or shearing force to the rectus sheath, **particularly in the setting of anticoagulation**. May present as an acutely tender mass that is more evident with tensing of the rectus muscles (**Fothergill's sign**). Diagnosis is clinical but can be confirmed with CT. Treat with **pressure to the hematoma** and **serial hematocrit (HCT)** evaluations. Consider emergent operative intervention or embolization for an enlarging hematoma, massive hemorrhage, or hemodynamic instability.

TABLE 13-4. Soft Tissue Neoplasms

Type	Demographics	Signs/Symptoms	Diagnosis	Treatment
Osteosarcoma	**Most common bone malignancy**. Affects **young adults** but can occur in patients > 40 years. Risk factors include history of radiation, Paget's disease, chemotherapy. Affects **metaphyseal regions of long bones**.	Bone pain with palpable mass. May present with **lung metastases.**	Extremity radiographs show **Codman's triangle** with cortical destruction (**sunburst sign**).	Neoadjuvant chemotherapy, WLE with 4 cm margins. If high-grade, limb salvage reconstruction or amputation.
Ewing's sarcoma	Primitive neuroectodermal tumor. Most commonly affects children **aged 5–15 years**. Affects pelvis, femur, humerus (diaphysis). **Due to chromosome 11–22 translocation.**	Malaise, fever, pain, edema.	Extremity radiographs show **onion skinning**.	Chemotherapy, radiation therapy, radical resection.
Rhabdomy-osarcoma	**Most common pediatric sarcoma**, affecting children 2–5 and 15–19 years. Arises as mesenchyme differentiates into skeletal muscle.	Palpable mass	Incisional biopsy, CT, and MRI to determine 1° site, extent, and histologic type.	Chemotherapy, WLE.
Kaposi's sarcoma	Associated with acquired immunodeficiency syndrome (AIDS), immunosuppression, chemotherapy, or human herpes virus-8. **Most common AIDS-related malignancy.**	**Red to purple nodule** on skin or mucosa.	Biopsy	Treat AIDS. Chemotherapy, radiation. Resection is reserved for lesions that interfere with vital functions.

▶ SAMPLE QUESTIONS

What gene is associated with Gardner's syndrome?	*APC* gene on chromosome 5. Gardner's syndrome is a variant of FAP.
A 35-year-old woman presents with a painful, subungual, bluish nodule of the index finger. Symptoms are exacerbated with cold weather and cold H_2O. How should she be managed?	Patient has a glomus tumor. Excise lesion via nail bed or via a lateral approach, if lesion is present on the nail margin.
A 69-year-old male has a biopsy consistent with an AK. What cancer is associated with AKs?	SCC.
A 72-year-old man presents with a brownish-black, "stuck-on" macule on his back. What is the most likely diagnosis?	SK.
A 1-year-old boy has a facial hemangioma. What is the correct management at this age?	Observation, as it will likely involute and not require further therapy.
A 38-year-old woman with UC has a necrotic ulcer with violaceous borders. What is the most likely diagnosis?	Pyoderma gangrenosum.
What is the treatment for a 3-mm BCC of the forehead?	Excision with 4-mm margins.
A 60-year-old male sustained a third-degree burn to his right lower extremity 25 years ago. He now presents with a chronic lesion at the site of the burn scar. What do you suspect?	SCC (Marjolin's ulcer).
What are the indications for SLNBx in the setting of melanoma?	SLNBx is indicated for melanomas > 1.0 mm thick without palpable lymph nodes or for high-risk lesions > 0.75 mm.
A 44-year-old male presents with pain and a palpable mass of the right lower extremity. Radiographs show a Codman's triangle. What is the next step in management?	This patient likely has osteosarcoma. Neoadjuvant chemotherapy followed by wide local resection is indicated.

A 82-year-old woman presents with a purple nodule of the right shoulder that stains + for NSE and neurofilament protein. What is the management of this condition?	WLE with a 3-cm margins for Merkel cell carcinoma. If lymph nodes are palpable, perform lymph node dissection.
An 80-year-old man who is anticoagulated for AF has the sudden onset of an expanding abdominal wall mass. What is the next step in management?	Apply pressure to the rectus sheath hematoma. Follow serial HCTs and check coagulation studies.

CHAPTER 14

Plastic and Reconstructive Surgery

Miguel A. Medina III, MD
Reviewed by William Gerald Austen, Jr, MD

▶ BASIC SCIENCE

Wound Healing

NORMAL WOUND HEALING

Phases of wound healing (see Figure 14-1) include

- **Inflammation**: Occurs from the time of injury until 3–4 days after injury. Includes **hemostasis** and **inflammation-sterilization** phases.
    - Hemostasis: Platelet aggregation and release of vasoconstrictive factors (eg, thromboxane, Factor V) and proinflammatory cytokines (eg, platelet-derived growth factor [PDGF], transforming growth factor [TGFβ], insulin-like growth factor [IGF-1], fibrinogen) → polymorphonuclear cell (PMN) recruitment.

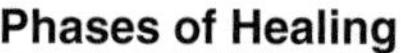

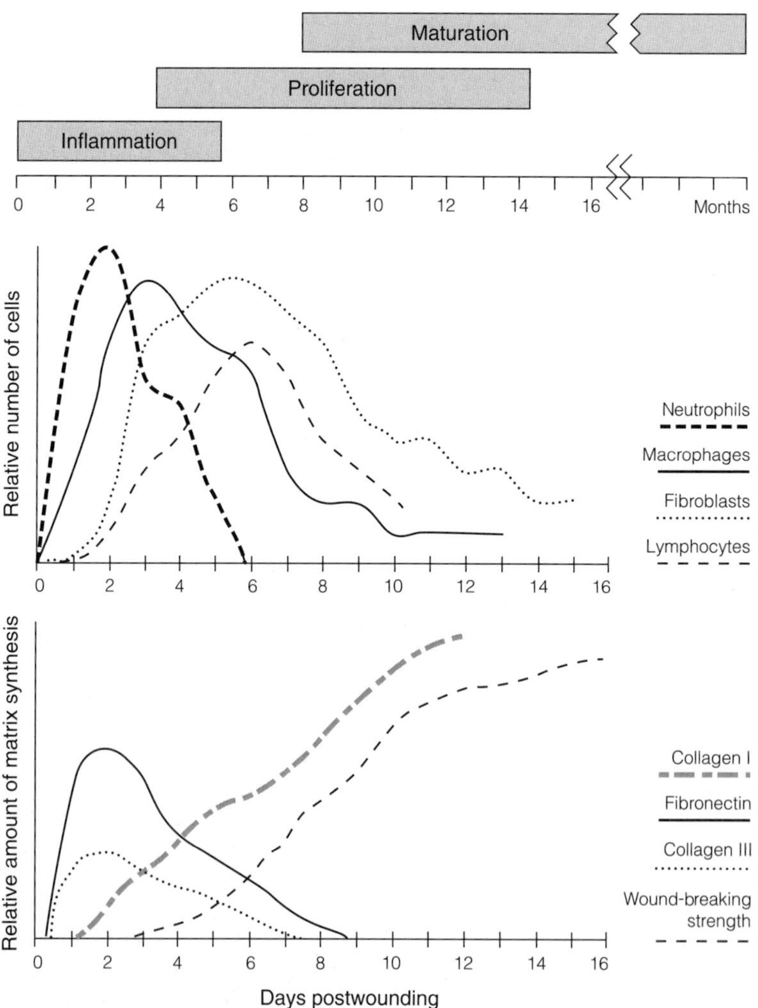

FIGURE 14-1. Phases of wound healing.

(Reproduced, with permission, from Brunicardi FC, et al. *Schwartz's Principles of Surgery*, 8th ed. New York: McGraw-Hill, 2005:225.)

- Inflammation-sterilization: PMNs induce vasodilation and recruitment of **macrophages**, lymphocytes, and fibroblasts. Superoxide and collagenase sterilize and degrade devitalized tissue.
- **Proliferation**: Begins 3–7 days after injury. Initial collagen matrix is laid down during this phase. Macrophages infiltrate and release cytokines → ↑ vascular permeability and angiogenesis. Lymphocyte activation → fibroblast response and epithelial cell migration.
  - Fibroplasia: Fibroblasts activated by macrophages (via epidermal growth factor [EGF], IGF-1) and platelets (via **PDGF**) lay down a disorganized collagen matrix (composed of collagen types I, II, and III).
  - Granulation: Collagen network provides scaffolding for vascular framework.
  - Epithelialization: Epidermal cells are activated and migrate over the granulating field to close the defect. The initial framework comprises the developing basement membrane.
- **Remodeling and maturation**: Following proliferation, this phase lasts 1 year after injury. Involves collagen remodeling and crosslinking → ↑ wound strength and ↓ vascularity. **Maximum wound strength is achieved by 1 year**. Complications can include:
  - Scarring: Scars are dense collagen matrixes that lack dermal appendages, such as hair follicles, or sweat glands. Tensile strength reaches **70–80% of original tissue**.
  - Contracture: By the sixth day, myofibroblasts contract and persist for 4–6 weeks in the wound. Final collagen crosslinking contributes to final scar contracture.

A number of cytokines are involved in wound healing process (see Table 14-1).

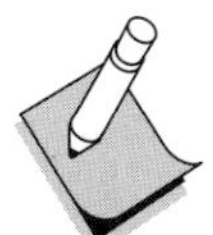

PDGF is the major chemoattractant for fibroblasts during the proliferation phase of wound healing.

Wounds reach 80% of overall healed strength by 30 days.

TABLE 14-1. Cytokines Involved in Wound Healing

Cytokine	Source	Target Cells	Function
IFNγ	Macrophages, T cells.	Fibroblasts, macrophages.	Activates macrophages, PMNs, fibroblasts. Induces collagenase activity.
IGF-1	Macrophages, fibroblasts.	Fibroblasts, keratinocytes, endothelial cells.	Triggers mitosis of fibroblasts and keratinocytes. Induces collagen production, ↑ vascular permeability.
IL1α, IL1β	PMNs, macrophages.	Fibroblasts, keratinocytes.	Recruits fibroblasts and keratinocytes. Induces collagen synthesis.
IL2	T cells.	Fibroblasts.	Recruits and triggers mitosis in fibroblasts.
PDGF	Macrophages, platelets, endothelial cells.	PMNs, macrophages, fibroblasts, endothelial cells.	Recruits PMNs, macrophages, and fibroblasts. Stimulates angiogenesis, ↑ vascular permeability.
TGFβ	Macrophages, platelets, fibroblasts.	Fibroblasts, keratinocytes, endothelial cells	Induces mitosis in fibroblasts and keratinocytes. Promotes angiogenesis, matrix production.
TNFα	PMNs.	Macrophages, fibroblasts.	Activates immune cells. Recruits macrophages. Induces cytotoxicity.
VEGF	Macrophages, keratinocytes.	Keratinocytes, endothelial cells.	Stimulates angiogenesis. Induces ↑ vascular endothelial permeability.

ABNORMAL WOUND HEALING

If major perturbations occur, impaired healing and the development of chronic wounds can occur. A robust blood supply is required for wound healing. Factors that impair healing are described in Table 14-2.

Ionizing radiation can cause severe wounds that are difficult to heal. **Rapidly dividing cell types (ie, fibroblasts, keratinocytes, basal epithelial cells) are the most susceptible to radiation injury.** Endothelial cell damage creates a hypoxic wound bed and severe inhibition of angiogenesis. Changes occur within 4-6 months of exposure, but fibrosis and hypovascularity are progressive. Ulceration may occur even decades after original injury. **If a patient**

PLASTIC AND RECONSTRUCTIVE SURGERY

TABLE 14-2. Local and Systemic Factors Inhibiting Wound Healing

FACTORS	MECHANISM
Local	
Ischemia	Oxygenases require a minimum tissue O_2 tension of ~20 mm Hg to function properly. Hyperbaric chambers and inhaled O_2 can ↑ levels > 100 mm Hg, potentially ↑ oxygenase activity. O_2 is also necessary for collagen crosslinking.
Infection	Chronic inflammation or high tissue bacterial burden causes an overabundance of cytotoxic oxidases, proteinases, and apoptosis. Can also lead to squamous neoplasms. **Bacterial load > 10^5 bacteria/g of tissue** or the presence of β-hemolytic *Streptococcus* prevents wound healing.
Radiation	Cytotoxic. Potent inhibitor of angiogenesis → poorly vascularized fibrotic wounds and inhibited fibroblast activity.
Previous trauma or scar	Scar tissue is cellularly depleted and poorly vascularized → ↑ susceptibility with repeat injury.
Venous insufficiency	Results in congested wounds with heavy drainage and poor immune cell/fibroblast wound localization. Can lead to hypoxic tissue.
Foreign bodies	Act as nidus for bacteria and cause fibrotic reactions in adjacent tissue → chronic inflammatory state.
Systemic	
Malnutrition	Catabolic protein state impairs wound healing. Vitamin C is involved in collagen synthesis (ie, crosslinking glycine residues from differing collagen bundles). Deficiency results in **scurvy**. Vitamin A (particularly retinol) is involved in bone growth and vision. Deficiency impairs monocyte activation, cell localization, and cell adhesion, resulting in **night blindness, xerophthalmia,** and **keratomalacia**.
Malignancy	Necrotic tumors can ulcerate and cause chronic wounds, requiring radical resection.
Diabetes mellitus (DM)	Impairs healing due to hypoxia, neuropathy, glycosylated protein malfunction, and impaired immune cell localization.
Corticosteroid use	Promotes a catabolic state and inhibits immune cell localization (ie, PMNs are suppressed). **Wound healing effects can be mitigated with topical vitamin A administration.**
Chemotherapy	↓ Rapidly dividing cell populations that would normally sterilize and repopulate wound. Antiangiogenesis therapy (eg, bevacizumab) is particularly detrimental.
Aging	Associated with a relative upregulation of matrix metalloproteinase (MMP)-2 and MMP-9 → ↓ collagen synthesis.

TABLE 14-3. Types of Collagen

TYPES	LOCATION	RELATED DISEASES	SPECIAL NOTES
Type I	Skin, bones, tendons.	Ehlers-Danlos syndrome, osteogenesis imperfecta, scurvy.	1° form in **healed wound.**
Type II	Cartilage.	Chondrodysplasias.	
Type III	Blood vessels, skin, granulation tissue.	Ehlers-Danlos syndrome.	1° form in **early phases of wound healing.**
Type IV	Basement membrane, lens of eye.	Alport's syndrome.	

presents with radiation-induced ulceration, confirm that ulceration is not a tumor recurrence. Complete excision of the radiated bed with regional flap or free flap reconstruction is necessary for closure of complex wounds and revascularization of wound bed. If a pedicled flap is used, donor vessel from nonirradiated tissue bed is preferred to minimize risk of flap necrosis.

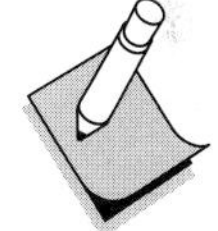

*Wounds with > $\mathbf{10^5}$ **bacteria/g** of tissue will not close and cannot support a skin graft.*

Collagen

Critical for wound healing. Types vary by location (see Table 14-3). Requires **vitamin C** for synthesis of repeating triplets of glycine-X-proline or glycine-X-lysine.

Skin Closure Techniques

Primary closure involves tissue re-approximation at time of injury. **Secondary closure** occurs when tissues are not initially closed (or are initially too extensive to close) and instead close via tissue proliferation at skin edges. **Tertiary (delayed 1°) closure** occurs when a wound is purposely left open or has remained open for > 6–8 hours (> 12-24 hours for highly vascular wounds such as the face, neck, and scalp) and is reapproximated at a later time.

Principal suture techniques include

- Simple interrupted: **Basic gold standard closure.** Enter perpendicular to the skin and follow the natural curve of the needle, creating a trapezoid loop with skin edge eversion. Staples are an alternative to simple interrupted closure.
- Vertical mattress: Used to ↑ skin eversion and to direct skin tension away from the wound edge and toward the distal suture line.
- Horizontal mattress: Has improved tissue eversion and better hemostatic properties. Most useful for thick skin (eg, hands, feet).
- Subcuticular running: Superficial closure of dermal-epidermal junction that minimizes external scars created by external sutures. **Not a load-bearing closure** and should be combined with external strips, adhesives, or deeper subdermal closure to reinforce.

Suture removal times–

Face: 3–5 days

Neck/scalp: 5–7 days

Trunk: 10–14 days

Extremities: 10–14 days

▶ CLINICAL SCIENCE

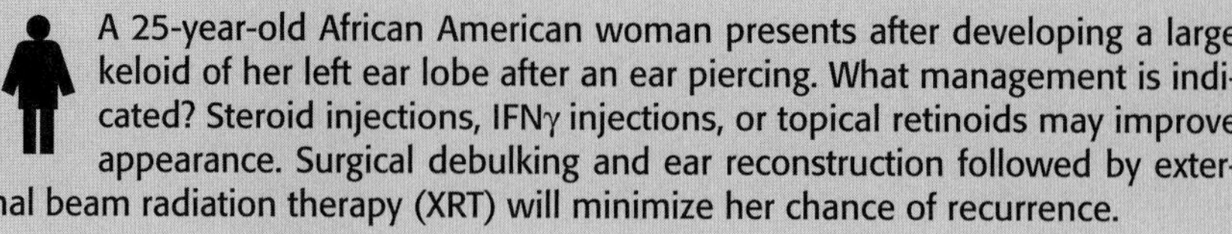

A 25-year-old African American woman presents after developing a large keloid of her left ear lobe after an ear piercing. What management is indicated? Steroid injections, IFNγ injections, or topical retinoids may improve appearance. Surgical debulking and ear reconstruction followed by external beam radiation therapy (XRT) will minimize her chance of recurrence.

Keloids and Hypertrophic Scars

KELOIDS

45-100% of keloids recur following surgical excision alone.

Locally aggressive scar in which **original scar tissue extends beyond the borders of the original wound. Collagen is inappropriately deposited** in adjacent tissue, possibly caused by dysregulation of collagen degradation and deposition (ie, fibroblast collagen synthesis is 20-fold normal). Found most frequently in genetically predisposed populations (eg, African Americans, Asians, Hispanics). Typically develop within 3 months of tissue injury. **Prevention** of keloid formation (ie, minimizing nonessential incisions on patients prone to keloids, performing tension-free repairs) is key. Keloids typically recur following excision (45–100% of cases). Nonsurgical treatment modalities include steroid injection, IFNγ injection, topical retinoids, silicone application, and pressure dressings. Surgical debulking followed by low-dose XRT (ie, fibroblast destruction) may be used in severe cases.

HYPERTROPHIC SCARS

Results from dysregulated collagen deposition that is **restricted to the original wound borders**. In contrast to keloids, hypertrophic scars have ↓ genetic predisposition and are related to chronic inflammation in the wound. Typically occur within 4 weeks of injury. Treatment is similar to keloids, though **hypertrophic scars have an improved response to surgical resection.**

Pressure Ulcers

Result from pressure necrosis of skin and underlying soft tissue. Will develop when external forces on the skin exceed capillary bed pressure for a period of time. In debilitated or immobilized patients, ulcers can occur within 2 hours. Most susceptible areas of a supine patient include the occiput, sacrum, and heels. Wounds are clinically staged stage I–IV (see Table 14-4).

As many as 10% of inpatients will develop pressure sores. Incidence ↑ to 20–30% in patients with spinal cord injuries.

Eliminate pressure source with airbed and frequent turns. Optimize nutrition. Control infection and reduce necrotic burden with debridement (eg, sharp, enzymatic, antimicrobial dressings). Culture wounds and initiate appropriate antibiotic therapy to maximize the chance of healing. Stage I and II lesions may heal secondarily with wound care. Stage III–IV lesions are amenable to vacuum-assisted closure (VAC) therapy (helps stimulate granulation and ↓ wound size) and if necessary, surgical closure (eg, musculocutaneous flap provides a robust blood supply and soft tissue padding over prominences).

TABLE 14-4. Pressure Ulcer Staging

Stage	Classification
I	Intact epidermis with nonblanching **erythema**. Typically heralds ulceration if pressure is not relieved.
II	Partial thickness epidermal-to-superficial dermal ulceration or blistering.
III	Full thickness loss of epidermis and dermis with necrosis or ulceration extending into subcutaneous tissue. Underlying fascia is not violated. Usually presents as a deep crater that is frequently superinfected.
IV	Full thickness skin loss with associated fascial loss, extensive soft tissue necrosis, and extension into underlying deep tissues. Exposed muscle or bone is evident on exam. Usually superinfected.

Wound Management

Depending on severity and complexity of wounds, wound management can include increasingly complex procedures: 1° closure, 2° closure, split thickness skin grafts (STSGs), full thickness skin grafts (FTSGs), random flaps, tissue expanders, pedicled flaps, or free tissue transfer.

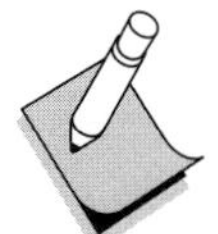

Basic premise of plastic and reconstructive surgery– *"Restoration of form and function"*

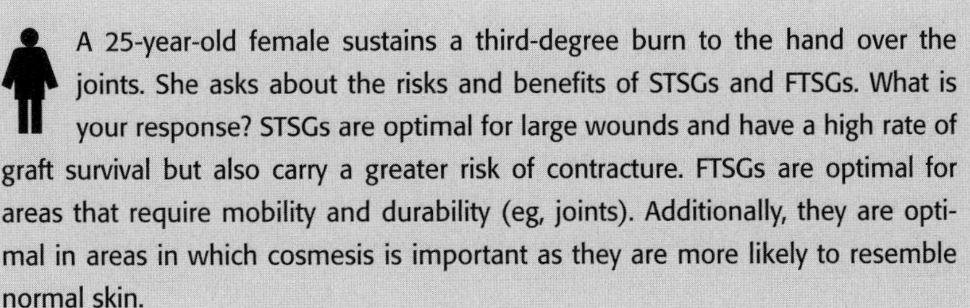

A 25-year-old female sustains a third-degree burn to the hand over the joints. She asks about the risks and benefits of STSGs and FTSGs. What is your response? STSGs are optimal for large wounds and have a high rate of graft survival but also carry a greater risk of contracture. FTSGs are optimal for areas that require mobility and durability (eg, joints). Additionally, they are optimal in areas in which cosmesis is important as they are more likely to resemble normal skin.

Skin Grafts

Used to cover wounds that cannot be closed primarily. Wounds must have a vascularized bed and allow for free transfer of partial or full thickness skin over the site to close the wound. Skin grafts will not adhere to bone, cartilage, or tendon without periosteum, perichondrium, or peritenon, respectively.

Four reasons for failed skin grafts—**P**oor **S**kin **H**ates **I**nfections:
Poor vascular supply
Shear (mechanical) forces
Hematoma
Infections

Split Thickness Skin Grafts

Most commonly taken at 1/100th of an inch including epidermis and a portion of dermis. Used for **large surface area wounds** (frequently burns) in which coverage is more important than function. Can be meshed to ↑ surface area. Associated with ↑ **contracture rate**. Donor site closes secondarily via re-epithelialization from upregulated dermal appendages. After closure, donor sites can be reharvested for additional grafts.

Imbibition provides nutrients to skin grafts during the first 24 hours after placement.

FULL THICKNESS SKIN GRAFTS

Includes epidermis and complete dermis. Used in places where mobility, sensation, or cosmesis are important (eg, over joints, digits, the face). Associated with ↓ **risk of contracture, improved movement, and greater sensation.**

Skin grafts initially adhere to the wound on a fragile fibrin scaffold within 72 hours of placement. In the first 24 hours, **imbibition** allows for direct nutrient supply to the new graft. Over the next 48 hours, **inosculation** (ie, graft vessels align and anastomose with the recipient bed) occurs and provides a blood supply until **angiogenesis** begins (~5–7 days).

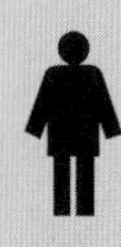

A 19-year-old man sustains a tibial fracture with extensive degloving. After debridement and external fixation, there is 30 cm of exposed tibia. His foot is neurovascularly intact. After initial wound care and stabilization, what wound closure options are available? Gracilis free flap with STSG of the muscular flap.

PLASTIC AND RECONSTRUCTIVE SURGERY

Reconstructive Flaps

Indications for wound closure with a skin flap include poorly vascularized wound beds, full thickness facial injuries (eg, eyelids, lip, ear, nose), deep soft tissue defects, or exposed tendons or bone. **Flaps have their own blood supply; unlike skin grafts, they do not depend on the wound bed for initial survival.**

LOCAL FLAP

Cutaneous flap used in areas where wounds cannot be closed primarily or where a skin graft would fail or result in unacceptable function or cosmesis. Flap blood supply derives from the dermal-subdermal plexus and direct cutaneous unnamed vessels. Locally elevated and rotated or advanced into wounds with 1° closure of the 2° defect.

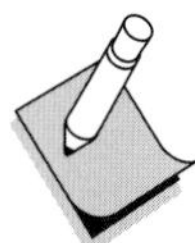

Most common cause of free flap failure—
Venous congestion.

PEDICLED FLAP

Fasciocutaneous or myocutaneous flap used in wounds in which the defect is too large for a local advancement (ie, unacceptable donor defect) or requires additional soft tissue bulk. Blood supply is based on named vessels or known cutaneous angiosomes. **Use of this flap is predominantly limited by the length of the donor vessel.**

FREE FLAP

Tissue transfer to a distant location. Used in wounds similar to pedicled flaps or in wounds requiring specialized tissues (eg, bone, nerve, enteral conduits). Reconstruction options are not limited by pedicle length or local tissue redundancy. Blood supply is derived from similar axial vessels as pedicled flaps; however, tissue **requires microvascular anastomoses of arterial and venous systems**. Major advantage is the lack of limitation on donor sites. Frequently used in head and neck reconstruction (eg, osteocutaneous fibular free flap), breast reconstruction (eg, free transverse rectus abdominus muscle [TRAM]), and limb salvage (eg, rectus, gracilis).

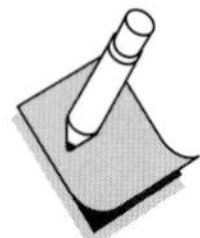

If ischemia is suspected, perform emergent re-exploration of flap.

A relatively thin 32-year-old female with a family history of breast cancer presents with a breast mass. She has had no prior surgical procedures and is in good health. Mammography suggests malignancy; biopsy confirms invasive ductal carcinoma with scattered foci of ductal carcinoma in situ. She is *BRCA1* +. After bilateral skin-sparing mastectomies, what are her reconstructive options? Autogenous reconstruction (eg, TRAM flap, TRAM variants) or implant reconstruction.

Breast Reconstruction

Reconstruction after mastectomy includes implant or autogenous tissue reconstruction. Preoperative reconstructive considerations include need for adjuvant therapies (eg, radiation), previous operations (eg, abdominal procedures), and microvascular risks (eg, tobacco use, DM).

Implant Reconstruction

Most common breast reconstruction technique. Almost all patients are candidates for implant reconstruction. Relative indications include need for bilateral reconstruction (though free tissue reconstruction is feasible), patient inability to tolerate extended operative time, and lack of adequate donor sites. **Relative contraindication is need for adjuvant radiation therapy.** Technically straightforward reconstructive option for immediate and delayed reconstruction: tissue expander followed by silicone or saline prosthesis is placed submuscularly with skin flaps closed primarily over the site. In select cases, single stage reconstruction with an implant may be performed.

Autogenous Reconstruction

Advantage includes using the patient's own tissue reconstruction with a single stage procedure. Immediate autogenous reconstruction with a skin-sparing mastectomy can provide a durable superior cosmetic result. Also provides an alternative reconstructive option for patients requiring adjuvant radiation. Common types include

- **TRAM flap and TRAM variants:** Most common autogenous reconstructive procedure performed. Myocutaneous tissue transfer based on the **epigastric artery** and includes abdominal adipose and skin. May be pedicled (based on superior epigastric artery) or harvested as a free flap (based on inferior epigastric artery). More recently, flaps based on the blood supply of perforators (eg, deep inferior epigastric perforator and superficial inferior epigastric artery flaps) have been employed. Perforator flaps require smaller fascial incisions and allow for the rectus abdominus to be left in situ. **Free TRAMs and their variants may have a more robust blood supply than the pedicled TRAM but do require a microvascular anastomosis** (usually to the internal mammary artery). **Contraindications to TRAM reconstruction include prior abdominoplasty and patient inability to tolerate an extended operative time or significant blood loss.** Relative contraindications include tobacco use (particularly for pedicled TRAMs), prior abdominal surgery, presence of significant ventral hernias, and obesity. Complications include postoperative abdominal wall laxity (20%), partial flap failure (20%), and complete flap failure (4%) in free flaps.

- **Latissimus dorsi flap:** Pedicled flap transposing the latissimus and its blood supply (ie, thoracodorsal artery) into the mastectomy defect. **Primary alternative to TRAM reconstruction in patients who have anatomic TRAM contraindications.** Well-suited to a single stage procedure, but an implant is usually necessary for additional bulk. Relative contraindications include nodal or axillary radiation, prior thoracotomy, and need for adjuvant radiotherapy.

Skin Substitutes

Though several major skin substitutes are approved, none replace autologous tissue at this time. Typically used to assist in closure of major burns or of chronic wounds with poor donor tissues. All constructs provide a neodermis through a collagen membrane (with or without fibroblasts) or an epidermis through cultured keratinocytes or an artificial silicone membrane.

- Allograft: Irradiated cadaveric skin used in burn closures or in abdominal wall reconstructions. Particularly useful in contaminated wounds such open abdomen closures after trauma.
- Biosynthetic dermal substitute made from silicone and nylon: Provides breathable closure where clot can form to facilitate deep tissue granulation.
- Bovine collagen crosslinked sheets with silicone outer layer: Promotes dermal healing and provides breathable barrier function.
- Keratinocyte sheets made from a patient's own cells: Patient's cells are cultured with mouse epidermal cells that supply proliferation signals.

▶ SAMPLE QUESTIONS

What are the first immune cells to arrive in a wound? Which cells predominate in the proliferative phase?	PMNs are first to arrive. Macrophages predominate the proliferative phase.
What are the major stages of wound healing and in what order do they occur?	Inflammatory → proliferative → remodeling/maturation.
When does a wound reach the majority of its tensile strength?	By 30 days, most wounds approach 80% of their overall healed strength.
What is the predominant type of collagen in early wound healing and in healed wounds (ie, scars)?	Early: Type III Scars: Type I
What wounds are amenable to 3° wound closure? What tissue provides an extended exception?	Tertiary closure (delayed 1°) is indicated for wounds that have been open for > 6–8 hours. Exceptions include facial injuries, which can remain open for 12–24 hours (highly vascular).
What is the typical recurrence rate for keloids with surgical therapy alone?	45–100% will recur. Surgical debulking with postoperative XRT ↓ recurrence rate to ~10–20%.
What is the most frequent complication resulting in free flap failure? Treatment?	Venous congestion leads to flap ischemia and failure. Treatment of acutely ischemic flaps is emergent exploration. Leech use can temporize congested flaps until they develop their own collateral venous drainage.
A 50-year-old woman undergoes a mastectomy and will require adjuvant radiation. What immediate reconstruction option is least likely to be successful?	Implant reconstruction.
What are advantages of free flaps compared to pedicled flaps? Disadvantages?	Advantages: Large number of donor sites, immediate defect closure, independent microcirculation. Disadvantages: Require anastomoses, lack collateral circulation.
A 30-year-old male is taken to the ED after he sustains an injury with a potentially contaminated wound. What is the preferred method of closure?	Interrupted suture (compared to subcuticular running) closure. ↓ Associated with a risk of infection.

PLASTIC AND RECONSTRUCTIVE SURGERY

A 27-year-old female undergoes bilateral mastectomies after developing breast cancer. She is *BRCA1* +. What is the benefit of a TRAM flap (versus a latissimus flap)?	TRAM flaps are suitable for patients who require bilateral reconstruction without needing additional implant placement.

CHAPTER 15

Cardiac

Danielle Gottlieb, MD, MS, MPH
Reviewed by Frederick Y. Chen, MD, PhD

Key embryonic vessels and functions–

Common cardinal veins: Return blood from body of embryo to heart of embryo.

Umbilical veins: Bring oxygenated blood from placenta to embryo.

Umbilical arteries: Bring deoxygenated blood from embryo to placenta.

Vitelline veins: Drain deoxygenated blood from the yolk sac.

Vitelline arteries: Bring partially oxygenated blood to the yolk sac.

Embryology

Derived primarily from **splanchnic mesoderm** and neural crest cells, heart development begins during the third week of gestation and includes

- Assembly: Two endocardial heart tubes fuse to form one.
- Chamber development: Genesis of primordial chambers (eg, sinus venosus [drainage site of the vitelline, umbilical, and common cardinal veins], primitive atria, primitive ventricle, bulbus cordis).
- Looping: Asymmetric growth of the primordial chambers results in bulboventricular loop. Blood circulation begins.
- Partitioning: Endocardial cushions fuse to create atrioventricular (AV) canals, which contribute to the atrial and intraventricular septum and partition left from right. Atrial separation begins with descent of the **septum primum** to close the **foramen primum.** Apoptosis of portions of the septum primum create the **foramen secundum** and a subsequent right-to-left shunt. **Septum secundum** forms adjacent to the septum primum, forming the **foramen ovale** (another site of right-to-left shunting). As respiration begins, ↑ left-sided pressures close the septum primum, compressing the septum secundum to close the valve (**fossa ovalis**).
- Initiation of conduction.

Fetal circulation includes the placental, vitelline, and embryonic arterial-venous systems (see Figure 19-1 in Chapter 19).

Adult equivalents to embryonic structures–

Obliterated umbilical vein → ligamentum teres.

Vitelline system → portal system.

Craniocaudal anatomy prior to the first heart beat–**TR**y **B**eating **V**ast **A**nd **S**low:
TRuncus arteriosus
Bulbus cordis
Ventricle
Atrium
Sinus venosus

Anatomy

Macroscopic Anatomy

Three-sided pyramidal shaped organ in the middle mediastinum. The AV valves (ie, mitral, tricuspid) separate the atria and ventricles. The semilunar valves (ie, aortic, pulmonic) separate the ventricles from the great vessels.

Conduction system of the heart is composed of the sinoatrial (SA) node, AV node, His bundle, and Purkinje fibers. Depolarization follows this pathway. HR is determined by the most rapidly depolarizing structure, typically the SA node.

Microscopic Anatomy

Cardiac muscle is composed of striated muscle arranged as sarcomeres. Thick filaments composed of myosin interact with thin, actin filaments. **Ca^{2+}-binding drives contraction** of cardiac muscle.

Blood Supply

Coronary anatomy is summarized in Figure 15-1. **Left main** coronary artery divides into the **left anterior descending (LAD)** and **circumflex** coronary arteries. LAD has two branching systems: **septal branches,** which supply the **interventricular septum,** and **diagonal branches,** which supply the **anterolateral left ventricle (LV)**. The **circumflex coronary artery** provides **marginal branches** supplying the **posterior and lateral LV**. The **right** coronary artery (RCA) provides blood supply to the **right ventricle (RV), the SA and AV nodes**, and the posterior and inferior LV.

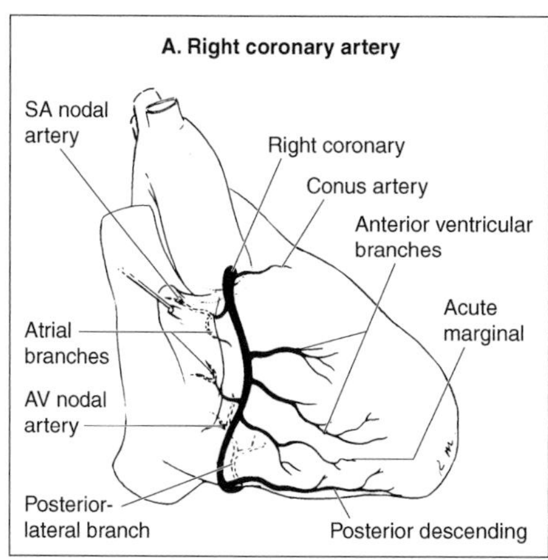

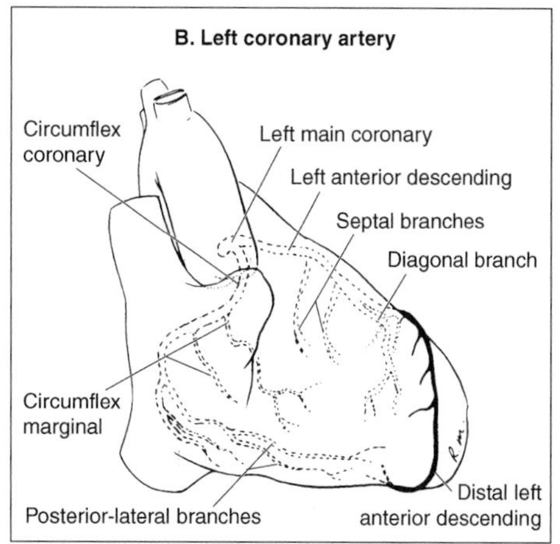

FIGURE 15-1. Anatomy of the coronary arteries.

(Reproduced, with permission, from Doherty GM, Way LW. *Current Surgical Diagnosis and Treatment*, 12th ed. New York: McGraw-Hill, 2006:391.)

Internal mammary artery is the first branch of the subclavian artery. The proximal portion of the internal mammary artery is closely associated with the phrenic nerve.

Dominance is determined by the coronary artery from which the posterior descending artery (PDA) originates. If the PDA originates from the RCA (85–90% of patients), the coronary circulation is called **right dominant**. Ten percent of patients have a left dominant circulation in which the circumflex gives rise to the PDA.

INNERVATION

Sympathetic nerves from T1-T4 function to ↑ HR, contractility, and conduction velocity. Parasympathetic innervation via the vagus nerve has the opposite effect.

Cardiac terminology–
End diastolic pressure: Determined by end diastolic volume (preload) and intrinsic myocardial wall stiffness.
End systolic pressure: Determined by contractility and afterload.
Stroke volume (SV): Function of end diastolic volume (Starling relationship) and end systolic volume.

Cardiac Physiology

HEMODYNAMIC PARAMETERS

Pressure-volume relationships are used to describe cardiac performance.

- Preload: Volume in the ventricle at end diastole.
- Afterload: LV wall tension during systole (determined by preload and the systemic vascular resistance [SVR]).
- Contractility: Intrinsic strength of ventricular myocardium.

Starling curve describes the relationship between preload and contractility. As sarcomeres are stretched within a physiologic range, the force and extent of ventricular contraction changes (see Figure 15-2).

A 60-year-old woman with a preoperative LV ejection fraction (LVEF) of 40% underwent coronary artery bypass grafting (CABG). Postoperatively, she demonstrates metabolic acidosis, oliguria, and poor oxygenation. Her extremities are pale, cool, and diaphoretic. You suspect low CO syndrome. Potential etiologies include abnormal preload, contractility, rhythm, HR, and afterload. What should this patient's workup include? Exam, hemodynamic measurements, serial blood gases, ECG, CXR, assess urine output and chest tube drainage, and echo.

Cardiac output (CO) = SV × HR

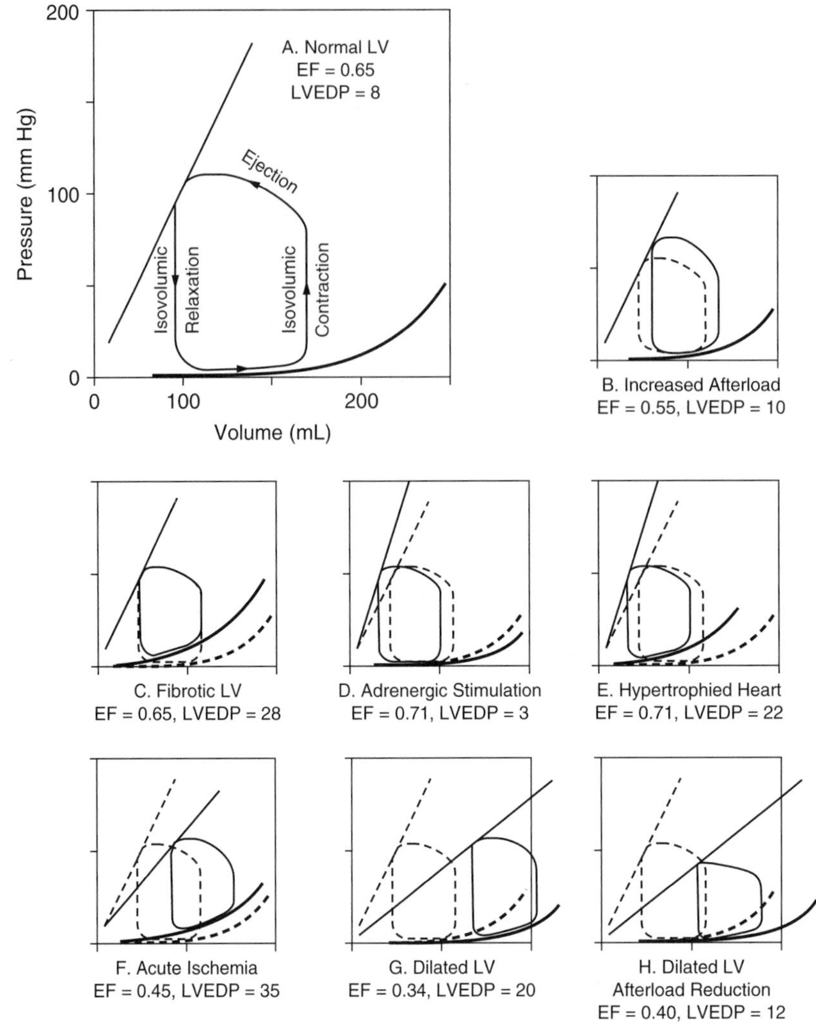

FIGURE 15-2. Left ventricular pressure-volume curve.

(Reproduced, with permission, from Cohn LH. *Cardiac Surgery in the Adult*, 3rd ed. New York: McGraw-Hill, 2007:65.)

Factors influencing myocardial O_2–**SaPPLY** and **USER** demand:

Sao_2	sq**U**eeze (contractility)
Pressure (coronary)	**S**tarting volume (preload)
Pressure (systemic)	**E**xit pressure (afterload)
Lack of RBCs (anemia)	**R**ate
Rh**Y**thm and rate	

O_2 delivery to the tissues is determined by–

Cardiac output

Hemoglobin

SaO_2

Oxygen Content and Extraction

Myocardium is very efficient at extracting O_2. O_2 delivery is a function of the blood's O_2 content and the rate of blood delivery (ie, CO). Relevant formulas include

- O_2 content = (Hgb × $Sa{O_2}$) (1.39) + ($Pa{O_2}$) (0.0031)
- O_2 extraction ratio = (O_2 content) – ([Hgb × $Sv{O_2}$] [1.39] + [$Pv{O_2}$] [0.0031])/ O_2 content

Myocardial O_2 consumption is not influenced by supply but is purely a function of myocardial work and basal metabolism. However, one needs to know the amount of O_2 going in and out to calculate how much O_2 the myocardium is using.

Pulmonary Artery Catheters

Pulmonary artery (PA) catheters are useful for quantifying hemodynamic parameters, as shown in Table 15-1. Allow for measurement of pulmonary capillary

TABLE 15-1. Pulmonary Artery Catheter Measurements According to Disease State

Measurement	Normal Values	Right Heart Failure	Left Heart Failure
CO	4–8 L/min	↓↓	↓↓
CI	2.5–4 L/min/m^2	↓↓	↓↓
SV	40–50 mL/m^2	↓	↓
PAP	15–30 / 8-15 mm Hg	↓	↓
PCWP	6–12 mm Hg	Nl/↓	↑
CVP	1–6 mm Hg	↑↑	Nl/↑
SVR	900–1200 dynes/cm^2	Nl/↑	↑

CI = cardiac index; PAP = pulmonary artery pressure; CVP = central venous pressure.

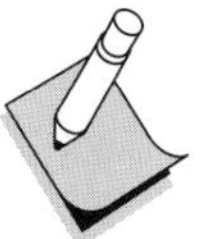

Estimate adequacy of tissue perfusion and oxygenation with mixed venous oxygen saturation (SvO_2) from a PA catheter sample.

Complications of PA catheters—**DISASTER:**
Dislodgement
Infection
Stop AV conduction (heart block)
Arrhythmia
Sick lung (pulmonary infarct)
Thrombosis
Entrapment
Rupture of the PA

wedge pressure (PCWP), which reflects LV preload in the absence of mitral valve insufficiency or stenosis (see Figure 15-3). While useful, a variety of serious complications can occur with their use. The most serious complications include heart block, thrombosis, catheter-related sepsis, and PA rupture.

You are called to see a 60-year-old woman just hours following CABG. Hemodynamic measurements show a CI 1.0, HR 95, SBP 95, CVP 12, PAP 50/28, SVR 1600. She has no known lung disease, and pulmonary vascular resistance (PVR) is normal. What is the next step in management? Low CI prompts you to look for ischemic changes (ie, ECG) and to support her LV function (ie, either by pharmacologic or mechanical means). The ischemic clamp period impairs LV function in patients but is typically inconsequential in those with a normal preoperative ejection fraction. The nadir of function occurs 4 hours after cardiopulmonary bypass (CPB).

Vasoactive Agents

Different vasoactive medications are used preferentially for different hemodynamic scenarios (see Table 15-2).

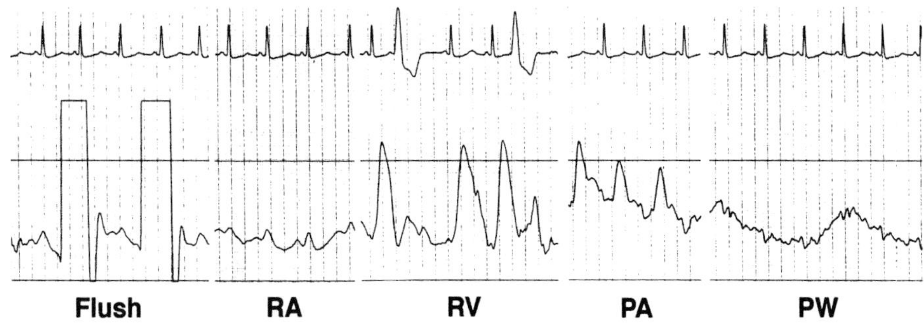

FIGURE 15-3. Pulmonary artery catheter tracings.

(Reproduced, with permission, from Hall JB, et al. *Principles of Critical Care,* 3rd ed. New York: McGraw-Hill, 2005:142.)

CARDIAC

TABLE 15-2. Commonly Used Vasoactive Agents and Their Properties

CATEGORY	AGENT	SITE OF ACTIVITY	HR	PCWP	CI	SVR	MAP
Inotropes	Dobutamine	β_1+, β_2+	↑↑	↓	↑	↓	↑↓
	Milrinone	Phosphodiesterase (PDE) → nitric oxide (NO) release	↑	↓	↑	↓↓	↓
Mixed	Epinephrine	β_1+, β_2+, α_1+	↑↑	↑↓	↑	↑	↑
	Norepinephrine	β_1+, β_2+, α_1+	↑↑	↑↑	↑	↑↑	↑↑
	Dopamine	Dopamine +, β_1+, β_2+, α_1+	↑↑	↑↓	↑	↑↓	↑↓
Vasopressors	Phenylephrine	α_1+	↔	↑	↔	↑↑	↑↑
	Vasopressin	Arginine vasopressin (AVP) +	↔	↔	↔	↑↑	↑↑
Vasodilator	Nitroglycerin	NO → smooth muscle relaxation	↑	↓↔	↔	↓	↓
	Nitroprusside	As above	↑↑	↓↔	↔	↓↓	↓↓

(Adapted, with permission, from Cohn LH. *Cardiac Surgery in the Adult*, 3rd ed. New York: McGraw-Hill, 2007:470.)

Physiologic Response to Cardiopulmonary Bypass

CPB results in microembolus formation, hypoperfusion, and the release of systemic inflammatory mediators. Sequelae of this insult are identified in every organ system (see Table 15-3).

TABLE 15-3. Organ Response to Cardiopulmonary Bypass

ORGAN	EFFECT	PRESUMED MECHANISM
Heart	Stunning, reperfusion injury.	Hypoperfusion, inflammatory mediators.
Brain	Cognitive impairment, neuropsychiatric symptoms, stroke.	Microemboli, hypoperfusion, inflammatory mediators.
Lung	Hypoxia, edema, infarct, acute respiratory distress syndrome (ARDS).	Atelectasis, hypoperfusion, inflammatory mediators, capillary leak, microemboli.
Kidney	Renal failure/insufficiency.	Hemoglobin precipitation in tubules, hypoperfusion (leads to antithrombin III release).
Liver	Transaminitis, hyperbilirubinemia.	Microemboli, hypoperfusion, inflammatory mediators.
Pancreas	Chemical or clinical pancreatitis	Ca^{2+} administration, hypoperfusion.
Blood	Heparin-induced thrombocytopenia (HIT), coagulopathy.	Heparin administration, inflammatory mediators, platelet dysfunction, clotting factor depletion, fibrinolysis.

Congenital Heart Disease

Often abnormal cardiac structural changes will result in shunting (see Table 15-4). Direction of aberrant blood flow results in characteristic pathologic symptoms. **Left-to-right** shunts cause **congestive heart failure** (CHF; ie, hepatomegaly, dyspnea, tachypnea, grunting, noisy breathing, retractions). Patients with **right-to-left** shunts display **cyanosis** (eg, clubbing, polycythemia), **failure to thrive** (FTT), and often **squat** to improve symptoms (↓ venous return → ↑ arterial pressure → ↓ right-to-left shunt → ↑ oxygenation).

BOOT-shaped heart of tetralogy of Fallot:
Big RV
Overriding aorta
Open ventricular septum (VSD)
Tiny pulmonic valve

TABLE 15-4. Congenital Defects Grouped by Shunt Direction

Disorder	Demographics	Signs/Symptoms	Diagnosis	Management
Left-to-Right Shunts				
Atrial septal defect (ASD)	**Most common adult congenital defect.** Secundum most common type. 1/1500 live births. More common in females.	Paradoxical emboli, atrial arrhythmias, CHF, systolic ejection murmur (SEM) with **fixed, split S2**.	Echo, catheterization, ECG.	Treat with digoxin, diuretics, percutaneous repair. Repair all primum, CHF cases, secundums that persist to school age.
Ventricular septal defect (VSD)	**Most common congenital heart defect.** Most close spontaneously by 6 months.	FTT, tachypnea, tachycardia, **pansystolic murmur.**	Monitor PVR by catheterization. If > 10–12 Wood's units, consider **Eisenmenger's syndrome**.	Treat with digoxin, diuretics, percutaneous devices. Repair at school age if still open, if PVR > 4–6 Woods units, or large defect.
Patent ductus arteriosus (PDA)	Common in premature infants.	Dyspnea, FTT, tachycardia, arrhythmias, **continuous machine-like murmur.**	Echo, CXR (cardiomegaly, pulmonary edema), ECG.	**Indomethacin** closes PDA; **PGE_2** keeps open. Operative ligation if no response to meds.
Right-to-Left Shunts				
Truncus arteriosus	Associated with 22q11 deletion (Di George's syndrome). 80% mortality in first year of life if CHF is present. Often associated with VSD.	Cyanosis at birth, CHF within weeks, SEM at left sternal border, SaO_2 ~80%.	Echo, CXR (cardiomegaly, pulmonary edema).	Optimize with diuretics, digoxin, fluid restriction, afterload reduction. Operative repair includes VSD repair, resection of PA from aorta (Ao), Ao repair, RV → PA conduit.

(Continued)

TABLE 15-4. Congenital Defects Grouped by Shunt Direction (*Continued*)

Disorder	Demographics	Signs/Symptoms	Diagnosis	Management
Transposition of the great vessels	**Most common cyanotic CHD occurring in first week of life.** Death prevented by shunts that mix blood: PDA, ASD, VSD, or combination.	FTT, tachypnea, syncope.	CXR (**"egg on a string"**), echo.	Optimize with PGE_1. Balloon atrial septoplasty is palliative. Operative repair includes arterial switch operation, closure of septal defects and PDA.
Tetralogy of Fallot	**Most common cyanotic heart defect.** More common in males. Associated with 22q11 (Di George's) and CATCH-22 syndrome. Fatal if untreated.	**Tet spells** (unpredictable acute hypoxic episodes caused by sudden ↑ right-to-left flow), growth retardation, SEM (varies with degree of RV outflow tract [RVOT] obstruction). **Squatting improves symptoms.**	CXR (**"boot-shaped heart"**), ECG, echo, catheterization.	Treat tet spell with β-blocker, phenylephrine, morphine (↓ PVR, ↑ SVR). **Blalock-Taussig shunt (systemic-to-pulmonary) is palliative.** Operative repair includes RVOT enlargement, VSD repair.
Other				
Tricuspid atresia	PDA, ASD, VSD present for mixing.	Cyanosis, tachypnea.	Echo.	Modified Blalock-Taussig shunt is palliative. Operative repair includes Fontan (single ventricle repair) procedure.
Total anomalous pulmonary venous return (TAPVR)	More common in males. PDA present for mixing.	Severe cyanosis, RV heave, **fixed, split S2, + S3.**	CXR (**"snowman sign"**), echo, catheterization.	PGE_1 is palliative (but can worsen cyanosis in some). Operative repair includes rerouting of pulmonary veins.
Hypoplastic left heart	Associated with aortic and mitral valve atresia.	Weak distal pulses, worsening CO as PDA closes.	Echo, catheterization.	PGE_1 is palliative. Operative repair includes transplant or Fontan procedure.
Aortic coarctation	Most common in Caucasian males. Associated with **Turner's (XO) syndrome, bicuspid aortic valve.**	Discrepancy in BP between right/left arms and upper/lower extremities, **SEM with weak and delayed distal pulses.**	CXR (**rib notching, "3 sign"**), MRA, catheterization, echo.	PGE_1 is palliative. Operative repair involves aortic patch plasty.

Acquired Valvular Cardiac Diseases

Pathologic valvular diseases result in either a ↓ (due to stenosis) or ↑ (due to insufficiency or regurgitation) in flow (see Table 15-5). If indicated, valve replacement options include:

- Mechanical (eg, St. Jude): Most durable. **Requires warfarin therapy**.
- Bioprosthetic (eg, porcine allograft, bovine pericardium): Less durable. Does not require anticoagulation in all cases.
- Cadaveric (eg, homograft): Least durable. Does not require anticoagulation.

Risk Factors for CAD—
CLOGGED:
Cholesterol
Lights up (+ tobacco use)
Obesity
Gender (male)
Got relatives (family history of CAD)
Excess BP (HTN)
Diabetes

Coronary Artery Disease and Ischemic Heart Disease

Demographics/Risk Factors

Atherosclerosis leads to clinical syndromes resulting in mismatched myocardial O_2 supply and demand. Plaque hemorrhage and rupture leads to acute

TABLE 15-5. Acquired Cardiac Valvular Disease

Diagnosis	Demographics	Signs/Symptoms	Diagnosis	Management
Aortic stenosis (AS)	**Most common acquired valve disease.** Valve calcification → LV outflow tract (LVOT) obstruction → pressure overload → LV hypertrophy → ↓ compliance, ↓ ejection fraction (EF).	**Syncope, CHF, angina,** sudden cardiac death. **Mid-SEM** that **radiates to the neck,** ↓ with standing/straining.	Determine aortic valve area by echo or catheterization. Perform coronary cath if angina or age > 40 years.	Replace valve if + symptoms or critical AS (aortic valve areas < 0.75 cm^2).
Aortic regurgitation (AR)	Associated with bicuspid aortic valve, aortic dissection, endocarditis.	CHF, angina, endocarditis, conduction abnormalities, **high-pitched, early diastolic decrescendo murmur ("blowing").**	Echo	Replace valve if + symptoms or if ↓ ventricular function/size. Can repair in certain select circumstances.
Mitral stenosis (MS)	Associated with **rheumatic fever.**	CHF, atrial thrombus, atrial fibrillation (AF), left parasternal heave. **Mid-diastolic/presystolic murmur preceded by opening click.**	Determine transvalvar gradient and valve area by echo or cath.	Percutaneous mitral valvuloplasty. Replace valve if + symptoms or critical MS (mitral valve area < 1 cm^2).
Mitral regurgitation (MR)	Associated with recent MI, endocarditis, idiopathic chordae rupture, myxomatous valve.	Acute, severe MR associated with CHF or cardiogenic shock. **Pansystolic murmur with short diastolic rumbling.** Mitral valve prolpase (MVP) has late SEM with click that ↑ intensity with squatting.	Echo	Optimize medically. Perform mitral valve repair or if not possible, replacement.

Sequelae of MI—**SAD PUMP:**
Shock (cardiogenic)
Aneurysm (LV)/**A**rrhythmia
Death
Pericarditis
Unending symptoms (chronic ischemic heart disease)
Mitral insufficiency
Papillary muscle rupture

coronary syndromes. Risk factors for ischemic heart disease are similar to those for atherosclerosis (see Chapter 17).

SIGNS/SYMPTOMS

Cornary artery disease (CAD) can lead to a range of symptoms from exertional shortness of breath (SOB) to unstable angina and MI with or without hemodynamic instability. **Substernal, persistent chest pressure radiating to the jaw and left arm** are classic MI symptoms. Other symptoms include nausea, vomiting, or heartburn. May be asymptomatic.

DIAGNOSIS

Suggested by clinical picture in conjunction with ECG and troponin levels. Specific ECG tracings will suggest involved coronary vessels. Confirm diagnosis with cardiac catheterization or coronary CT angiography (CTA).

Durability of bypass conduits (with 1 year patency)—
LIMA (95%) > saphenous vein (80%) > radial artery (70%)

TREATMENT

May be medical, percutaneous, or surgical. Medical optimization consists of β-blocker, angiotensin-converting enzyme (ACE) inhibitor, and nitrates. Percutaneous coronary interventions (PCI) includes balloon angioplasty and stenting. Surgical treatment is CABG, which is indicated for

- ST elevation MI (STEMI) with failed PCI, hemodynamic instability, ventricular arrhythmia, cardiogenic shock, or other MI complications
- Low EF due to ischemia
- Life-threatening ventricular arrhythmia
- Unstable angina
- Left main coronary artery disease
- Three-vessel disease
- Two-vessel disease with proximal LAD disease and EF < 50%
- One- or two-vessel disease with disabling symptoms or arrhythmia.

Left internal mammary artery (LIMA) is the preferred graft to the LAD, if possible. One-year patency rate of the LIMA is ~95%, which is superior to greater saphenous vein (80%) and radial artery (70%) patency rates. CABG complications include bleeding, infection, pericarditis, or continued infarction due to graft failure.

BIG complications associated with CABG:
Bleeding
Infection (superficial/deep sternal wound)/ **I**nflammation (postpericardiotomy syndrome)
Graft failure → ischemia/infarct

Idiopathic Hypertrophic Subaortic Stenosis

Also known as **hypertrophic obstructive cardiomyopathy (HOCM)**. Autosomal dominant syndrome caused by functionally impaired myocardial sarcomere components. Causes **asymmetric hypertrophy (most commonly of the interventricular septum), resulting in dynamic LVOT obstruction.** Commonly presents as dyspnea, syncope, or angina; **may be undiagnosed until sudden death.** Diagnosis is suspected by exam (nonradiating SEM that ↑ in intensity with maneuvers that ↓ LV volume) and abnormal ECG (LV strain pattern). Confirm diagnosis with echo, cardiac catheterization, and ventriculography. Treat surgically with **septal resection**.

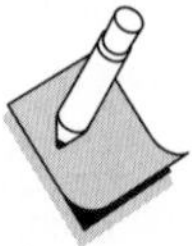

Idiopathic hypertrophic subaortic stenosis (IHSS) is the leading cause of sudden death in children and adolescents.

Endocarditis

Disease begins with an initial endocardial injury → platelet aggregation and nonbacterial valvular vegetations. Transient bacteremia of any source seeds the vegetation, and bacterial overgrowth ensues. Pathogens differ by valve type, but most commonly include *Streptococcus viridans*, *Staphylococcus aureus*, *Staphylococcus epidermidis*, and *Enterococcus*. High-risk patients include patients with native valve disease, prosthetic valves, congenital heart disease, or rheumatic heart disease as well as IV drug users.

Patients present with myalgias, weight loss, and anorexia. Exam shows petechiae, splinter hemorrhages, Roth's spots (vasculitis of retinal arteries), Osler's nodes (indurated palmar nodules), Janeway lesions (red macules on distal extremities), and distal septic emboli. Confirm diagnosis with blood cultures and transesophageal echo visualization of valvular vegetations. Treat initially with antimicrobials. Valve replacement is indicated for CHF, embolic events, persistent sepsis, or abscess. Valve replacement options are discussed in above.

Common organisms in endocarditis–

NATIVE VALVE:

S. viridans *(most common)*

S. aureus

Enterococcus

PROSTHETIC VALVE:

S. epidermidis *(early)*

S. viridans *(late)*

Cardiac Myxomas

Most common 1° tumor of the heart. Typically affect women in the third to sixth decade of life. Usually involve the left atrium. Subsequent symptoms mimic MS (eg, dyspnea on exertion, paroxysmal noctural dyspnea). Diagnose with echo. Treatment includes resection.

Streptococcus bovis (viridans *group) is associated with occult colorectal malignancy.*

Cardiac Transplantation

Indicated only after conventional therapies have failed for patients with end-stage heart failure, ischemia, arrhythmia, and IHSS. Donor and recipient are matched for ABO blood group and organ size. Graft can tolerate ischemic time of only **4–6 hours**, necessitating coordination of donor and recipient teams. After transplant, rejection is usually asymptomatic until late in the course. RV endomyocardial biopsies are routinely performed for surveillance. Complications of transplantation are described in Chapter 20. Mortality is 7% at 30 days, and 1-year survival approaches 85%.

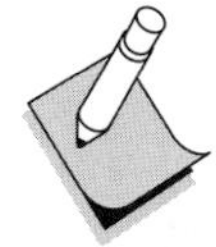

Indications for valve replacement in endocarditis–

*When the heart is **weak** (CHF),*

*The outlook is **bleak** (embolic events),*

*Bugs are on a **winning streak** (abscess, persistent abscess)*

Mechanical Circulatory Support Devices

Ventricular Assist Device

Mechanically decompresses the ventricle(s) while perfusing systemic or pulmonary vasculature. Can be used as a bridge to transplantation, myocardial recovery, or as destination therapy. Provides time for metabolic and functional recovery of supported ventricle(s).

Intra-aortic Balloon Pump

Provides hemodynamic support and improves coronary artery perfusion. Balloon is timed to ECG or arterial waveform and deflates immediately before systole → mechanically ↓ afterload. Balloon reinflates in diastole, forcing blood into coronary arteries and augmenting perfusion. Improves myocardial O_2 supply–demand ratio.

Most common cardiac tumors–

*The most common **benign** cardiac tumor → myxoma*

*The most common **malignant** cardiac tumor → metastatic disease*

▶ SAMPLE QUESTIONS

A child has considerable CHF during the first year of life and is diagnosed with a large VSD. You are consulted with regard to closure of the VSD as the patient's CHF symptoms have improved. What is your prognosis?	Grave. CHF in the first year of life followed by resolution of symptoms is consistent with Eisenmenger's syndrome. As pulmonary HTN worsens, a left-to-right shunt becomes right-to-left shunt. Most patients die from Eisenmenger's in their late teens or early 20s.
A 75-year-old has undergone aortic valve replacement for AS. You are called because she is hypotensive. Vital signs show a HR 100 in normal sinus rhythm, BP 86/54. PA catheter shows a CVP 4, PAP 11/7, CI 1.7, and a normal PCWP. What will you do?	Give volume. Hypovolemia can cause significant hemodynamic compromise following aortic valve replacement for AS due to ↓ ventricular compliance and dependence on euvolemia. As patients rewarm after bypass, they vasodilate and become functionally hypovolemic.
Following five vessel CABG, a patient has an amylase of 84 and lipase of 1251. He is hemodynamically stable. The patient remains intubated. What do you suspect?	Chemical pancreatitis without clinical significance. Follow with abdominal exams after extubation and serial enzymes. Consider imaging if symptomatic.
Coming off bypass, a patient has a HR 48 and is hypotensive with a low CO. What do you do?	Use pacing wires to pace at a faster rate and then reassess.
Following an MI, a patient has acute CHF and is found to have acute MR. What is the mechanism?	Ruptured mitral valve papillary muscle.
Seven years s/p CABG, a patient presents to the ED with substernal chest pain and ST elevation in the lateral leads. What is the likely mechanism of MI?	Progressive atherosclerosis in the graft and/or native coronary arteries.
A 60-year-old patient with bacterial endocarditis is found to have a splenic abscess. She is hemodynamically stable. What is the correct management?	As patient is stable, place on antibiotics and observe closely. If the patient does not stabilize, surgery is indicated.
Following left atrial myxoma resection, a patient has chest pain, fever, and tachycardia. ECG shows ST segment elevation in all leads. What is the most likely diagnosis?	Postpericardiotomy syndrome. Treat with NSAIDs. Obtain CK-MB to ascertain diagnosis.

A 75-year-old has undergone aortic valve replacement for AS. You are called because she is hypotensive. Vitals show a HR 100 in normal sinus rhythm, BP 86/54. PA catheter shows a CVP 19, CI 1.7, and PCWP 20. Chest tubes have minimal output. What are possible diagnoses?	Consider tamponade as well as low CO syndrome.
A 65-year-old man is preoperative for a CABG. What factors predict a greater risk of postoperative MI?	↑ Creatinine, ischemic changes on Holter monitor, ↓ activity level, claudication.
A newborn is found to have a continuous, machinery-like murmur. What is the likely diagnosis?	PDA.

CHAPTER 16

Thoracic

Timothy M. Millington, MD
Reviewed by Dean M. Donahue, MD

▶ BASIC SCIENCE

Embryology

Lung Development

Begins at 3-4 weeks from ventral foregut groove (ie, laryngotracheal groove). Bronchial tree develops by 16 weeks with true alveoli by 26–28 weeks. Alveoli development continues after birth (20 million at birth, roughly 300 million by 8 years of age).

> **Innervation of the diaphragm:**
> C3-4-5 keeps the diaphragm alive.

Diaphragm Development

Develops from cervical hypaxial muscle in neck and descends into lower thorax, carrying motor neurons (eg, phrenic nerve) from cervical plexus.

Anatomy

Macroscopic Anatomy of the Tracheobronchial Tree

Includes the trachea, major lobar bronchi, and segmental bronchi.

Macroscopic Anatomy of the Lung

The right lung has three lobes that contribute **55% of lung volume**: upper (apical, posterior), middle (anterior, lateral, posterior), and lower (superior, medial basal, anterior basal, lateral basal, posterior basal). Azygous lobe is found in 0.5% of people; this aberrant lobe is associated with an aberrant position of the azygous vein near the lung hilum. Though its development is independent from the rest of the lung, it is **not** considered a separate segmental bronchus. The right lung has a minor (horizontal) fissure between the upper and middle lobes and a major (oblique) fissure between the middle and lower lobes. The left lung has two lobes that contribute **45% of lung volume**: upper (apical posterior, apical anterior, superior lingular, inferior lingular) and lower (superior, anteromedial basal, lateral basal, posterior basal). The left lung has only an oblique fissure.

Macroscopic Anatomy of the Mediastinum

Includes anterior (with superior), middle, and posterior compartments.

Microscopic Anatomy of the Upper and Lower Airways

Cartilaginous walls are ciliated with goblet cells and submucosal glandular cells. The **mucociliary escalator** defends against and removes particulate matter. Distal, noncartilaginous terminal bronchioles have mast cells and neuroendocrine cells. There are four main cell types in lung tissue:

- **Type I pnemocytes** make up 40% of pulmonary cells but 90% of the alveolar lining. Participate in **gas exchange**.
- **Type II (granular) pneumocytes** manufacture **surfactant** (dipalmitoyllecithin makes up 50% of the phospholipid concentration).
- **Clara cells** are found in the terminal and respiratory bronchioles and are involved in **lung defense** and surfactant production.
- **Alveolar macrophages** are involved in phagocytosis of certain bacteria, viruses, and particles.

Oxygen must cross five layers to get from air to blood: alveolar epithelium, basement membrane, ground substance, basal membrane, capillary epithelium. **Kohn pores** allow O_2 exchange between alveoli.

***Hilar anatomy*–**
pulmonary arterial branches are ventral to bronchi. Superior pulmonary veins are ventral to bronchi. Inferior pulmonary veins are dorsal to bronchi.

Blood Supply

Dual blood supply includes transport of deoxygenated blood via the pulmonary arteries and oxygenated blood via bronchial arteries (arising from thoracic aorta and intercostal arteries). Venous return occurs through the azygous-hemiazygous (deoxygenated) and pulmonary venous (oxygenated) systems.

Innervation

There is no nerve supply to pulmonary parenchyma. Parietal pleura has a rich somatic nerve supply.

Phrenic nerve = anterior to hilum.
Vagus nerve = Posterior to hilum.

Lymphatic Drainage

Arising in the abdomen as the **cisterna chyli**, the **thoracic duct** enters the thorax between the aorta and right crus, initially running to the right of midline between the azygous and aorta, then crossing to the left at T5 to drain into the **junction of the left internal jugular and left subclavian veins**.

Pleural fluid is generated mainly by the parietal pleura in the less dependent zones and is reabsorbed by the parietal pleura in the dependent zones. One to two liters of pleural fluid are made daily. Production follows the **Starling equation** and depends on the interactions between hydrostatic and colloid pressures and permeability.

***Starling equation*–**
$Q_f = K_f([P_c - P_{is}] - \delta[\pi_{pl} - \pi_{is}])$
Q_f = *Net flow*
K_f = *Filtration coefficient (permeability of capillary wall to fluid)*
δ = *Osmotic reflection coefficient (permeability of capillary wall to protein)*
$(P_c - P_{is})$ = *Capillary filtration pressure*
$(\pi_{pl} - \pi_{is})$ = *Capillary absorptive pressure*

Physiology of Breathing

Normal negative pressure of the pleural space (**–5 mm Hg**) varies from –15 mm Hg in inspiration to 0–2 mm Hg in expiration. Results from the outward elastic recoil force of the chest wall and the inward elastic recoil of the lungs. **Diaphragm** is the 1° muscle involved in normal inspiration.

Changes in lung volume (and thus, pressure) are governed by compliance, resistance, and alveolar ventilation distribution.

- Compliance: **Δ Volume/Δ Pressure**. Inverse of elasticity. Greater at low volumes.
- Airway resistance: Resistance to air flow is greatest in small, long airways as per **Poiseuille's law**.
- Alveolar ventilation distribution: Apical lung regions have greater transpulmonary pressure gradients, greater volume, and less compliance. These are less likely to have volume changes during normal respiratory mechanics.

Ventilation-Perfusion Relationships

Alveolar ventilation is minute ventilation minus anatomic dead space. Usually 4–6 L/min. The normal ventilation/perfusion (V/Q) ratio is 0.8–1.2.

Normal regional differences in lung perfusion and ventilation are present (see Figure 16-1).

Poiseuille's law–

$R = 8\eta L / \Pi r^4$

See Chapter 17 for a description of Poiseuille's law.

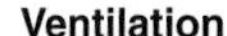

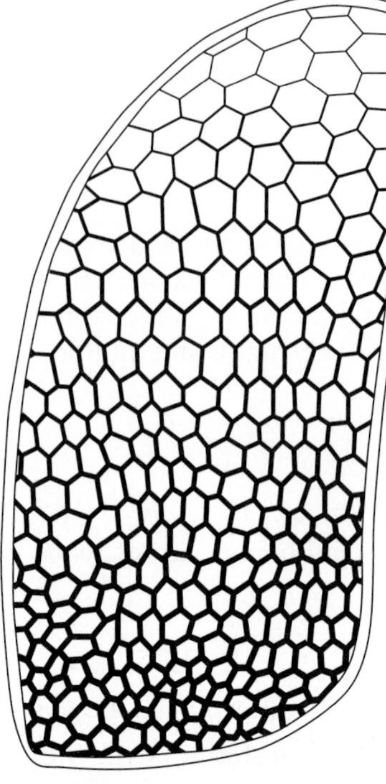

FIGURE 16-1. Ventilation-perfusion regional distribution.

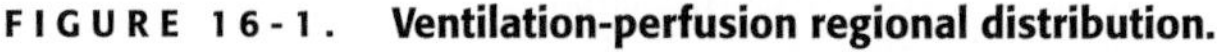

(Reproduced, with permission, from Levitzky MG. *Pulmonary Physiology,* 7th ed. New York: McGraw-Hill, 2007:125.)

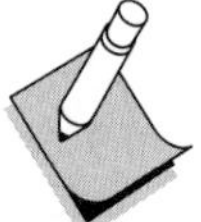

Be able to use the alveolar gas and O_2 content equations for the ABSITE.

Unless otherwise stated, use the following constants:

- P_b (barometric pressure) = 760 torr
- PH_2O (*H_2O pressure at 100% humidity) = 47 torr*
- *RQ* (respiratory quotient) = 0.8

Equations that reflect alveolar ventilation and ventilation-perfusion relationships include:

- **Alveolar gas equation**: $P_AO_2 = FiO_2(P_b - PH_2O) - (P_ACO_2/RQ)$
- **O_2 content**: $CaO_2 = (Hgb \times 1.34 \times SaO_2) + (0.0003\ [PaO_2])$
- **A-a gradient**: $P_AO_2 - PaO_2$

Hemoglobin-O_2 dissociation is ↑ with ↓ pH, ↑ temperature, and ↑ 2,3-DPG. Dissociation is ↓ by ↑ pH, ↓ temperature, and ↓ 2,3-DPG.

Hemoglobin-O_2 dissociation curve–

↑ O_2 delivery: ↓ pH, ↑ temperature, ↑ 2,3-DPG

↓ O_2 delivery: ↑ pH, ↓ temperature, ↓ 2,3-DPG

Pulmonary Function Tests

Assessing lung volumes can help differentiate between obstructive and restrictive pulmonary pathologies and is a crucial part of the preoperative assessment (see Figure 16-2).

> A 67-year-old man has a solitary lesion noted incidentally on CXR. Chest CT confirms a 5-mm noncalcified nodule. He has no prior history of malignancy and is a nonsmoker. What is the next appropriate step? Follow-up CT in 3 months. After 3 months, the lesion has doubled in size. What is the next step? Percutaneous biopsy or video-assisted thoracoscopic surgery (VATS) biopsy.

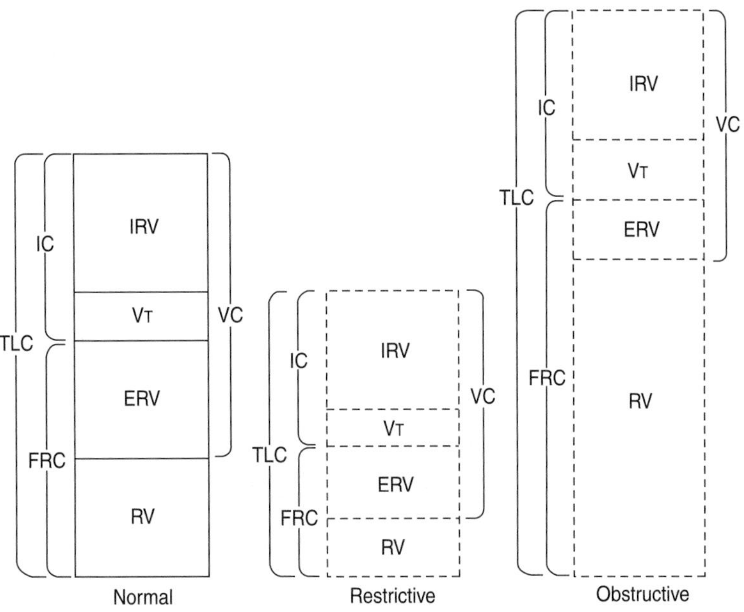

FIGURE 16-2. Lung volumes and the impact of lung pathology.

(Reproduced, with permission, from Levitzky MG. *Pulmonary Physiology*, 7th ed. New York: McGraw Hill, 2007:55.)

Lung volume vocabulary–

RV (residual volume) = Volume in lung at maximal expiration

ERV (expiratory reserve volume) = Volume that can be expired after normal expiration

TV (tidal volume) = Volume that moves into lung with normal inspiration (~500 mL)

IRV (inspiratory reserve volume) = Volume that can be inspired, beyond TV, with maximal inspiration

TLC (total lung capacity) = IRV + TV + ERV + RV

FRC (functional residual capacity) = RV + ERV

VC (vital capacity) = IRV + TV + ERV

IC (inspiratory capacity) = IRV + TV

▶ CLINICAL SCIENCE

Solitary Pulmonary Nodule

DEMOGRAPHICS/RISK FACTORS

Defined as a single circumscribed lesion < 3 cm in diameter, surrounded by normal lung parenchyma. Present on 0.1–0.2% of CXRs and associated with malignancy in 20–40% of all patients and > 50% of those who smoke. Risk factors for malignancy include smoking, prior malignancy, age > 35 years, and history of hemoptysis.

SIGNS/SYMPTOMS

Look for lymphadenopathy (particularly supraclavicular) and evidence of extrapulmonary 1° neoplasms (eg, breast, rectal, testicular).

DIAGNOSIS

Differential diagnoses are summarized in Table 16-1.

Imaging can include CT or positron emission tomography (PET).

- Thin section CT scan can identify multiple nodules. Characteristic CT features suggesting malignancy include **lobulations, irregularities, corona radiata sign (spiculations on CXRs), and size > 2 cm** (see Figure 16-3). Smooth calcifications are associated with benign disease.
- PET scanning is highly sensitive, but false + scans can occur with inflammatory diseases.

Obstructive versus restrictive disease physiology–

Obstructive: ↑ TLC, ↑ FRC, ↓ FEV_1, ↓ FEV_1/FVC

Restrictive: ↓ TLC, ↓ FRC, ↓ FEV_1, nl FEV_1/FVC

Probability of malignancy in solitary pulmonary nodule–
In all patients: 20-40%
In smokers: > 50%

TABLE 16-1. Differential Diagnoses of a Solitary Pulmonary Nodule

LESION TYPE	ETIOLOGY
Benign	
Infectious	Granuloma (TB, fungus), PCP, bacteria (abscess, pneumonia), viruses (measles, CMV).
Neoplastic	Hamartoma (**"popcorn lesion"**), chondroma.
Other	Infarct, arteriovenous fistula or malformation, amyloidosis, sarcoidosis.
Malignant	
1°	Bronchogenic carcinoma, bronchial carcinoid, lymphoma.
Metastatic	Most common 1° malignancies: **Colorectal, breast, renal cell, testicular, melanoma, sarcoma.**

Obtain pathologic diagnosis with biopsy. Bronchoscopic biopsy is 20-80% sensitive (higher if lesion is close to bronchial tree and if pretest probability is high). Transthoracic biopsy is up to 95% accurate, but there is a 30% rate of iatrogenic pneumothorax (PTX). **Thoracoscopic resection** may be a better option than biopsy for patients with low surgical risk.

A 53-year-old woman has a right-sided lung mass noted on CXR. She is a smoker with no cancer history. Chest CT confirms an irregular 4-cm mass and a right paratracheal node measuring 1.9 cm. Percutaneous biopsy of the lung mass confirms a bronchogenic adenocarcinoma. What must be done before choosing further treatment? Mediastinoscopy and lymph node biopsy.

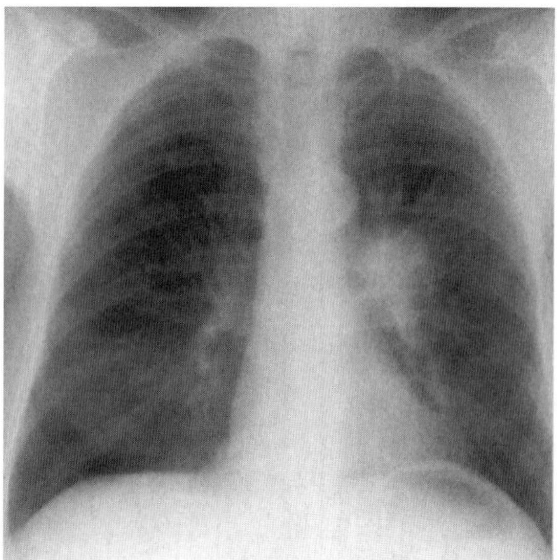
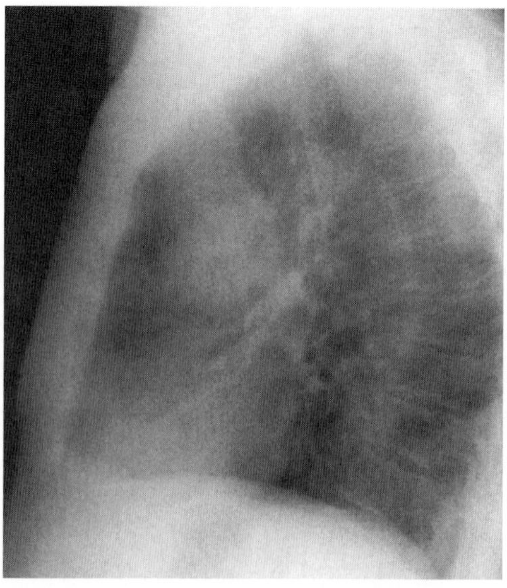

FIGURE 16-3. Radiographic appearance of lung cancer. See also color insert.

(Reproduced, with permission, from Chen MYM, et al. *Basic Radiology*. New York: McGraw-Hill, 2004:92.)

A 72-year-old male smoker presents with a biopsy-proven 1.5-cm squamous cell carcinoma (SCC) of the lower lobe of the right lung. There is no radiographic evidence of lymph node involvement; mediastinoscopy is negative. What is the next appropriate step? Right lower lobectomy. What surgical treatment is indicated if the patient has poorly controlled chronic obstructive pulmonary disease (COPD) and cannot walk more than a city block without severe dyspnea? Limited wedge resection or radiotherapy.

Relative risks of developing lung cancer–

Current smoker: ↑ 16-fold

1-9 years after quitting: ↑ 6-20 fold

10-19 years after quitting: ↑ 2-6 fold

20+ years after quitting: ↑ 2-3.7 fold

Lung Cancer

Demographics/Risk Factors

Leading cause of cancer deaths in the United States (30% of all cancer deaths). Majority (85–90%) of cases are attributed to tobacco use with an ↑ number of cases in former smokers. Smokers with asbestos exposure have a 50- to 100-fold ↑ risk. Head and neck cancers, smoking-related COPD, sarcoidosis, and possibly TB are also associated with an ↑ lung cancer risk.

Types

Histologic categories are summarized in Table 16-2.

40% of lung cancer patients have metastases at time of presentation.

Signs/Symptoms

Symptoms include cough, dyspnea, hemoptysis, fatigue, and weight loss. Physical exam may demonstrate supraclavicular or scalene lymphadenopathy or focal neurologic deficit if brain metastases are present. Paraneoplastic syndromes

TABLE 16-2. Histologic Categories of Lung Cancer

Histologic Category	% of Lung Cancer Cases	Notes
Small cell lung cancer (SCLC; oat cell)	20–25	Neuroendocrine origin. Associated with **paraneoplastic syndromes**. Often local or distant metastases present at time of presentation. **Central** location.
Non–SCLC	75–80	
Squamous cell carcinoma	25–35	From bronchial epithelium. Characteristic **keratin pearls. Central** location. **Tumor growth rate is slower and metastases** are less common than in other types.
Adenocarcinoma	25–35	From mucous glands. **Peripheral** location. Includes **bronchoalveolar type**. Increasing incidence.
Large cell carcinoma	10	**Central or peripheral location.**

TABLE 16-3. **Paraneoplastic Syndromes**

Paraneoplastic Syndrome	Associated Cancer	Signs/Symptoms
Hypertrophic pulmonary osteoarthropathy	Adenocarcinoma	Periostitis of fibula, tibia, radius, metacarpals, metatarsals; clubbing.
Hypercalcemia	SCC	↑ Ca^{2+} due to PTHrP.
SIADH	SCLC, thymoma	High urine osmolarity in spite of low serum osmolarity (see Chapter 12).
Cushing's syndrome	SCLC, thymoma	Results from ACTH analogue production. Patient will fail dexamethasone suppression test.
Eaton-Lambert syndrome	SCLC	Caused by antibodies against Ca^{2+} channels. Causes weakness that improves with repeated effort. **Neostigmine is NOT effective**.

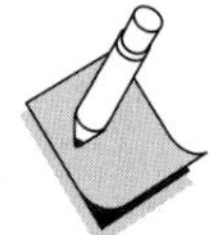

Signs of Pancoast tumors–

Ptosis, miosis, anhydrosis

or local obstructive syndromes (eg, superior vena cava [SVC] syndrome) may be present (see Table 16-3). **A Pancoast tumor** is a superior sulcus tumor affecting the brachial plexus and the sympathetic trunk causing **ptosis**, **miosis**, and **anhydrosis**.

Diagnosis

CXR may show a nodule or mass, persistent infiltrate, atelectasis, hilar or mediastinal lymphadenopathy, or pleural effusion. **Chest CT** is the best noninvasive tool for identifying mediastinal lymph node metastases; specificity is 70%. Other noninvasive staging options are PET, endoscopic ultrasound, and bronchoscopic fine needle aspiration (FNA). **Gold standard remains mediastinoscopy.** Perform biopsy of suspicious masses and lymph nodes and obtain cytologic evaluation of suspicious effusions.

Treatment

Based on stage of disease.

- **Stage I and II: Anatomic resection (eg, lobectomy) has a clear survival advantage over wedge resection.** Other operations include sleeve resection (if adequate bronchial margin cannot be obtained by conventional lobectomy) and pneumonectomy (for large, centrally located tumors or bulky, extracapsular N1 nodal spread). Tumors involving the chest wall and diaphragm are resected en bloc. Though mortality is significantly higher, consider a limited surgical resection (wedge resection) or 1° radiotherapy for poor operative candidates. Adjuvant and neoadjuvant regimens for early stage disease are under investigation.

- **Stage III (locoregionally advanced disease)**: In patients with limited lymph node involvement or anatomically accessible tumors, surgical resection continues to play a role. In stage IIIA patients, cisplatin-based neoadjuvant chemotherapy followed by surgical resection is the standard. Stage IIIB patients are not generally operative candidates (except for tumors involving the SVC, carina, or vertebral bodies with N0 or N1 disease). Most locoregionally advanced cases are treated with cisplatin-based chemoradiation (concurrent or sequential).
- **Stage IV (metastatic disease): Chemotherapy** is the mainstay of therapy. Select patients with a single brain metastasis can be treated with surgical excision of both the 1° and metastatic tumor.

Absolute indication for mediastinoscopy = nodes > 1 cm on chest CT. Relative indications for mediastinoscopy = centrally located tumor, T2 or T3 1° tumor, adenocarcinoma, or large cell pathology (higher rate of metastasis).

Perform preoperative risk stratification for surgical candidates. Relative contraindications to lung surgery due to high morbidity include **preoperative FEV_1 < 0.8 L, predicted postoperative FEV_1 < 0.8 L, $Paco_2$ > 45 mm Hg, Pao_2 < 50 mm Hg, and maximum voluntary ventilation < 50%.** For indeterminate cases, qualitative V/Q scans can predict who will tolerate a lobar resection. Diffusing capacity of lung for CO (DLCO) < 60% is also associated with ↑ mortality. Additional guidelines include:

- Functional status: If a patient walks three flights of stairs, he/she will tolerate a pneumonectomy. If he/she walks two flights, he/she will tolerate a lobectomy. If he/she walks one flight, he/she will tolerate a wedge resection.
- Ability to walk > 1000 feet in 6 minutes predicts an uncomplicated postoperative course.

STAGING/OUTCOME

Tumor, node status, metastasis (TNM) categories include

- T: T1 (< 3 cm, completely intraparenchymal), T2 (> 3 cm, involving main bronchus > 2 cm distal to carina, disease invading visceral pleural, or disease causing local [segmental] obstruction), T3 (involves chest wall, proximal main bronchus, diaphragm, parietal pleura, or complete [lobar] obstructive atelectasis), T4 (involves mediastinum, heart, trachea, or esophagus *or* results in malignant effusion *or* associated with ipsilateral satellite lesion)
- N: N0 (– lymph nodes), N1 (+ ipsilateral peribronchial, hilar, or intraparenchymal nodes), N2 (+ ipsilateral mediastinal or subcarinal nodes), N3 (+ ipsilateral supraclavicular, scalene, or contralateral pulmonary nodes)
- M: M0 (metastatic disease absent), M1 (metastatic disease present)

Staging includes

- Stage I: T1N0M0 *or* T2N0M0
- Stage II: T1N1M0 *or* T2N1M0 *or* T3N0M0
- Stage III: T1N2M0 *or* T2N2M0 *or* T3N0M0 *or* T3N1M0 *or* T3N2M0 *or* T4, any N, M0 *or* Any T, N3M0
- Stage IV: Any T, any N, M1

Five-year survival varies from 75% for stage I disease, to 35% for stage II, 10-25% for stage III, and < 5% for stage IV.

Pneumothorax

Air in the pleural space caused by a pleural (eg, parietal, visceral) insult.

SPONTANEOUS PTX

Most common etiology is **bleb rupture**. Risk factors include tobacco use, male gender, young age, and **tall, thin body habitus**. Treatment begins with chest tube insertion. If leak is present ≥ 3 days, treat persistent PTX with pleurodesis (eg, mechanical, talc). Risk of ipsilateral recurrence is up to 30% at 6 months and 50% at 2 years. Consider wedge resection of blebs and mechanical pleurodesis for recurrence.

TENSION PTX

A ball-valve effect allows air into the pleural space, which is then trapped. Positive pressure ventilation can convert a simple PTX into a tension PTX. Results in respiratory distress, tracheal deviation, muffled, ipsilateral breath sounds, distended neck veins, and ultimately, **shock** (due to impaired filling of right ventricle). Treat with emergent chest tube placement, with or without preprocedure needle decompression.

Removal of aerated but poorly perfused emphysematous regions in lung volume reduction surgery should improve pulmonary mechanics.

Chronic Obstructive Pulmonary Disease

Fourth leading cause of United States deaths; affects 32 million Americans. Types include chronic bronchitis, emphysema, and asthma. Emphystematous blebs carry a high incidence of spontaneous PTX. Medical treatment includes supplemental O_2, bronchodilater therapy, and steroids. Consider lung volume reduction surgery in patients with **heterogeneous emphysema with apical predominance**. Compared to medically managed patients, select surgically managed patients have improved exercise capacity and quality of life. Operative mortality is ~17%; after 2 years, patients begin to decline toward baseline status.

Lung Transplantation

INDICATIONS

Most common indications are **COPD, idiopathic pulmonary fibrosis (IPF), 1° pulmonary HTN, and cystic fibrosis (CF). Pulmonary function test** (PFT) criteria include FEV_1 < 25% of predicted or in IPF patients, FVC < 60%, or DLCO < 50% of predicted. Concurrent cardiac transplant is indicated for uncorrectable congenital heart disease (eg, Eisenmenger's syndrome) or ventricular failure. Consider bilateral lung transplant in patients with pulmonary failure due COPD or CF.

COMPLICATIONS

Early mortality is most commonly due to **ischemia reperfusion injury** (1° graft failure). Signs include edema, hypoxia, and V/Q mismatch. Management is similar to that of acute respiratory distress syndrome. Long-term mortality can be caused by **bronchiolitis obliterans syndrome** (BOS; chronic rejection), which is associated with progressive cough and dyspnea on exertion. See Chapter 20 for additional transplant-related complications.

OUTCOMES

Summarized in Table 16-4.

TABLE 16-4. Graft and Patient Survival After Lung Transplantation

Time After Transplant (years)	Graft Survival (%)	Patient Survival (%)
1	76	77
5	41	59
10	18	23

Massive Hemoptysis

Greater than 600 mL of blood loss over 24 hours. Causes include acute (eg, necrotizing pneumonia) or chronic (eg, TB, CF) inflammatory processes as well as neoplastic lesions. Results from ↑ pressure in or erosion into pulmonary or bronchial circulation. Diagnosis is clinical. Workup, when patient stabilizes, includes CXR, chest CT, bronchoscopy (flexible or rigid), or if necessary, diagnostic angiography. Emergent management for persistent, massive hemorrhage includes **airway control** (via occlusion of mainstem bronchus on bleeding side with double-lumen endotracheal tube, bronchial blocker in bleeding side), rigid bronchoscopy with cannulation of nonbleeding site, and iced saline lavage of bleeding site. Nonemergent management for persistent, submassive hemorrhage includes **Trendelenburg positioning with affected side down**, aerosolized epinephrine, IV vasopressin, and correction of coagulopathy. Bronchoscopy (with epinephrine lavage) and angiography (with embolization) can be both diagnostic and therapeutic. Though few patients require emergent operative correction, indications for urgent operative intervention include fungus ball, abscess, cavitary disease, and uncontrolled bleeding. Associated with up to 60% recurrence (after embolization) and up to 50% mortality.

Rasmussen's aneurysm—*Erosion of a blood vessel into a cavitary TB lesion, forming a pocket of blood*

A 58-year-old woman presents with dyspnea. CXR reveals a large left pleural effusion. Thoracentesis yields bloody pleural fluid. What are the three most likely causes, and how can they be evaluated? Occult malignancy (evaluate with pleural fluid cytology and chest, abdomen, and pelvis CT), pulmonary embolism ([PE]; evaluate with spiral chest CT), and TB (evaluate with acid fact bacteria [AFB] stain of pleural fluid as well as [AFB] stain and culture of induced sputum).

Pleural Effusion

Demographics/Risk Factors

Fluid collection in pleural space. Most commonly associated with congestive heart failure (CHF), pneumonia, PE, and malignancy. Malignant pleural effusions suggest advanced disease and are associated with a mean survival of 3–11 months. Most common malignant causes in men are lung cancer (50%) and lymphoma; breast (37%) and gynecologic (20%) sources are more common in women.

TABLE 16-5. Transudative and Exudative Pleural Effusion Differentiation

Diagnostic Criteria	Transudative Effusion	Exudative Effusion
Pleural fluid protein/Serum protein	< 0.5	> 0.5
Pleural fluid LDH/Serum LDH	< 0.6	> 0.6
Pleural fluid LDH level	< 2/3 of upper limit for serum LDH level	> 2/3 of upper limit for serum LDH level

Types

May be **transudative or exudative**. Etiologies vary by type.

- Transudative (protein-poor): CHF, cirrhosis.
- Exudative (protein-rich): Parapneumonic effusion, malignant effusion, PE, viral infection, postsurgical and posttraumatic.

Signs/Symptoms

Associated with fever, cough, and dyspnea.

Diagnosis

Determination of effusion type is based on the pleural fluid-to-serum protein and lactate dehydrogenase (LDH) levels (see Table 16-5). Exudative effusions may also be associated with fluid that has ↑ hematocrit (HCT; eg, malignancy, trauma, PE), ↑ white blood cell (WBC) counts (eg, malignancy, TB), ↑ amylase (eg, acute pancreatitis, pseudocyst, esophageal rupture), and ↓ glucose (ie, < 60 mg/dL).

Treatment

Drain and pleurodese symptomatic effusions.

Empyema

Purulent pleural effusion. Most common in elderly, debilitated, and immunocompromised patients. Due to **extension of lung or mediastinal infection**; hematogenous spread or traumatic or iatrogenic inoculation can occur. Most common organisms are ***Streptococcus pneumoniae*, *Staphylococcus aureus*, and Gram - bacteria** (eg, *Escherichia coli, Klebsiella pneumoniae, Pseudomonas aeruginosa*). Three disease phases include **exudative (acute), fibrinopurulent, and organizing (chronic)**. Associated with fever, chest pain, and dyspnea. Confirm diagnosis with thoracentesis of **purulent** pleural fluid that has a **pH** < 7.2 and **glucose < 40 mg/dL**. If tube thoracostomy does not re-expand lung, VATS decortication or open thoracotomy with decortication may be required.

> Phases of empyema pathology—**EXUDATING FIBRIN ORGANIZES:**
> Acute **exudative**: Pus accumulation, mobile lung
> **Fibrin**opurulent: Loculation of fluid, trapped lung
> Chronic **organizing**: Scar formation, fixed lung

Mediastinal Masses

Mediastinal masses vary by mediastinal compartment and patient age (see Table 16-6).

TABLE 16-6. **Mediastinal Masses**

Adult Population		Pediatric Population	
Type of Mass	**Compartment**	**Type of Mass**	**Compartment**
Neurogenic tumor	Posterior	Neurogenic tumor	Posterior
Benign cyst	Any	Lymphoma	Anterior/Middle
Thymoma	Anterior	Benign cyst	Any
Lymphoma	Anterior/middle	Germ cell tumor	Anterior
Germ cell tumor	Anterior	Mesenchymal tumor	Any

THYMOMA

Common in adults 40–60 years of age. Circulating **antibodies against acetylcholine receptor** are found in up to 50% of patients and result in **myasthenia gravis;** < 10% of myasthenia patients have a thymoma. May be associated with paraneoplastic syndromes (eg, Cushing's, SIADH) and compression. Requires complete surgical resection usually with chemoradiation.

NEUROGENIC TUMORS

Most arise from the nerve sheath and require resection, if possible.

LYMPHOMA

Most common malignancy of the mediastinum. Treat with radiation and chemotherapy.

GERM CELL TUMORS

Majority are **teratomas** and can be resected with a good prognosis. **Seminoma** is usually discovered when advanced disease causes compressive symptoms. Treatment includes neoadjuvant cisplatin-based chemotherapy with etoposide or vinblastine followed by resection of residual mass. Treat **nonseminomatous germ cell tumors** similarly.

MEDIASTINAL CYSTS

Bronchogenic cysts arise from abnormal foregut or tracheobronchial tree buds. Resect if found in symptomatic adult or asymptomatic children (because of risk of enlargement, airway compression, infection, malignant transformation). **Enteric cysts** should be removed due to possible complications from enlargement. Other cysts (eg, 1°, pericardial, thymic) should be resected if symptomatic or if malignancy is suspected.

Chest Wall Tumors

Consider these to be malignant unless proven otherwise (see Table 16-7).

Excisional biopsy for tissue diagnosis is preferred if wound can be closed primarily. Treatment is lesion-specific.

TABLE 16-7. Chest Wall Tumors

TYPE	TUMOR TYPE	NOTES
Benign	Chondroma	Affects children and young adults. Can grow very large. Excise with 2-cm margins.
	Fibrous dysplasia	Rarely painful. May be associated with **trauma**. Excise with 2-cm margins.
	Osteochondroma	**Most common benign bone tumor**. Carries some malignant potential. Excise with 2-cm margins.
	Eosinophilic granuloma	Benign osteolytic lesions. Can be locally excised.
	Desmoid tumor	Fibroblastic tumors. May form at site of old incisions. Should be locally excised with 2- to 4-cm margins. **High recurrence rate.**
Malignant	Chondrosarcoma	**Most common 1° chest wall malignancy.** Requires 4-cm margins. No benefit associated with chemoradiation.
	Osteosarcoma	Treat with neoadjuvant chemotherapy followed by excision with 4-cm margins.
	Other chest wall tumors	Primitive neuroectodermal tumors, Ewing's sarcoma, plasmacytoma.

Tracheostomies

Indications include **prolonged intubation, mechanical ventilation, pulmonary toilet, and impaired airway reflexes.** Complications include wound infection, large vessel erosion (**tracheoinnominate fistula**), tracheal stenosis, recurrent laryngeal nerve injury, PTX, and pneumomediastinum. Major hemorrhage from a tracheoinnominate fistula is usually preceded by a **herald bleed**. Treatment includes rapid diagnosis, airway stabilization, rigid bronchoscopy, and immediate fistula resection.

▶ SAMPLE QUESTIONS

What are possible causes of a pleural effusion with low LDH and protein?	Cirrhosis, CHF.
What are the causes of an effusion with high LDH and protein?	Parapneumonic effusion, malignant effusion, postsurgical or posttraumatic causes.
What are the stages of the following lung cancers? (a) 3.5 cm mass confined to the parenchyma of the lung without lymphatic spread. (b) 2 cm mass associated with a pleural effusion containing malignant cells. (c) 5 cm mass firmly adherent to the diaphragm without nodal involvement. (d) 2 cm mass with spread to the ipsilateral peritracheal nodes.	(a) IIA (b) IIIA (c) IIB (d) IIIB
What is the difference in pathophysiology between Eaton-Lambert syndrome and myasthenia gravis?	Eaton-Lambert = antibody against voltage-gated Ca^{2+} channel. Myasthenia = antibody against acetylcholine receptor.
How can Eaton-Lambert syndrome be distinguished from myasthenia gravis by physical exam?	Weakness with myasthenia gets better with rest. Weakness improves with repeated effort in Eaton-Lambert.
What agent is used to test for myasthenia gravis?	Edrophonium (tensilon test).
Are the following tumors likely to be resectable or unresectable? (a) 3.5 cm mass invading the chest wall. (b) 2 cm mass with an ipsilateral pleural effusion. (c) 2 cm adenocarcinoma with solitary brain metastasis. (d) 3 cm tumor with metastasis to a contralateral scalene node.	(a) Resectable. Requires en bloc resection of involved chest wall. (b) Check cytology. Unresectable if it is a malignant effusion. Otherwise, resectable. (c) Resectable if both 1° tumor and solitary metastatic lesion can be removed. (d) Unresectable. Contralateral scalene nodal disease counts as M1 disease.
Name the paraneoplastic syndromes commonly associated with SCLC.	Cushing's syndrome, SIADH, Eaton-Lambert syndrome.
What radiographic features suggest that a solitary lung nodule is benign?	Smooth calcifications, doubling time < 20 days or > 450 days, size < 2 cm.

What radiographic features suggest that a solitary lung nodule is malignant?	Lobulations, corona radiata sign, doubling time 30–450 days, size > 2 cm.
What cancers should be specifically ruled out in smokers with lung cancer?	Head and neck cancer, esophageal cancer.
What diseases should be suspected in a 60-year-old woman with a bloody pleural effusion?	Occult malignancy (ovarian cancer), PE, TB, occult trauma.
What common cause of mediastinal mass should be suspected in adults but not children?	Thymoma.

CHAPTER 17

Vascular

Andrew J. Meltzer, MD
Reviewed by James H. Balcom IV, MD

The Bernoulli principle is the basis for using duplex ultrasonography to evaluate the extent of carotid stenosis.

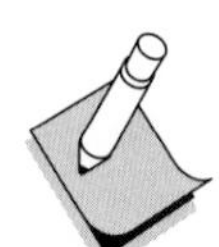

Poiseuille's law—
$F = \pi pr^4/8\ \mu L$

Poiseuille's law explains why short, peripheral IVs are preferable to long, central lines for rapid resuscitation.

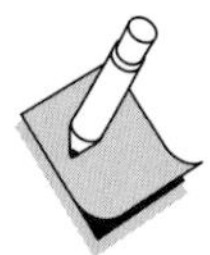

Law of Laplace—
Wall tension is proportional to pressure × radius

▶ BASIC SCIENCE

Principles of Hemodynamics

BERNOULLI PRINCIPLE

For an ideal fluid, ↑ **velocity occurs in conjunction with ↓ pressure** (or potential energy). Therefore, as the diameter of a blood vessel ↓ (ie, stenosis), blood flow velocity ↑ and BP ↓.

POISEUILLE'S LAW

Describes laminar flow through a cylindrical tube. States that flow is

- Directly related to pressure gradient.
- Directly related to the vessel radius raised to the fourth power (r^4).
- Inversely related to length.

LAW OF LAPLACE

Arterial aneurysms rupture when tangential stress exceeds tensile wall strength. Law of Laplace states that **wall tension ↑ as intravascular pressure and vessel diameter ↑**. When applied to aneurysm pathophysiology, this law leads to two conclusions:

- Aneurysm size (ie, diameter) is a predictor of risk and should dictate timing of operative intervention.
- BP control (ie, ↓ intravascular pressure) reduces risk of rupture.

Anatomy

MACROSCOPIC ANATOMY

Anatomy of the abdominal arterial and venous systems is depicted in Figure 17-1.

MICROSCOPIC ANATOMY

Systemic arteries are more muscular than pulmonary vessels or systemic veins due to high pressure flow. There are three major layers of the arterial wall:

- Tunica externa: Outermost layer. Composed of collagen.
- Tunica media: Middle layer. Composed of smooth muscle cells and elastic tissue.
- Tunica intima: Innermost layer. Composed of a single layer of endothelial cells and an internal elastic lamina basement membrane.

Veins also have three layers, though connective tissue and smooth muscle mass is less than in arteries. Medium and large veins have valves to prevent retrograde blood flow. Unlike arteries, veins are highly distensible, and significant changes in volume do not translate into significant changes in pressure (ie, veins are **capacitance vessels**).

Pathophysiology of Atherosclerosis

Atherosclerosis is the 1° cause of luminal narrowing and ↓ arterial flow. Follows a defined pathophysiologic course: endothelial injury → monocyte accumulation

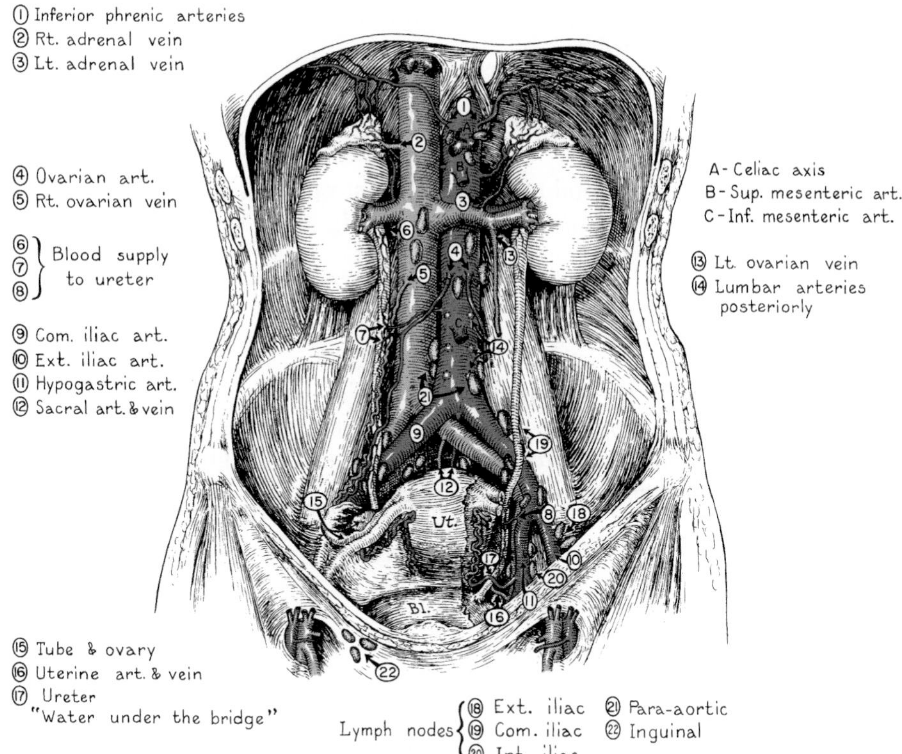

FIGURE 17-1. Anatomy of the abdominal arteries and veins. See also color insert.

(Reproduced, with permission, from Zollinger RM Jr, Zollinger RM Sr. *Zollinger's Atlas of Surgical Operations*, 8th ed. New York: McGraw-Hill, 2003:19.)

→ macrophage accumulation of lipid (foam cell) → fatty streak → smooth muscle cell proliferation → endothelial disruption → atheroma → fibrous plaque → complex plaque → rupture.

Risk factors for developing atherosclerotic disease are summarized in Table 17-1.

Noninvasive Monitoring of Vascular Disease

Duplex Ultrasound

Noninvasive, noncontrast visualization of arterial anatomy. Duplex functionality permits measurement of peak systolic and end diastolic velocities.

TABLE 17-1. Risk Factors for Atherosclerotic Arterial Disease

Risk Stratification	Risk Factors
Major	Tobacco use, ↑ age, diabetes mellitus (DM), hyperlipidemia, HTN, + family history, homocysteinemia, hyperfibrinogenemia, ↑ lipoprotein A
Minor	Obesity, sedentary lifestyle, male gender, hypercoagulable states, non-white race, excessive alcohol use, ↑ C-reactive protein

(Adapted, with permission, for Doherty GM, Way LW. *Current Surgical Diagnosis and Treatment*, 12th ed. New York: McGraw-Hill, 2006:795.)

Velocities allow measurement of stenosis through application of the Bernoulli principle.

SEGMENTAL PRESSURE MEASUREMENT

Measurement of systolic blood pressure (SBP) at various sites along extremity. **Intersegmental systolic drop of > 20 mm Hg may identify the site of occlusion.**

ANKLE-BRACHIAL INDEX

SBP at the ankle/SBP the brachial artery. Ankle-brachial index (ABI) ≥ 1 → normal. ABI 0.5-1 → moderate disease. ABI < 0.5 → severe disease. **Highly calcified vessels are noncompressible, so ABI is falsely high.** Important clinical correlations can be made based on ABI values:

- ABI 0.5–0.7: Claudication
- ABI 0.3–0.5: Rest pain
- ABI < 0.3: Gangrene

PULSE VOLUME RECORDING

Also known as plethysmography. Measures dynamic volume changes of a limb. **Assesses presence or absence of pulsatile blood flow.** Does not depend on compressibility of vessels and, therefore, is particularly useful in patients with calcified vessels.

CT ANGIOGRAPHY AND MR ANGIOGRAPHY

Permit three-dimensional analysis of vessels following iodine-based contrast (CTA) or gadolinium (MRA) injection.

DIGITAL SUBTRACTION ANGIOGRAPHY

Invasive test that remains the gold standard for assessment of vascular anatomy and disease in extremities.

Reperfusion Injury

Damage to tissues that occurs after blood flow is resumed in a previously ischemic extremity. White blood cells arrive with restored circulation and release inflammatory cytokines and O_2 free radicals in response to damaged tissue. Xanthine oxidase converts molecular O_2 to the highly reactive superoxide and hydroxyl radicals. **Superoxide** and **O_2 free radicals** damage cellular proteins, DNA, and the plasma membrane. The massive inflow of leukocytes may cause capillary bed occlusion and further ischemic insult.

Complications might include hypotension, **metabolic acidosis**, **hyperkalemia** with subsequent arrhythmias, **myoglobinuria** with subsequent acute tubular necrosis, and compartment syndrome. Recognize early, and treat with aggressive hydration, normalization of electrolytes, support of renal blood flow (e.g., mannitol), alkalinization of urine (e.g., HCO_3^-), and pressor support, if necessary.

▶ CLINICAL SCIENCE

Carotid Disease

DEMOGRAPHICS/RISK FACTORS

Manifestation of atherosclerotic disease. Risk factors are summarized in Table 17-1.

SIGNS/SYMPTOMS

Atherosclerosis of the internal carotid artery may present as an **asymptomatic carotid bruit (most common)**, transient neurologic or ophthalmologic deficit(s) lasting < 24 hours (transient ischemia attack [TIA]), or persistent (> 24 hours) motor and sensory deficit (cerebrovascular accident [CVA]). TIAs are most commonly due to emboli rather than to hypoperfusion.

DIAGNOSIS

Severity of luminal narrowing is based on velocity criteria as measured by Doppler ultrasound. **Velocity ↑ with luminal narrowing.** Arteriography, CTA, and MRA are adjunctive imaging modalities.

TREATMENT

Carotid endarterectomy (CEA) removes atherosclerotic plaque at the carotid bifurcation (see Figure 17-2). Indications differ based on the presence or absence of symptoms. In the setting of recent CVA, recommend CEA 4–6 weeks after recovery.

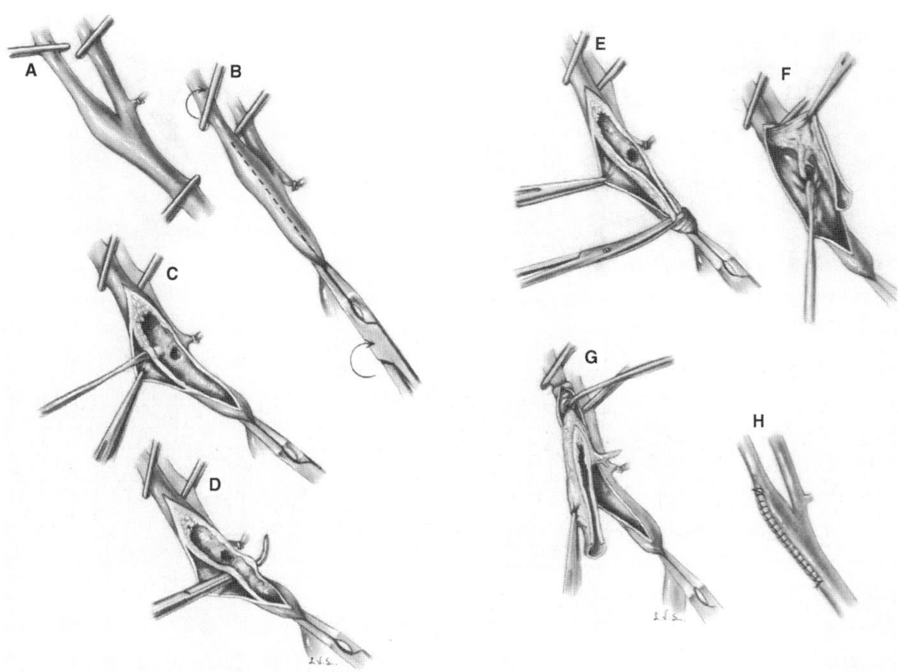

FIGURE 17-2. Technique of carotid endarterectomy.

(Reproduced, with permission, from Doherty GM, Way LW. *Current Surgical Diagnosis and Treatment,* 12th ed. New York: McGraw-Hill, 2006:795.)

- **North American Symptomatic Carotid Endarterectomy Trial**: For **symptomatic patients with carotid stenosis ≥ 70%**, performing CEA significantly ↓ the incidence of ipsilateral CVA. Patients with moderate (50–69%) stenosis also benefit from CEA. Patients with mild stenoses (< 50%) do not benefit from surgery and should be medically managed.
- **Asymptomatic Carotid Atherosclerosis Study:** Five-year CVA risk is **significantly ↓ in asymptomatic patients managed with CEA who have ≥ 60% stenosis**. For those with stenosis < 60%, medical management is indicated.

Aortic Dissection

DEMOGRAPHICS/RISK FACTORS

Involves an aortic intimal tear allowing separation from the medial layer and escape of blood from the true lumen. Affects ~5–10 patients per million annually. Risk factors are similar to that of other arterial diseases but also include the presence of **connective tissue disorders** (e.g., Marfan's or Ehlers-Danlos syndromes), aortitis, bicuspid aortic valve, medial degenerative disease, aortic injury, pregnancy, and cocaine and amphetamine use.

TYPES

Stanford and DeBakey classification systems define the type of dissection (see Figure 17-3).

Stanford classification of aortic dissections–
Type A: Ascending aorta (regardless of origin)
Type B: Descending aorta

DeBakey classification of aortic dissections–
Type I: Ascending aorta, arch, descending aorta
Type II: Ascending aorta only
Type III: Descending aorta, distal to the subclavian

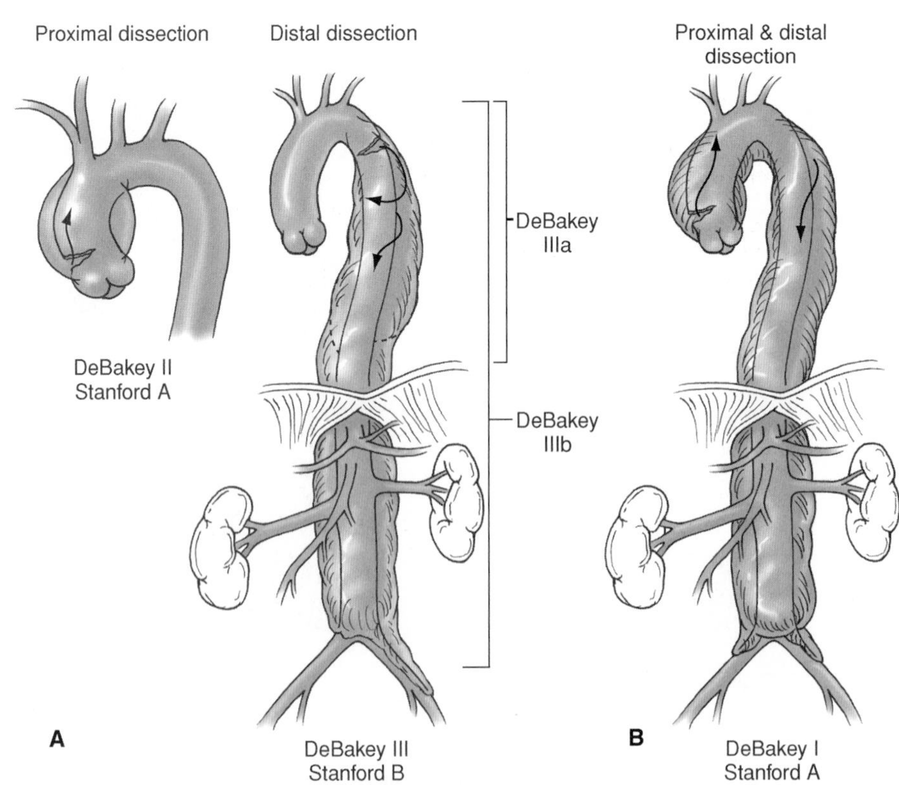

FIGURE 17-3. Classifications of aortic dissections.

(Reproduced, with permission, from Brunicardi FC, et al. *Schwartz's Principles of Surgery*, 8th ed. New York: McGraw-Hill, 2005:704.)

SIGNS/SYMPTOMS

Presents with **acute onset of chest or back pain** with maximal intensity at onset. Pain migrates as flap moves distally, resulting in a tearing sensation. May secondarily cause heart failure, aortic insufficiency, myocardial infarction (MI), CVA, or other end-organ failure.

Classic aortic dissection findings–

Discrepancy in pulse or BP among extremities

DIAGNOSIS

History and physical examination should raise suspicion for this diagnosis. CXR may show **widened mediastinum**. CT, MRI, or transesophageal echo (TEE) are used for definitive diagnosis. Duration of study may preclude use of MRI; operator-dependence limits use of TEE.

TREATMENT

Initial management of suspected or confirmed aortic dissection is **aggressive BP control** (β-blockade followed by nitroprusside). Continuous BP monitoring using the right radial artery is preferred. The **rate of change in BP (Δ Pressure/Δ time) is of particular importance.** Operative management (e.g., open or endovascular grafts) aims to obliterate the false lumen and **is indicated urgently in acute type A dissections**. Type B dissections are managed nonoperatively; surgical repair is indicated for aortic rupture, ↑ periaortic or pleural fluid, rapidly expanding aortic diameter, uncontrolled HTN, and persistent pain despite adequate medical therapy. Operative intervention carries a mortality rate of > 15%. Immediate postoperative concerns include MI, paralysis, and extremity ischemia. Patients have ↑ long-term risk of distal aortic aneurysmal dilation and therefore should be followed with annual imaging.

Thoracic Aortic Aneurysm

DEMOGRAPHICS/RISK FACTORS

Isolated thoracic aortic aneurysms (TAAs) are less common than abdominal aortic aneurysms (AAA). Classified as atherosclerotic (i.e., wall remodeling and dilation) or degenerative (i.e., abnormal collagen metabolism). Causes of degenerative aneurysms include Marfan's syndrome, Ehlers-Danlos syndrome, cystic medial degeneration, and infection (e.g., mycotic aneurysm).

SIGNS/SYMPTOMS

Often asymptomatic and diagnosed incidentally after CXR or CT. When present, symptoms are related to compression of adjacent structures (esophageal compression → dysphagia; tracheal compression → stridor; recurrent laryngeal nerve compression → vocal cord paralysis), leak, or frank rupture.

DIAGNOSIS

History may reveal symptoms of connective tissue diseases, HTN, or prior aortic infection. CXR may show a **prominent aortic knob**. CT is more specific for anatomy and extent of dilation; MRA provides high-resolution images of the aorta and is particularly useful for assessing involvement of branch vessels.

TREATMENT

Determined by maximal aortic diameter and the presence of symptoms.

- Asymptomatic patients with TAAs < 5 cm require aggressive control of BP.
- Repair TAAs if > 6 cm, enlarging > 1 cm/year, or symptomatic.
- Manage patients with connective tissue diseases with a lower threshold for intervention.
- Ascending and arch aneurysms require open repair via a median sternotomy with cardiopulmonary bypass.
- Descending aneurysms (distal to the left subclavian artery) may be repaired via a left thoracotomy with single lung ventilation. Careful attention is given to preserving spinal cord circulation or spinal cord cooling.
- Endovascular repairs are being performed with increasing frequency.

Complications include spinal cord ischemia (5–7%), renal failure (4–7%), pulmonary failure, vocal cord paralysis, esophageal injury, and death (5% for ascending repairs, 5–10% for descending repairs).

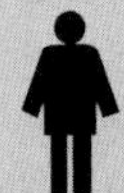

A patient undergoes an open AAA repair. Postoperatively, he has increasing abdominal pain, bloody diarrhea, and leukocytosis. What is the next step to confirm his likely diagnosis? A bedside colonoscopy will reveal colonic ischemia.

Abdominal Aortic Aneurysm

DEMOGRAPHICS/RISK FACTORS

Exist in 2% of the elderly male population. **Rupture is a leading cause of death** (see Figure 17-4). HTN and tobacco use are significant risk factors, though family history also confers ↑ risk. The involved aortic segment is typically below the takeoff of the renal arteries.

TYPES

Classified according to location, severity, and etiology. Examples include:

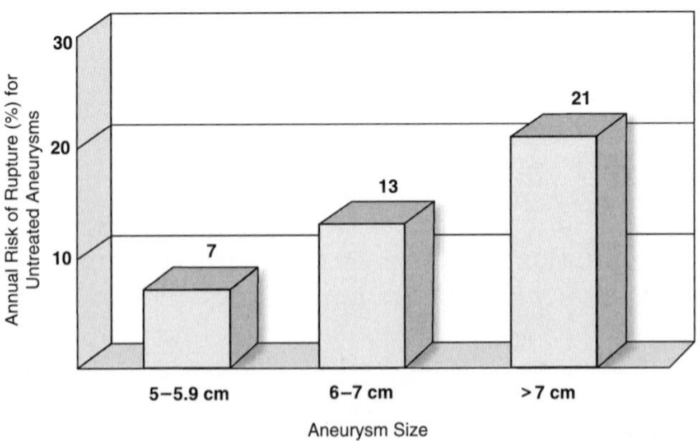

FIGURE 17-4. Risk of AAA rupture based on size.

(Reproduced, with permission, from Brunicardi FC, et al. *Schwartz's Principles of Surgery*, 8th ed. New York: McGraw-Hill, 2005:732.)

- **Suprarenal:** Uncommon. Located proximal to renal arteries. Low risk of rupture until > 6–7 cm. Ruptures usually leak to the left posterolateral space.
- **Infected (mycotic):** Bacterial contamination of preexisting aneurysm. Gram infections result in ↑ rupture rates.

SIGNS/SYMPTOMS

Contained AAAs are usually asymptomatic. Leaking or ruptured AAAs are classically associated with **abdominal pain, back pain, a pulsatile abdominal mass, and hypotension.**

DIAGNOSIS

Perform serial ultrasounds for small aneurysms to assess changes in size. Perform CT and MRA preoperatively for detailed anatomy. Aortography is rarely needed.

TREATMENT

Dictated by risk of rupture, which is in turn related to aneurysm size. **Repair (e.g., open, endovascular) is indicated for AAAs > 5.5 cm or those that are rapidly enlarging.** Open repair consists of AAA resection and replacement with tubular or bifurcated prosthetic graft. May be performed via transperitoneal or retroperitoneal approach. For suprarenal AAAs, use a thoracoabdominal approach and reimplant the celiac, superior mesenteric artery (SMA), and renal arteries. Ruptured AAAs require emergent surgery with **proximal control being the first priority.** For mycotic lesions, excise the AAA and perform an extra-anatomic bypass; long-term antibiotics are necessary. For inflammatory AAA, do not dissect the duodenum from the AAA.

General rule of thumb for AAA repair–

> 5.5 cm or enlarging > 0.5-1 cm/year → surgical repair

< 5.5 cm → serial ultrasounds.

Endovascular repair may be employed for AAAs with limited aortic tortuosity and an appropriate neck (i.e., proximal to the AAA and distal to the renal arteries) conducive to stent placement.

Immediate postoperative complications include bleeding, renal failure, MI, infection, colonic ischemia, extremity ischemia, and erectile dysfunction. Morbidity is 5–10%; operative mortality with open repair is 2–4%. **Paraplegia** is a rare complication due to an aberrantly low artery of Adamkiewicz. **Colonic ischemia** may occur due to ↓ inferior mesenteric artery perfusion. Diagnosis is confirmed with colonoscopy; if full thickness necrosis is present with systemic illness, perform urgent colectomy.

Delayed postoperative complications include **aorto-enteric fistula** (< 1%) in which the proximal graft erodes into the duodenum. May present with a **herald bleed** prior to massive hemorrhage. Perform prompt esophagogastroduodenoscopy (EGD) to confirm diagnosis in the stable patient. Treat with duodenal repair, graft excision, and extra-anatomic bypass.

Postoperatively endovascular patients should be screened annually with CT to assess for **endoleak.**

- Type I endoleak: Ineffective proximal or distal sealing. **Requires immediate correction.**
- Type II endoleak: Results in persistent flow through the aneurysm via low pressure collaterals. Does not warrant repair unless aneurysm is enlarging.
- Type III endoleak: Involves a leak between components of a modular graft. Requires intervention.

An 80-year-old female with atrial fibrillation (AF) has the sudden onset of midabdominal pain out of proportion to exam. She is hemodynamically unstable, and labs reveal leukocytosis with a left shift and lactic acidosis. What is the next step in management? Start fluid resuscitation, broad spectrum antibiotics, and proceed emergently to the OR with a presumptive diagnosis of acute mesenteric ischemia.

Mesenteric Ischemia

Demographics/Risk Factors

Rare disorder involving ↓ perfusion and reperfusion injury. Most commonly affects elderly who have diseases leading to embolic activity (e.g., AF).

Types

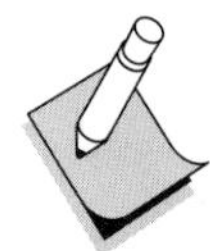

Embolic versus thrombotic mesenteric ischemia–
Embolic: Emboli lodge in SMA distal to middle colic artery. Spares proximal jejunum and transverse colon.
Thrombotic: Lesion present at SMA origin. Involves entire small intestine, right colon, and transverse colon.

Acute arterial mesenteric ischemia is divided into embolic, thrombotic, and nonocclusive forms.

- Embolic: 30–50% of cases. Emboli arise from left atrium or left ventricle. Most common site of occlusion is the **SMA, distal to the middle colic artery.**
- Thrombotic: Most commonly found at the **origin of SMA**. Results from thrombosis superimposed on area of atherosclerosis. More proximal the occlusion → more bowel at risk.
- Nonocclusive: Found in critically ill patients. Commonly related to vasopressor administration and low-flow states that result in **vasoconstriction of the mesenteric vessels**. Weak arterial pulsation may be present, and any area of bowel may be affected.

Acute venous occlusion occurs in patients with **hypercoagulable states**, and most commonly involves the SMV. Chronic mesenteric ischemia is most common in middle-aged women, resulting in a gradual ↓ in blood flow caused by atherosclerotic disease of ≥ 2 mesenteric vessels.

Signs/Symptoms

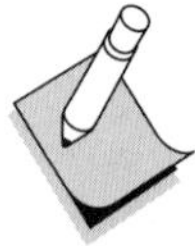

Classic finding in acute mesenteric ischemia–
Pain out of proportion to exam.

Acute disease is associated with a **sudden onset** of midabdominal pain, **out of proportion to exam,** and diarrhea. Exam shows hemodynamic instability, irregular HR (particularly with embolic type), abdominal distension, peritonitis, and melena or hematochezia.

Chronic disease results in chronic postprandial abdominal pain, resulting in "**food-fear**" and weight loss. Exam might be nonspecific.

Diagnosis

Labs in acute disease might reveal leukocytosis with left shift, electrolyte abnormalities, and lactic acidosis. Venous occlusion might be associated with abnormal coagulation studies (e.g., PT, PTT); workup of a hypercoagulable state should ensue. If the patient is hemodynamically stable, CT scan with oral and IV contrast may reveal **calcifications, absence of contrast flow, and**

stranding and wall thickening around ischemic portions. Though mesenteric angiography is the gold standard, patients often are not stable enough for this procedure. MRA with gadolinium is becoming increasingly useful.

Labs in chronic disease might be nonspecific. Radiographic imaging includes CTA, MRA, or angiography and may show collateral development.

TREATMENT

Expeditious identification and management is the key to minimizing morbidity and mortality. Infarction can occur within 6 hours. Fluid resuscitation, broad spectrum antibiotics, and heparin (for venous occlusion) should be started. Hemodynamic instability, peritonitis, and perforation warrant emergent operative intervention.

- Embolic: First perform revascularization (i.e., embolectomy, bypass). Bowel with marginal blood supply will then declare itself. If patient can tolerate, resect areas of infarction. "Second-look" operations may be necessary for bowel of questionable viability.
- Thrombotic: Similar to treatment for embolic disease.
- Nonocclusive: Intra-arterial papaverine and cessation of vasoconstricting agents. Laparotomy and resection if peritonitis and infarction develop.
- Venous: Anticoagulation with heparin followed by coumadin. Laparotomy and resection if peritonitis and infarction develop.

Chronic disease is generally treated with transaortic endarterectomy (for ostial lesions) or mesenteric artery bypass. Endovascular therapy is becoming increasingly utilized.

Delayed diagnosis and treatment significantly ↑ morbidity and mortality. In addition to the complications associated with other abdominal vascular procedures, **short bowel syndrome** may occur after extensive resection (see Chapter 9). The prognosis is generally poor (30–45%), with the nonocclusive subgroup exhibiting the highest mortality (80–90%).

Renal Artery Stenosis

DEMOGRAPHICS/RISK FACTORS

Common cause of 2° HTN (5% of HTN patients), particularly in young patients with refractory HTN and elderly men with peripheral vascular disease (PVD). Most common cause is atherosclerosis, though **fibromuscular dysplasia,** arterial dissection, renal artery aneurysm, Takayasu's arteritis, or restenosis after stenting may also be involved.

SIGNS/SYMPTOMS

Generally asymptomatic, though patients will have **HTN refractory to multiple medications** and later, chronic renal insufficiency. Exam may reveal abdominal bruit.

DIAGNOSIS

Duplex renal ultrasound demonstrates a velocity ratio > 3.5 compared to aorta. Angiography or MRA in patients with fibromuscular dysplasia may show "**string of beads.**" Catheter-directed venous sampling demonstrates **discrepant renin levels between renal veins** (ratio > 1.5 is diagnostic).

Treatment

Though **angiotensin converting enzyme (ACE) inhibitors may initially be effective, they will accelerate renal failure and should be avoided.** First-line therapy includes balloon angioplasty with or without stent placement. Surgical revascularization should be considered for recurrent cases.

Acute Limb Ischemia

Demographics/Risk Factors

Surgical emergency due to the sudden occlusion of a previously patent artery after an embolic or thrombotic event. Embolic sources are nearly always cardiac in origin (e.g., AF, MI with mural thrombus, left ventricular aneurysm, dilated cardiomyopathy, and valvular vegetations).

Signs/Symptoms

> **Six P's** of acute limb ischemia:
> **P**ain
> **P**allor
> **P**aralysis
> **P**aresthesias
> **P**ulselessness
> **P**oikilothermia

Patients with acute ischemia classically present with the **six "P's" of a threatened limb. Pain is the most reliable indicator,** but **its absence is not sufficient to rule out ischemia.** In contrast to thrombotic disease, those with an embolic source will have a contralateral extremity without stigmata of chronic ischemia. Patients with an acute embolus usually recall the exact time of symptom onset. Those with acute thrombosis report a history of claudication, which has recently become worse. **"Water-hammer" pulses** are palpable proximal to the occlusion.

Diagnosis

Generally a clinical diagnosis. Doppler ultrasound can help delineate the exact location of the occlusion.

Treatment

As soon as diagnosis is considered, administer heparin bolus and infusion. A high-risk patient with mild disease and distal occlusion should be treated with catheter-directed thrombolysis. Most patients, though, should be treated with **embolectomy**. The entire leg should be prepped in case bypass is required. Intraoperatively, use angiography to confirm the obstruction and restoration of flow. Retrieved clot should be sent to pathology to rule out atrial myxoma. **Fasciotomy** may be required after a long ischemic period.

Compartment Syndrome

Ischemia followed by reperfusion causes capillary leak. This volume, when added to a fascial compartment, causes ↑ tissue pressure and ↓ venous outflow. Eventually, inflow of O_2 and nutrients is halted, and the patient experiences **pain on passive movement** (typically the earliest sign) and loss of sensation in the extremity. In spite of palpable pulses, lower extremity compartment syndrome can be diagnosed clinically by **numbness in the first webspace (innervated by the deep peroneal nerve)**. Confirm the diagnosis with measurement of compartment pressures (**> 25 mm Hg is abnormally high**). Treat with compartment fasciotomy (four compartment fasciotomy of the lower leg). Hyperkalemia and lactic acidosis may follow in the washout period.

A 26-year-old male presents to the ED complaining of pain and swelling in his left arm. He has occasional numbness in his fingers. He is healthy but reports a recent auto accident. No atrophy of the intrinsic hand muscles is noted, and electromyography (EMG) tests are within normal limits. The arm appears somewhat blue, and radiographs do not demonstrate cervical ribs. Duplex ultrasound with the arm abducted confirms external compression of the subclavian vein by an edematous scalene muscle. What is the appropriate management? Rest, elevation, and nonsteroidal anti-inflammatory drugs (NSAIDs) can lead to symptom resolution.

Thoracic Outlet Syndrome

Demographics/Risk Factors

Abnormal compression of the neurovascular bundle (i.e., brachial plexus, artery, and vein), which exits the thoracic cavity and innervates the arm. Though all structures may be compressed, **neurologic symptoms are usually prominent.** May be due to **enlarged scalene muscle, cervical rib,** acute neck trauma, or repetitive stress injury. Women are affected more often than men (except for venous syndrome), with symptoms most commonly occurring in the fourth decade of life.

Signs/Symptoms

Presentation depends on which structure is primarily involved. **Pain and paresthesias are the most common neurologic symptoms.** Symptoms will be most prominent after movements that stretch the nerve roots (i.e., **holding arms above head**). Exam may show **tenderness over the anterior scalene muscle** or **↑ paresthesias while tilting the head away from the affected side.** A supraclavicular bruit, pulsatile mass, signs of microemboli, or unilateral edema (consistent with venous disease) may be noted. Hand atrophy and EMG changes are only seen in extreme cases.

Diagnosis

Cervical spine radiographs can rule out cervical ribs. Digital artery occlusion in a young patient should prompt angiography in neutral position and with arm abducted.

Treatment

For symptoms caused by edematous scalene muscles, treat with postural correction, rest, and physical therapy (e.g., limb elevation). **First rib resection may be required in some cases.** Venous symptoms may be treated with directed thrombolysis and rib resection, if necessary.

Peripheral Vascular Disease

Demographics/Risk Factors

Commonly caused by atherosclerosis. Affects the lower extremities more often than the upper extremities. Risk factors are identical to those for atherosclerosis.

Approximately 5% of men and women > 65 years of age will have symptomatic disease with ~10% eventually requiring amputation. Patients with DM or tobacco use have a significantly ↑ incidence.

Signs/Symptoms

Most common presenting symptom is claudication. Pain initially is noted with exercise; as disease progresses, patients develop pain at rest. Rest pain will eventually progress to ulceration and tissue loss if not treated. Characteristic symptoms of PVD are

Leriche's syndrome—

Claudication of calf, thigh, and buttocks

Impotence

Diminished femoral pulses

- Decreased pulses: Obstruction is proximal to level of ↓ pulses.
- Foot pallor: Pallor when elevated and rubor when dependent suggests advanced arterial insufficiency. Helpful to differentiate venous stasis from ischemia. **Venous stasis is associated with purple discoloration in any position, while the ischemic foot is pallid on elevation.**
- Intermittent claudication: Cramping, pain, or fatigue in the lower extremities **caused by walking and relieved by rest.**
- Rest pain: Burning pain usually **localized to the forefoot**. Aggravated by elevation of the diseased limb and may inhibit sleep. Patients may dangle leg off the bed, using gravity to augment blood flow.
- Leriche's syndrome: Aorto-iliac disease → impotence, diminished femoral pulses, and claudication of the calf, thigh, and buttocks.
- Nonhealing wounds: Minor trauma causes severe wounds that do not heal. Wounds are frequently deep and lack evidence of granulation.
- Necrosis and atrophy: Effects start distally and progress proximally. Dry gangrene becomes wet gangrene after superinfection.

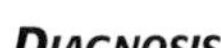

Diagnosis

Primarily based on history and exam, but noninvasive tests (see Noninvasive Monitoring of Vascular Disease section) are useful adjuncts. In addition to the modalities discussed above, serial BP measurements before and after exercise are informative. An **ankle SBP ↓ > 20% after exercise is abnormal.** Angiography remains the gold standard.

Treatment

Intervention should be designed to halt disease progress, relieve symptoms, and maintain bipedal gait. Conservative treatment consists of risk factor reduction (i.e., smoking cessation, tight glucose control, control of hyperlipidemia), exercise rehabilitation (e.g., muscle conditioning), foot care, and pharmacotherapy (i.e., **aspirin, clopidogrel, cilostazol, pentoxifylline**).

Indications for surgical intervention include rest pain, inability to maintain functional status, tissue loss, and gangrene. Options include endovascular versus reconstructive (bypass) revascularization.

- Open endarterectomy: Used for occlusive disease involving the common femoral and profunda femoral arteries. Not used for superficial femoral artery disease due to the high rate of restenosis.
- Femoropopliteal bypass: Used for disease limited to the femoropopliteal segment. **Autologous saphenous vein is preferred** and may be left in situ or resected and reversed. Polytetrafluoroethylene (PTFE) grafts may also be used for bypass to the above knee popliteal artery. **Below knee PTFE conduits yield lower patency rates and should be avoided.** Five-year patency rates

range from 60–80%. Bypass procedures distal to the trifurcation are usually performed only for limb salvage due to low patency rate (< 50%).

- Endovascular revascularization: Usually limited to short segment disease in large vessels. Drug eluting stents are being used in ongoing trials.
- Amputation: Often the procedure of last resort. The goal is removal of diseased tissue, relief of pain, and construction of a stump that will permit the most useful function. Indications for 1° above knee amputation include contracture at the knee and nonviable calf muscle or skin. Frequent failure of healing of below knee amputation and the high surgical morbidity in this population make 1° above knee procedures the preferred technique.

Venous Insufficiency and Lower Extremity Ulcers

Due to incompetent valves in the deep venous system. Chronic venous insufficiency affects over 500,000 patients annually. If left untreated, will result in edema, varicose veins, **hyperpigmentation**, and **venous ulceration**. Typically a clinical diagnosis, though duplex ultrasound confirms and evaluates segmental reflux. The 1° treatment is compression therapy (e.g., stockings, boots) with local wound care. Endoscopic ligation of perforator veins is the surgical therapy of choice for perforator reflux.

Varicose Veins

Dilated and tortuous veins, most commonly affecting overweight females with a family history of varicosities. Common symptoms include pain and fatigue of the affected extremity. Symptoms are exacerbated with legs in a dependent position and are alleviated with elevation. Majority of patients are treated conservatively with compression stockings. Surgical intervention is indicated for cosmesis or after failure of compression to alleviate symptoms. Interventions include sclerotherapy (i.e., destruction of endothelium), saphenous vein stripping, laser ablation, or catheter-directed radiofrequency ablation.

Superficial Thrombophlebitis

Thrombophlebitis can affect any vein but usually affects varicosities or veins with indwelling catheters. Diagnosis is confirmed by exam, which reveals erythema, warmth, tenderness to palpation, and **fibrosis ("cord")**. Ultrasound can evaluate extension of thrombosis into the deep venous system. Treat with compression, heat, and anti-inflammatory medications. Thrombophlebitis due to indwelling catheters is often associated with infection (i.e., **suppurative thrombophlebitis**) and may require vein excision.

Types of 1° lymphedema–

Congenital lymphedema: Presents at birth.

Lymphedema praecox: Most common. Presents in childhood and teenage years.

Lymphedema tarda: Presents with ↑ age, typically later than praecox.

Lymphedema

Typically an acquired condition due to disruption of lymphatic vessels (e.g., surgery, radiation). Less frequent causes include filariasis, occult malignancy, or 1° forms (e.g., congenital lymphedema, lymphedema praecox, lymphedema tarda). Patients complain of limb heaviness and fatigue. Diagnosis is confirmed by history and exam. Classic findings include fluctuations in limb diameter, hyperkeratotic skin, **skin "weeping,"** and **recurrent cellulitis.** While no cure exists, treatment with compression and extremity elevation may help relieve symptoms. Skin care, compression, and massage help reduce the risk of recurrent cellulitis.

▶ SAMPLE QUESTIONS

As the radius of an occluded carotid artery ↓, what happens to the velocity blood flow?	↑.
A 12-year-old female with a tibial plateau fracture complains of increasing pain upon dorsiflexion of the foot. Pedal pulses are equal bilaterally. What is the diagnosis? Treatment?	Compartment syndrome can be present even in the setting of normal pulse exam. Measure compartment pressures. Four compartment fasciotomy is necessary.
A 60-year-old male smoker presents with claudication of the right leg. What is his expected ABI?	ABI 0.5–0.7.
What is the incidence of transient cranial nerve injury after CEA?	10%.
A patient with chest pain and diminished pulses in the left upper extremity should undergo radial artery catheterization (for monitoring) in which extremity?	Patients with arch dissection should have arterial monitoring on the right (unaffected) side so as not to undertreat the HTN.
A 67-year-old otherwise healthy male presents with a TAA. What are the indications for repair?	TAA > 6 cm; TAA in a symptomatic patient (e.g., aortic insufficiency); TAA growth rate > 1 cm/year; TAA > 5 cm in the setting of a connective tissue disorder.
A 70-year-old male who underwent an open AAA 1 year prior presents with an aorto-enteric fistula? What are possible management options?	Extra-anatomic bypass or antibiotic-saturated graft.
What is the treatment of superficial thrombophlebitis?	NSAIDs, heat, elevation, compression wraps. If symptoms persist > 2 weeks, excision or systemic anticoagulation is warranted.
What is Leriche's syndrome?	Claudication of calf, thigh, and buttock muscles, impotence, and diminished femoral pulses associated with aorto-iliac occlusive disease.
What are the six P's of acute limb ischemia?	Pain, pallor, paralysis, paresthesias, pulselessness, poikilothermia.

A 42-year-old male in a motor vehicle collision has a right knee dislocation that is reduced and splinted in the field. What further evaluation is necessary?	Doppler studies if pulses are normal as popliteal artery dissection and thrombosis is highly associated with knee dislocation. In case of diminished pulses, obtain arteriogram. If the leg is pulseless, proceed emergently to the operating room for an on-table arteriogram and exploration of the popliteal artery.

CHAPTER 18

Trauma, Burns, and Critical Care

Elizabeth A. Sailhamer, MD, MMSc
Reviewed by Hasan B. Alam, MD

▶ BASIC SCIENCE

Mortality After Trauma

Mortality follows a trimodal distribution.

- 0–30 minutes: 50% of deaths. Due to lacerations to the aorta, heart, or central nervous system (CNS).
- 30 minutes to 4 hours: 30% of deaths occur in the "golden hour." Due to traumatic brain injury (TBI; 50%) and hemorrhage (50%).
- Days to weeks: 20% of deaths. Due to infection, sepsis, and multisystem organ failure.

Shock

Inadequate tissue perfusion with end organ dysfunction as evidenced by lactic acidosis, ↑ HR, ↑ RR, altered mental status (AMS), ↓ urine output, and ↓ BP. Can result from ↓ preload (ie, hypovolemic), ↓ afterload (ie, septic, neurogenic), or impaired contractility (ie, cardiogenic; see Table 18-1).

Hemorrhagic shock is classified according to the degree of blood loss (see Table 18-2).

Ventilator Management

Trauma patients with depressed mental status (Glasgow Coma scale [GCS] ≤ 8) may require intubation and mechanical ventilation for airway protection or for respiratory failure in the acute (eg, flail chest, pulmonary contusion) or chronic (eg, acute respiratory distress syndrome [ARDS], pneumonia) settings. Ventilation

TABLE 18-1. Classification of Types of Shock

VARIABLES	HYPOVOLEMIC	CARDIOGENIC	SEPTIC	NEUROGENIC
Mechanism	↓ Preload	↓ Contractility	↓ Afterload	↓ Afterload
Etiology	Hemorrhage, dehydration.	Myocardial ischemia/infarction, contusion with ventricular dysfunction.	Hyperdynamic cardiac function, loss of vascular tone.	Spinal cord injury, loss of sympathetic tone.
HR	↑	↑	↑	↑
CO	↓	↓	↑	↑
Signs/ symptoms	↓ JVD, cool feet, pallor.	↑ JVD, cool feet, angina, ECG changes.	↓ JVD, warm feet, fever, ↑ WBC count.	↓ JVD, warm feet, cervical/thoracic spine fracture, paraplegia.
Treatment	Crystalloid +/– blood products.	Dobutamine, levophed.	Crystalloids, antibiotics, +/– vasopressin or levophed.	Crystalloids +/– phenylephrine.

TABLE 18-2. Classification of Classes of Hemorrhage

VARIABLES	CLASS I	CLASS II	CLASS III	CLASS IV
Blood loss (% blood volume)	< 750 mL (< 15%)	750–1500 mL (15–30%)	1500–2000 mL (30–40%)	> 2000 mL (> 40%)
HR	Nl	> 100 bpm	> 120 bpm	> 140 bpm
Pulse pressure	Nl	↓	↓	↓
BP	Nl	Nl	↓	↓
Mental status	Nl	Anxious	Confused	Lethargic
Resuscitation	Crystalloid	Crystalloid	Crystalloid and blood	Crystalloid and blood

modes are either volume-controlled, pressure-controlled, or neither. **Fraction of inspired oxygen (FiO_2)** and **positive end-expiratory pressure (PEEP) control oxygenation** (O_2); **tidal volume** and **RR control ventilation** (CO_2; see Table 18-3).

To adjust O_2 → Change FiO_2 or PEEP
To adjust CO_2 → Change tidal volume, pressure support, or RR

TABLE 18-3. Modes of Positive Pressure Ventilation

VENTILATION MODE	SET PARAMETER	DESCRIPTION
Continuous mandatory ventilation	Volume	Fixed volume, fixed rate. Patient cannot initiate own breaths. Typically used in OR.
SIMV	Volume	Fixed volume and rate. Patient can take unassisted breaths. Ventilator breaths are synchronized with unassisted patient breaths (avoids breath stacking).
Assist control ventilation	Volume	Fixed volume delivered by the ventilator after patient-initiated breath. No set rate, so backup rate (SIMV) required.
Pressure control ventilation	Pressure	Fixed pressure delivered by the ventilator. Initiated by patient. Backup rate (SIMV) must be set. Volume determined by lung compliance (Δ volume/Δ pressure).
Pressure support ventilation	Pressure	Fixed pressure delivered by the ventilator. Initiated by patient. Volume is determined by compliance (Δ volume / Δ pressure). No set rate so not appropriate for fully passive patients.
Continuous positive airway pressure	None	Ventilator delivers constant pressure to facilitate patient's own inspiratory efforts.

ABCDs of cardiac arrest resuscitation:
Airway
Breathing
Circulation
Defibrillation
Differential diagnosis

See Chapter 15 for summary of vasoactive medications.

The **5 H's** and **5 T's** of PEA arrest:
Hypovolemia
Hypoxia
↑ **H**⁺ (acidosis)
Hyper- or **H**ypo-kalemia
Hypothermia
Tablets (drug overdose)
Tamponade (cardiac)
Tension pneumothorax (PTX)
Thrombosis (coronary)
Thrombosis (pulmonary embolism)

▶ CLINICAL SCIENCE

Evaluation and Resuscitation of a Cardiac Arrest Patient

According to the 2002 Advanced Cardiac Life Support (ACLS) protocols, cardiac arrest resuscitation includes 1° and 2° survey (see Table 18-4).

For **pulseless electrical activity (PEA)** and asystole, management includes epinephrine 1 mg IV push every 3–5 minutes and atropine 1 mg IV push every 3–5 minutes; there is **no role for defibrillation**. For **ventricular fibrillation (VF) and pulseless ventricular tachycardia (VT)**, administer epinephrine 1 mg IV push every 3–5 minutes or vasopressin 40 IU × 1, followed by defibrillation × 1 (360 J) within 30–60 seconds of medication. Amiodarone, lidocaine, Mg^{2+}, and procainamide may be used. Some evidence supports the induction of mild hypothermia (ie, 33–34°C) after return of normal cardiac activity (following VF arrest) to improve outcome.

Evaluation and Resuscitation of a Trauma Patient

According to the 1997 Advanced Trauma Life Support (ATLS) protocols, trauma resuscitation is divided into 1° and 2° surveys.

PRIMARY SURVEY

Intended to identify life threatening injuries that require immediate intervention (see Table 18-5). Many can be definitively treated in the trauma bay with intubation or chest tube drainage. ABCDEs include

- Airway control with cervical spine stabilization: Inspect airway for foreign body. Secure airway with chin lift or jaw thrust (**use jaw thrust with suspected cervical spine [C-spine] injuries**) and tracheal intubation, if indicated. Place a surgical airway (eg, cricothyroidotomy) if oro- or nasotracheal intubation is unsuccessful.
- Breathing and ventilation: Assess for presence of equal breath sounds, tracheal shift, percussion asymmetry.
- Circulation and hemorrhage control: Assess HR, skin color, temperature, and level of consciousness. Control external bleeding with direct manual

TABLE 18-4. ACLS Primary and Secondary Surveys

PRIMARY SURVEY	SECONDARY SURVEY
Airway: Open airway. **B**reathing: Positive pressure ventilation (bag mask 100% O_2). **C**irculation: Assess HR, start chest compressions. **D**efibrillation: Assess rhythm, shock × 3 (200 Joules [J], 200-300 J, 360 J) if ventricular fibrillation (VF) or pulseless ventricular tachycardia (VT).	**A**irway: Secure airway (eg, endotracheal tube). **B**reathing: Confirm airway device placement. **C**irculation: Obtain IV access, place monitors, administer vasoactive medications, defibrillate. **D**ifferential diagnosis: Identify/treat reversible causes.

TABLE 18-5. Diagnosis and Management of Acute Life-Threatening Injuries

INJURY	DIAGNOSIS	MANAGEMENT
Airway obstruction	Apnea or stridor, maxillofacial trauma.	Definitive tracheal intubation (oro- or naso-tracheal) or cricothyroidotomy.
Flail chest	Paradoxical chest wall motion.	Positive pressure ventilation.
Tension PTX	Respiratory distress, tracheal deviation, hypotension, distended neck veins, absent unilateral breath sounds, hyperresonant percussion.	Needle decompression (second interspace, midclavicular line) followed by placement of chest tube (fourth interspace, anterior axillary line).
Open PTX	Open wound into chest → **"sucking chest wound."**	Sterile gauze secured on three sides, placement of chest tube.
Massive hemothorax	**≥ 1500 mL initial output or ≥ 200 mL/h × 4 hours.** Absent breath sounds, dullness to percussion, hypotension.	Chest tube placement. **Massive hemothorax necessitates thoracotomy.**
Cardiac tamponade	Distended neck veins, muffled heart sounds, hypotension **(Beck's triad)**, pulsus paradoxus.	Pericardiocentesis (or emergency thoracotomy if pulseless).

compression, close pelvic volume, obtain large bore IV access, and restore circulating blood volume with 2 L of warmed crystalloid fluid and blood products, if necessary.

- Disability (including neurologic evaluation): Assess gross level of consciousness and determine GCS (see Head Trauma section).
- Exposure/Environment control: Expose patient for complete 2° survey. Keep patient warm.

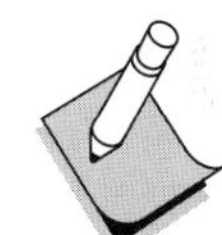

Massive hemothorax and indications for thoracotomy–

- *≥ 1500 mL on insertion of chest tube*
- *≥ 200 mL/h × 4 hours*

SECONDARY SURVEY

The 2° survey includes a head-to-toe evaluation to identify other injuries. Adjuncts include CXR, anterior–posterior (AP) pelvis radiograph, Focused Assessment by Sonography in Trauma (FAST) exam, labs, arterial blood gas, ECG, as well as placement of a nasogastric tube (NGT) and urinary catheter. Further radiologic studies may be indicated in stable patients. Unstable patients may need a diagnostic peritoneal aspiration (DPA) to determine source of bleeding.

Evaluation and management of the hemodynamically unstable trauma patient summarized in Table 18-6. **Hemorrhage is the most common reason for hypotension in a trauma patient,** but other etiologies must be considered.

Take an **AMPLE** history during 2° survey:
Allergies
Medications
Past medial history
Last meal
Events associated with injury

TABLE 18-6. Workup and Management of the Unstable Trauma Patient

Etiology	Diagnosis	Management
Hemorrhagic Shock		
Chest	Breath sounds, CXR.	Chest tube(s); thoracotomy when indicated (see Chest Trauma).
Abdomen	Abdominal exam, FAST, diagnostic peritoneal lavage (DPL) or DPA.	Laparotomy
Retroperitoneum	AP pelvis radiograph.	Angiographic embolization versus extraperitoneal pelvic packing +/– laparotomy.
Extremity/Thigh	Palpate for hematoma, extremity radiograph.	Reduce/Splint; operative control of bleeding if necessary.
External	Ongoing bleeding from a wound, report of blood at the scene.	Direct manual compression.
Compressive Shock		
Tension PTX	Auscultation, percussion, dilated neck veins, tracheal deviation (does **not** require CXR for diagnosis).	Needle decompression, chest tube.
Cardiac tamponade	Beck's triad on exam, + FAST (cardiac view)	Pericardiocentesis (ED thoracotomy for pulselessness).
Cardiogenic Shock		
Cardiac contusion	History of blunt anterior chest trauma, **ECG ectopy**, echo, cardiac enzymes.	Vasoactive agents
Myocardial infarction	ECG changes.	Vasoactive agents, cath lab if STEMI.
Neurogenic Shock	Neurologic exam, spine radiographs, CT.	C-spine immobilization. 2 liters crystalloid +/– phenylephrine. Steroids if < 8 hours from injury.

Head Trauma

Demographics

TBI is the leading cause of morbidity and mortality in trauma patients. Primary injury may be focal (eg, hematoma; see Table 18-7) or diffuse (eg, diffuse axonal injury).

TABLE 18-7. Types of Intracranial Hemorrhage

TYPE	LOCATION	CT FINDINGS	MANAGEMENT
Epidural hematoma	**Middle meningeal artery**.	**Lens-shaped (convex)** hyperdensity. May cross midline but not suture lines.	Emergent craniotomy, evacuation of hematoma.
Subdural hematoma	Bridging veins.	**Crescent-shaped (concave)** hyperdensity. Crosses suture lines but not midline.	May require craniotomy if midline shift (> 5 mm) or if exam deteriorates.
Intraparenchymal hematoma	Parenchymal hematoma.	Discrete hyperdensity +/– mass effect.	May require craniotomy if mass effect or exam deteriorates.
Subarachnoid hemorrhage	Blood in subarachnoid space.	Hyperdensity in subarachnoid space (base of brain, along cerebral gyri).	Prevention of 2° injury.
Intraventricular hemorrhage	Blood in ventricles.	Hyperdensity in ventricles.	Prevention of 2° injury.
Cerebral contusion	Parenchymal contusion.	Patchy opacities (coup or contracoup).	Prevention of 2° injury.

SIGNS/SYMPTOMS

AMS or focal neurologic deficits may be present. A full neurologic exam should be performed as soon as possible. GCS is a useful, quick prognostic assessment (see Table 18-8).

DIAGNOSIS

If TBI is suspected, order an **immediate head CT without contrast** to assess for mass lesions requiring neurosurgical decompression.

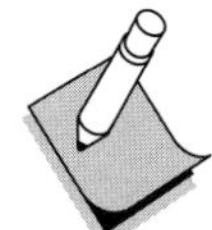

Severe TBI/coma–

GCS ≤ 8 → indication for intubation and intracranial pressure (ICP) monitoring

TREATMENT

Prevent 2° injury and ischemia.

- If unable to follow clinical exam (GCS ≤ 8), intubate and perform ICP monitoring.
- Treat ↑ ICP aggressively with **goal ICP < 20 mm Hg** (see Table 18-9).
- If indicated, perform decompressive craniectomy and hematoma evacuation.
- Avoid hypotension. Administer fluids or pressors to optimize cerebral blood flow (CBF) keeping **cerebral perfusion pressure (CPP) > 60 mm Hg**.
- Avoid hypoxia.
- Avoid hypo- or hyperventilation.
- Avoid hyponatremia. Administer isotonic or hypertonic fluids.
- Treat fevers.
- Provide seizure prophylaxis (eg, phenytoin for 1 week).

Formula for CPP–

CPP = Mean arterial pressure (MAP) – ICP

Goal CPP > 60 mm Hg

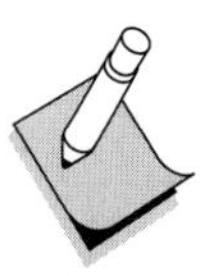

Criteria for brain death–

1. *Known cause of coma or documented irreversible structural injury*
2. *Other causes (hypotension, hypoxia, hypothermia, drugs, metabolic) excluded*
3. *Absence of cortical function or brainstem reflexes:*
   - *No respirations with $Paco_2$ = 60 mm Hg (apnea test)*
   - *Absent brainstem reflexes (pupillary, corneal, oculocephalic [doll's eyes], oculovestibular [cold water caloric], or gag)*

TABLE 18-8. GCS Scoring

Category	Assessment	Score
Eye opening	Spontaneously	4
	To voice	3
	To pain	2
	Closed	1
Verbal response	Oriented	5
	Confused	4
	Words or phrases	3
	Sounds	2
	No sounds	1
Motor response	Follows commands	6
	Localizes to painful stimulus	5
	Withdraws from painful stimulus	4
	Arm flexion (decerebrate posturing)	3
	Arm extension (decorticate posturing)	2
	No movement	1

Neck Trauma

Demographics

Can include penetrating or blunt cervical wounds that can penetrate the platysma.

TABLE 18-9. Management of Elevated Intracranial Pressure

Intracranial Compartment	Management	Rationale	Precautions
Blood	Straighten neck.	↑ Venous drainage.	C-collar may impair drainage.
	Head of bed at 30°.	↑ Venous drainage.	Thoracolumbar fractures.
	Treat pain/anxiety (eg, propofol).	↓ CBF.	Avoid hypotension.
	Neuromuscular paralysis.	↓ CBF.	Unable to follow exam.
	Hyperventilation (partial pressure of carbon dioxide [$Paco_2$] = 30–35 mm Hg).	Arterial vasoconstriction, ↓ CBF.	Temporizing. Excessive hyperventilation → ischemia.
Cerebrospinal fluid (CSF)	Ventriculostomy drainage.	Remove CSF.	Bleeding, infection.
Brain	Mannitol (0.25–1 g/kg bolus).	↓ Cerebral edema.	Hypovolemia can cause hypotension. Follow serum Na^+ and osmolality.

TABLE 18-10. Evaluation and Management of the Penetrating Neck Wound

Zone of Neck	Anatomic Location	Management: Hemodynamically Unstable	Management: Hemodynamically Stable	
			+ Signs/Symptoms	– Signs/Symptoms
Zone 1	Clavicle to cricoid.	Emergent exploration.	Selective management.	Selective management.
Zone 2	Cricoid to angle of mandible.	Emergent exploration.	Urgent exploration.	Selective management.
Zone 3	Angle of mandible to base of skull.	Emergent exploration.	Selective management.	Selective management.

Signs/Symptoms

Definitive signs and symptoms vary by injured structure.

- Carotid: Active hemorrhage, **expanding or pulsatile hematoma**, thrill, bruit, neurologic deficit (stroke).
- Esophagus/Pharynx: **Crepitus**, dysphagia or odynophagia, hemoptysis or oropharyngeal bleeding.
- Trachea/Larynx: **Subcutaneous emphysema, "bubbling" wound, stridor,** dyspnea, dysphonia, hoarseness.

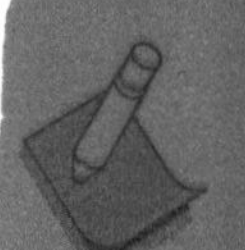

Never probe a neck wound or enter a neck hematoma without proximal and distal vascular control.

Diagnosis

Stable patients can be evaluated with **selective management (ie, aortogram, esophagoscopy with esophagogram,** and **bronchoscopy and laryngoscopy).** This is especially important in zones 1 and 3 because of the difficulty with exposure. In recent years, high resolution CT angiography (CTA) has been used as an adjunct for diagnosis.

Treatment

Exsanguination or an expanding, pulsatile mass necessitate immediate surgical exploration (see Table 18-10).

Maxillofacial Trauma

Injuries affect the face, orbit, base of skull, or nose. Diagnose facial fractures with high-resolution facial CT with axial and coronal reconstructions. Rule out an associated C-spine fracture. Major life-threatening risk is **airway obstruction** (ie, oropharyngeal bleeding, soft tissue swelling). Ensure airway patency; may require surgical airway.

Le Fort Fracture

Summarized in Figure 18-1. On exam, Le Fort I fractures present with upper teeth movement; Le Fort II demonstrate upper tooth and nose movement; and Le Fort III demonstrate upper tooth, nose, orbit, and zygoma movement.

Mandible Fracture

Usually associated with **malocclusion**. Confirm with panographic films. Treat with maxillomandibular or internal fixation.

Le Fort fractures—
Le Fort I: Maxillary fracture (separates upper jaw/maxilla from face).
Le Fort II: Nasomaxillary fracture (separates nasomaxillary complex from upper face).
Le Fort III: Craniofacial separation (separates entire face from base of skull).

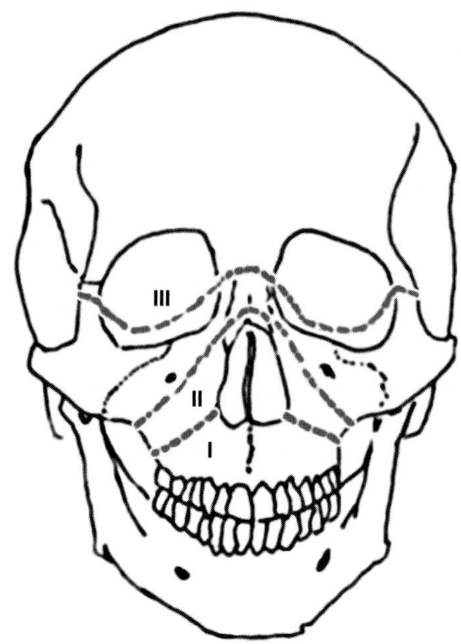

FIGURE 18-1. Le Fort fractures.

(Reproduced, with permission, from Brunicardi FC, et al. *Schwartz's Principles of Surgery*, 8th ed. New York: McGraw-Hill, 2005:1808.)

ORBITAL "BLOWOUT" FRACTURE

Associated with an intact orbital rim with fractures of the floor and medial wall. **Diplopia and limited ocular movement** suggest **nerve entrapment.**

BASILAR SKULL FRACTURE

Presents with **raccoon eyes, Battle's sign** (ie, mastoid ecchymoses), hemotympanum, CSF rhinorrhea, or otorrhea. **Avoid NGT use.**

NASAL FRACTURE

May be associated with deformity and bleeding. Treat with nasal packing if actively bleeding. **Septal hematoma** necessitates incision and drainage to prevent cartilage necrosis and saddle nose deformity.

Chest Trauma

Six acute, life-threatening injuries (ie, airway obstruction, tension PTX, open PTX, flail chest, massive hemothorax, cardiac tamponade) involve the airway and chest and must be diagnosed and treated during the 1° survey (see Table 18-5). Other common thoracic injuries should be diagnosed during the 2° survey and treated based on specific etiology.

CHEST WALL INJURIES

- Rib fracture: First rib fractures (high mechanism of injury) are associated with other intrathoracic injuries (eg, **aortic injury**). Lower rib fractures are associated with intra-abdominal solid organ injury (eg, liver, spleen).

- Sternal fracture: Indicates high mechanism of injury and often **associated with intrathoracic injury** or **myocardial contusion**. Manage conservatively; fixation rarely indicated.
- Scapular fracture: Indicates high mechanism of injury. Treat with sling immobilization.
- Clavicle fracture: Relatively common. Associated with tenderness, deformity, and crepitus on exam. Look for concurrent PTX or subclavian artery injury. Treat with sling immobilization.

PULMONARY INJURIES

- Simple PTX: Lung collapse due to pleural injury; not associated with hemodynamic instability. Often associated with rib or clavicle fractures. Exam might reveal **absent breath sounds**. Confirm with CXR. Generally treated with chest tube placement.
- Hemothorax: Bleeding into the pleural space from **intercostal or internal mammary arteries** or from pulmonary parenchyma. Associated with ↓ breath sounds and dullness to percussion. Treat with chest tube, serial hematocrits (HCTs), and blood transfusions, if needed.
- Pulmonary contusion: Injury to lung parenchyma resulting in alveolar edema with blood collection. CXR reveals nonanatomic parenchymal opacity, often with overlying rib fractures or flail chest. Typically blossoms on posttrauma day 1–2. Treat with supportive care: chest physical therapy, O_2 supplementation, pain control, and minimization of fluid resuscitation.

TRAUMA, BURNS, AND CRITICAL CARE

MEDIASTINAL INJURIES

- Esophageal injury: Usually due to penetrating trauma to the cervical esophagus. Presents with crepitus, chest pain, dysphagia, hematemesis, or signs of mediastinitis. CXR may demonstrate **hydropneumothorax or pneumomediastinum.** Esophagography and upper endoscopy identify the location of perforation. Treat like Boerhaave's syndrome (see Chapter 4).
- Tracheobronchial injury: Partial or complete laceration of the tracheobronchial wall, most commonly occurring at the carina or main bronchi; rarely found as an isolated entity. CXR demonstrates pneumomediastinum and PTX. Confirm diagnosis with bronchoscopy. **Have a high index of suspicion for this injury as chest tubes may have large air leaks and worsen respiratory distress.** For tracheal injuries, **definitive airway is a priority** but should be placed under direct visualization over a bronchoscope in the operating room (if possible).

Use H_2O-soluble contrast agents when evaluating a suspected esophageal injury.

CARDIOVASCULAR INJURIES

- Aortic injury: Responsible for ~15% of deaths after motor vehicle collisions (MVC). Due to rapid deceleration resulting in **disruption at points of aortic fixation (eg, ligamentum arteriosum).** Patients may die before reaching the hospital, may be hemodynamically unstable, or may be asymptomatic. Radial pulses may be unequal if subclavian takeoff is involved. CXR classically demonstrates **widened mediastinum, loss of aortic knob, and presence of a pleural cap.** However, a normal CXR does not rule out the injury. Diagnosis is confirmed with aortogram or CT of the chest with contrast. Complete aortic transection is immediately lethal. Manage contained aortic disruption with permissive hypotension and IV β-blockers to minimize Δ pressure/Δ time until definitive surgical repair (eg, aortic stent graft, open resection with graft) is performed.

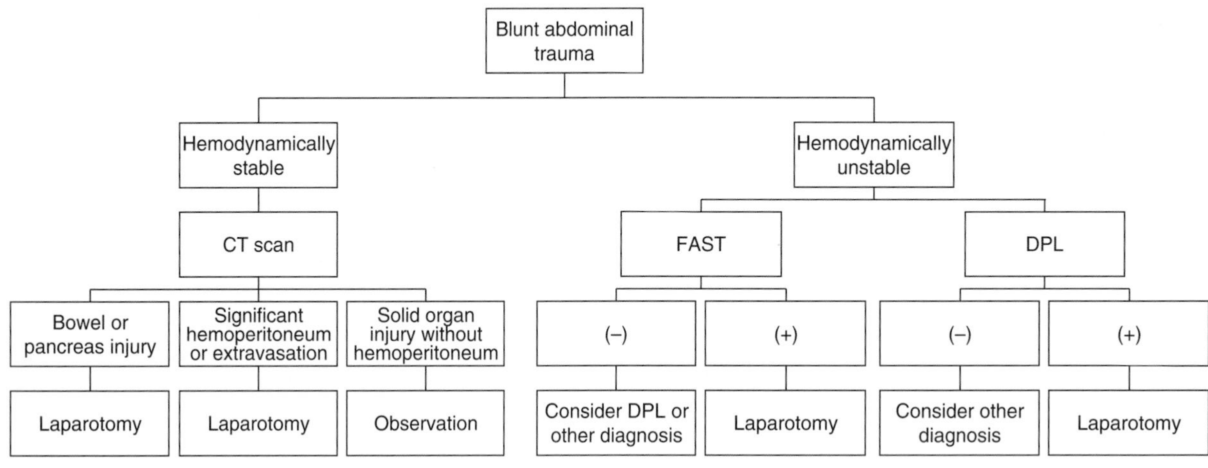

FIGURE 18-2. Algorithm for blunt abdominal trauma.

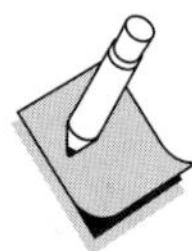

Emergency thoracotomy–

Left anterolateral thoracotomy at the fourth interspace:

1. *Open pericardium (anterior to phrenic nerve) to relieve tamponade.*
2. *Deliver heart and start open cardiac massage.*
3. *Control intrathoracic hemorrhage.*
4. *Aortic cross clamp (↑ blood to heart/brain, ↓ intra-abdominal bleeding).*

- Penetrating cardiac injury: Suspect after penetrating trauma to the precordium or epigastrium. **Right ventricle** is most commonly injured. Most survivable injuries are from stab wounds, which the thick ventricular muscle can seal; gun shot wounds (GSW) are often lethal. Cardiac injury often presents with **tamponade,** which can be temporarily treated with pericardiocentesis (if early) or emergency thoracotomy (for cardiac arrest).
- Blunt cardiac injury: Myocardial contusion, cardiac rupture, or injury to valves, papillary muscles, chordae tendinae after blunt trauma to the precordium (eg, bent steering wheel, sternal fracture). Evaluation may reveal new murmur, ECG ectopy, or ↑ **cardiac enzymes**; these mandate echo. Management is controversial, though generally patients are admitted for serial enzymes and cardiac monitoring.

Abdominal Trauma

Subdivided into injuries of the diaphragm, solid organs, hollow viscera, and retroperitoneal vessels. Exam may be unreliable. Mechanism of injury (blunt versus penetrating) and hemodynamic stability determine diagnostic tests and management (see Figures 18-2 and 18-3).

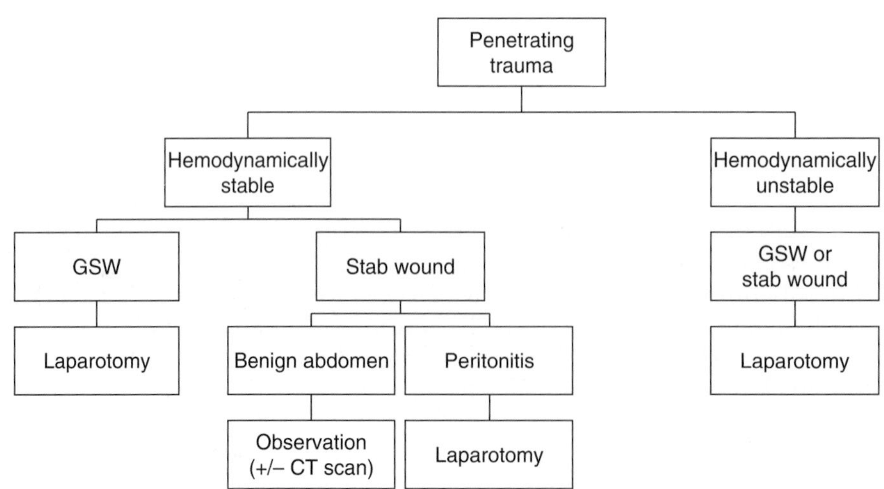

FIGURE 18-3. Algorithm for penetrating abdominal trauma.

Specific tests include

- **FAST**: Bedside ultrasound exam in hemodynamically unstable trauma patients to detect hemoperitoneum. Rapid, portable, noninvasive, and reproducible. However, can be operator-dependent, have a low sensitivity (falseexam with hemoperitoneum < 500 mL), or **fail to evaluate the retroperitoneum**.
- **DPL/DPA**: Technique to evaluate intra-abdominal blood in patients unable to tolerate CT scan. Place catheter into the peritoneum via a midline, **infraumbilical** approach; place **supraumbilically in pregnant women and patients with suspected pelvic hematomas**. Perform after NGT and urinary catheter decompression. **Test is "grossly +" for aspiration of 10 mL blood or aspiration of any biliary or enteric contents. Test is "microscopically +" for red blood cell (RBC) ≥ 100,000/mm^3, WBC ≥ 500/mm^3, or bile after lavage with 1 L saline**. Does not evaluate the retroperitoneum.
- **Abdominal CT scan**: Ideal test in a stable patient to evaluate the peritoneal cavity and **retroperitoneum**. Limited ability to detect bowel and pancreatic injury (good + predictive value but low – predictive value). Triple contrast CT (ie, IV, oral, rectal contrast) is optimal to evaluate retroperitoneal injury after flank wounds.

Specific injury types and their management are discussed below. Severe abdominal trauma and hemorrhage can lead to the lethal triad of **acidosis, hypothermia, and coagulopathy**. The goals of **damage control laparotomy** are hemostasis and containment of enteric contamination, followed by temporary abdominal closure and ICU management (eg, resuscitation, rewarming) until definitive repair.

Diaphragmatic Injuries

Penetrating thoracoabdominal and blunt abdominal trauma may cause diaphragmatic injuries. Traumatic rupture can result in herniation of abdominal contents into the chest. **CXR may show a coiled NGT in the left hemithorax;** confirm with diagnostic laparoscopy. **Repair left diaphragm injuries** to prevent abdominal herniation; small, right-sided injuries do not generally herniate due to the liver.

Solid Organ Injuries

Most commonly injured in **blunt abdominal trauma.** Grades of injuries are summarized in Table 18-11.

- Hepatic injury: May be asymptomatic or present with peritonitis and hemodynamic instability. FAST or CT confirm diagnosis. Majority of injuries are managed nonoperatively (ie, serial exams, serial HCTs, bedrest, monitoring). Ongoing hemorrhage requires **angiographic embolization or laparotomy**. During laparotomy, perform Pringle maneuver (≤ 60 min), liver packing, vessel ligation, or partial hepatectomy with or without drainage.
- Splenic injury: Similar to hepatic injuries in terms of presentation. **Kehr's sign** (ie, diaphragmatic irritation → left shoulder pain) may be present. May be managed nonoperatively (similar to hepatic injuries), but perform splenectomy or splenorrhaphy for hemodynamic instability. Administer vaccines prior to discharge or at follow-up, if splenectomy is performed.
- Pancreatic injury: May present asymptomatically even with transection. Diagnosis may be difficult. Follow **serum amylase (be suspicious if persistently increasing)** and check CT abdomen, endoscopic retrograde cholangiopancreatography (ERCP), or intraoperative pancreatogram. **Management is related to involvement of pancreatic duct:** if no ductal injury is present, drain the injury, but if major pancreatic duct disruption

TABLE 18-11. **Grades of Solid Abdominal Organ Injuries**

GRADE	LIVER	SPLEEN	PANCREAS
I	*Hematoma:* Subcapsular < 10% surface area (SA). *Laceration*: Capsular tear, < 1-cm parenchymal depth, - bleeding.	*Hematoma*: Subcapsular < 10% SA. *Laceration*: Capsular tear < 1-cm parenchymal depth.	*Hematoma:* Minor contusion, – duct injury. *Laceration:* Superficial laceration, – duct injury.
II	*Hematoma:* Subcapsular 10–50% SA or intraparenchymal < 10 cm diameter. *Laceration:* Capsular tear plus bleeding, 1 to 3-cm parenchymal depth, or < 10-cm length.	*Hematoma:* Subcapsular 10–50% SA, < 5-cm diameter. *Laceration:* 1 to 3-cm parenchymal depth not involving trabecular vessel.	*Hematoma:* Major contusion, – duct injury/tissue loss. *Laceration:* Major laceration, – duct injury/tissue loss.
III	*Hematoma:* Subcapsular > 50% SA or expanding; ruptured subcapsular hematoma with bleeding; intraparenchymal hematoma > 10 cm or expanding. *Laceration:* > 3 cm parenchymal depth.	*Hematoma:* Subcapsular expanding or > 50% SA; ruptured subcapsular or parenchymal hematoma; > 5 cm or expanding intraparenchymal hematoma. *Laceration:* > 3 cm parenchymal depth or + trabecular vessel involvement.	*Laceration:* Distal transection/ parenchymal injury, + duct injury.
IV	*Hematoma:* Ruptured intraparenchymal hematoma with bleeding. *Laceration:* Parenchymal disruption 35–75% of one lobe or 1–3 Couinard segments in one lobe.	*Laceration:* Injury to segmental/hilar vessel with major devascularization.	*Laceration:* Proximal transection/parenchymal injury.
V	*Laceration:* Parenchymal disruption > 75% of one lobe or > three Couinard's segments in one lobe. *Vascular:* Juxtahepatic venous injury.	*Laceration:* Shattered spleen. *Vascular:* Hilar vessel disruption (devascularized spleen).	*Laceration:* Major disruption of pancreatic head.
VI	*Vascular:* Hepatic avulsion.	N/A	N/A

is present, resect affected region with or without closed drainage to create controlled pancreatic fistula.

HOLLOW VISCUS INJURIES

Most commonly injured in **penetrating abdominal trauma.** Grades of injuries are summarized in Table 18-12.

- Stomach injury: May present with chemical peritonitis (due to spillage of HCl), blood in NGT, or free air on CXR. While most (grades I–II and possibly III) can be closed primarily, others require partial gastrectomy (grade IV) or total gastrectomy (grade V). If pylorus is injured, perform pyloroplasty.

TABLE 18-12. Grades of Hollow Viscus Organ Injuries

GRADE	STOMACH	DUODENUM	SMALL INTESTINE
I	*Hematoma:* Contusion/Hematoma – devascularization. *Laceration:* Partial thickness, – perforation.	*Hematoma:* One portion of duodenum. *Laceration:* Partial thickness, + perforation.	*Hematoma:* Contusion or hematoma. *Laceration:* Partial thickness.
II	*Laceration:* < 50% circumference.	*Hematoma:* > One portion of duodenum. *Laceration:* < 50% circumference.	*Laceration:* < 2 cm involving GEJ/pylorus; < 5 cm involving proximal 1/3 of stomach; < 10 cm involving distal 2/3 of stomach.
III	*Laceration:* ≥ 50% circumference, – transection.	*Laceration:* 50-75% circumference of D2, 50-100% circumference of D1, D3, or D4.	*Laceration:* > 2 cm involving GEJ/ pylorus; ≥ 5 cm involving proximal 1/3 of stomach; ≥ 10 cm involving distal 2/3 of stomach.
IV	*Laceration:* + SI transection.	*Laceration:* > 75% circumference of D2; common bile duct or ampulla injury.	*Laceration:* Tissue loss. *Vascular:* Devascularization < 2/3 of stomach.
V	*Laceration:* + SI transection, tissue loss. *Vascular:* Devascularized segment.	*Laceration:* Major disruption of duodenopancreatic complex. *Vascular*: Duodenal devascularization.	*Laceration:* Tissue loss. *Vascular:* Devascularization > 2/3 of stomach.

- Duodenal injury: Associated with complications in up to 60% of cases and death in up to 25%. Diagnosis is with serum amylase, CXR (free air or "stack of coins" with hematoma), and CT with oral contrast (assess for retroperitoneal air and hematoma). Hematomas may be managed nonoperatively with NGT. However, exploration and 1° closure (grades I–II) or pyloric exclusion, duodenoduodenostomy, or duodenojejunostomy (grades III–IV), or Whipple (grade V) may be necessary. Vast majority of duodenal injuries (80%) are suitable for 1° closure.
- Nonduodenal small intestine (SI) injury: Difficult to diagnose. Requires high index of suspicion (eg, **seatbelt sign**). CT scan is unreliable but may demonstrate **free air, free fluid, bowel thickening or enhancement, contrast leak or extravasation.** Perform 1° repair (grades I–III) or resection with anastomosis (grades IV–V).
- Colorectal injury: Colonic injuries are generally amenable to 1° repair or resection with anastomosis. Reserve colostomy for delayed diagnosis and inflammation. Treat rectal injuries with diverting colostomy and presacral drainage.

RETROPERITONEAL VASCULAR INJURIES

Location of injury determines management:

- Zone I (central hematoma): Injury to aorta, inferior vena cava (IVC), celiac axis, proximal superior mesenteric artery or vein, or renal artery or vein. Explore for blunt or penetrating trauma.

Always obtain proximal and distal control before exploring a vascular injury.

Unstable trauma patient
↓
Exam of the thigh compartments, CXR, FAST/DPL, AP pelvic radiograph
↓
+ FAST → laparotomy
– FAST, + pelvic fracture → angiography.

TRAUMA, BURNS, AND CRITICAL CARE

- Zone II (upper lateral hematoma): Injury to kidney and renal artery or vein. Explore for penetrating trauma; **do not explore for blunt trauma unless hematoma is expanding.**
- Zone III (pelvic hematoma): Injury to iliac artery or vein. Often involves diffuse venous bleeding associated with a pelvic fracture. **Explore only in penetrating trauma.**
- Portal-retrohepatic region: May involve portal vein, IVC, hepatic artery, or hepatic vein. Associated with hemodynamic instability if active hemorrhage present. Because of the risk of massive bleeding if tamponade is released, explore only if ruptured or rapidly expanding.

The classic indications for exploration of retroperitoneal hematomas (as listed above) are changing rapidly with the widespread use of high-resolution CT scans. Stable patients with hematomas resulting from venous injuries (and selected arterial injuries) are observed regardless of location.

Genitourinary Trauma

Involved in about 10% of traumatic injuries. Diagnosis and management are injury–specific.

Renal Injuries

Most commonly associated with blunt trauma (see Table 18-13). May present with **hematuria**, flank ecchymoses, or costovertebral angle tenderness. Labs may reveal **blood in the urinalysis** with or without anemia; check a baseline BUN and creatinine. The presence of hematuria necessitates an intravenous pyelogram (IVP) or abdominal CT (with contrast and delayed images). **Always perform an IVP to evaluate the contralateral kidney if trauma nephrectomy is considered.** Nonoperative management and renal salvage is indicated for grade I–IV injuries; grade V requires partial or complete nephrectomy.

TABLE 18-13. Grades of Renal Injuries

Grade	Kidney
I	*Contusion:* Microscopic or gross hematuria; normal studies. *Hematoma:* Subcapsular, nonexpanding, – parenchymal laceration.
II	*Hematoma:* Nonexpanding perirenal hematoma; confined to renal retroperitoneum. *Laceration:* < 1 cm parenchymal cortical involvement, – urinary extravasation.
III	*Laceration:* > 1 cm parenchymal cortical involvement, – urinary extravasation/collecting system involvement.
IV	*Laceration:* Renal cortex, medulla, collecting system involvement. *Vascular:* Injury to main renal artery or vein; contained.
V	*Laceration:* Shattered kidney. *Vascular:* Devascularized kidney with hilar avulsion.

URETERAL INJURIES

Similar to renal injuries but should be repaired immediately with 1° repair or reconstruction.

BLADDER INJURIES

Rupture may occur after penetrating or blunt trauma; **associated with pelvic fracture. Gross hematuria** is almost always present. CT cystogram demonstrates intra- or extra-peritoneal leak. Manage **extraperitoneal injuries with urinary catheter drainage** (2–3 weeks); **intraperitoneal injuries require immediate 1° repair**.

URETHRAL INJURIES

Anterior (ie, straddle injury) and posterior (ie, pelvic ring fractures) injuries are suggested by **blood at urethral meatus**, inability to void, or **"high-riding" prostate on rectal exam**. Confirm with retrograde urethrogram. **Do not attempt urinary catheter placement.** Treatment can include suprapubic drainage with early or delayed repair (based on type and degree of injury).

Vertebral and Spinal Cord Trauma

DEMOGRAPHICS

Not only are C-spine fractures more common than thoracolumbar injuries, but they are also associated with a different age distribution: C-spine fractures affect the young and elderly rather than the middle-aged population. About 1% of spinal fractures have subsequent spinal cord injury.

TYPES

Pertinent C-spine fractures include

- C1 (Jefferson fracture): Fracture of anterior and posterior arches with lateral displacement due to **axial loading**. Treat with halo brace.
- C2 (Hangman's fracture): Bilateral pedicle fracture due to hyperextension. Treat with halo brace.
- C2 (odontoid fracture): Type I (tip of dens) is stable. Types II (base of dens) and III (body of C2) are unstable and require halo placement or open reduction with internal fixation (ORIF) or fusion.

Thoracolumbar spine fractures can involve any of three columns. Fracture or ligamentous injury to 2–3 columns results in an unstable spine. Fractures include

- Compression fracture: Stable fracture involving anterior column due to hyperflexion. Treat with TLSO brace for comfort.
- Burst fracture: Unstable fracture involving anterior and middle columns often with retropulsion into spinal canal; due to axial loading. Requires ORIF.
- Chance fracture: Transverse fracture through vertebral body, pedicles, and lamina due to hyperflexion and distraction (ie, **lap belt injury**). Treat with ORIF.
- Facet fracture: Injury to all three columns due to rotational forces. Treat with ORIF.

SIGNS/SYMPTOMS

Associated with pain, tenderness, and **step-off deformity**. Spinal cord injury can present with numbness, tingling, and a partial or complete loss of function (motor and sensory). High cervical injuries can result in diaphragm compromise and death (eg, asphyxia), while quadriplegia and paraplegia result from cervical and thoracic cord injuries, respectively. **Injuries above T6 cause autonomic instability**.

DIAGNOSIS

Selected patients (ie, alert, normal exam) may have their C-spines cleared without radiographs. In all others, thin cut C-spine CT can rule out fracture. **MRI or flexion-extension fluoroscopy can assess ligamentous injury.** Assess thoracolumbar spine clinically or with CT scan with sagittal and coronal reformats.

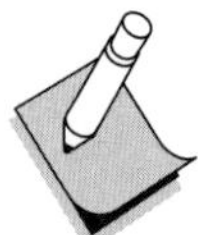

Steroids are indicated for spinal cord trauma (within 8 hours) but not brain injury

TREATMENT

Spinal fractures or dislocations require closed (axial traction) or open reduction. Achieve permanent stabilization with external orthosis (eg, C-collar, halo) or internal fixation (eg, spinal fusion).

For **spinal cord injuries, start high-dose methylprednisolone (30 mg/kg bolus over 45 minutes, followed by 5.4 mg/kg/h × 24–48 hours) within 8 hours of injury to improve outcome.**

Pelvic ring fractures– *Major source of hemorrhage in unstable patients*

Orthopaedic Trauma

Specific injuries are summarized in Table 18-14

Acute Respiratory Distress Syndrome

DEMOGRAPHICS/RISK FACTORS

Diffuse lung injury (alveolar-capillary leak) → low pressure pulmonary edema and acute hypoxemic respiratory failure. Occurs after systemic insults (eg, trauma, massive transfusion, sepsis, severe pancreatitis) or local injury (eg, pneumonia, aspiration, contusion).

Acute limb ischemia and compartment syndrome are discussed in Chapter 17

SIGNS/SYMPTOMS

Initial, exudative phase is characterized by the acute onset of respiratory failure, tachypnea, hypoxemia, and low lung compliance (usually within 24–48 hours of insult). This phase is followed by fibroproliferative (> 10 days; patient improves or symptoms become persistent) and fibrosis phases.

Fat embolus syndrome– *AMS, petechiae, and acute lung injury (ARDS). Associated with long bone fractures. Treat supportively.*

DIAGNOSIS

Clinical diagnosis is based on three criteria:

1. Hypoxia refractory to O_2 supplementation ($PaO_2/FiO_2 \leq 200$ mm Hg)
2. Presence of bilateral infiltrates (CXR, chest CT)
3. Absence of left heart failure (pulmonary capillary wedge pressure [PCWP] < 18 mm Hg, normal left ventricular function on echo, normal central venous pressure [CVP])

TABLE 18-14. Common Orthopaedic Injuries and Associated Traumatic Injuries

INJURY	PERTINENT POINTS	MANAGEMENT
Shoulder dislocation	Anterior (most common) → axillary artery/nerve injury. Posterior (eg, electrocution, seizure) → radial artery injury.	Closed reduction, immobilization.
Humeral head fracture	**Brachial artery, axillary nerve, brachial plexus injuries.**	Immobilization. Based on location/type may require fixation.
Humeral shaft fracture	Radial nerve injury (**wrist drop**, loss of thumb abduction).	Immobilization. Surgical repair for open fracture or vascular compromise.
Supracondylar fracture	Brachial artery injury → **Volkmann's contracture.**	Closed reduction, percutaneous pinning.
Posterior hip dislocation	Avascular necrosis.	Early reduction.
Hip fracture	**Foreshortened, externally rotated leg.** High rate of avascular necrosis, fracture nonunion.	ORIF with parallel pinning of the femoral neck. Hemiarthroplasty for elderly patients with displaced fractures.
Femur fracture	Foreshortened, internally rotated limb. Risk of **fat embolism.**	Intramedullary nailing.
Knee dislocation	Popliteal artery injury (dissection) and thrombosis → neurovascular compromise.	If acute limb ischemia, repair/bypass popliteal injury with knee reduction and fixation.
Tibial fracture	High risk of open fracture, compartment syndrome.	Open reduction with fixation (internal/external).
Pelvic ring facture		
Lateral compression	↓ Pelvic diameter/volume → usually **no** associated vascular injury.	Supportive management.
AP compression	Widening of the pelvic diameter (**"open book" fracture**) with pubic symphysis diastasis or sacroiliac joint disruption. ↑ Pelvic volume → + vascular injury, severe hemorrhage. Usually retroperitoneal venous bleeding but also can see **arterial "contrast blush"** on CT.	↓ Pelvic volume (bedsheet wrap, external fixation) followed by angiographic embolization. Never open a pelvic hematoma from blunt trauma. ORIF of pelvic fracture only after hemorrhage is controlled and other injuries identified.
Vertical shear	Usually involves all ligaments of a hemipelvis. Always an **unstable fracture** with major vascular injury.	See above.
Open fracture	Suspect with skin laceration adjacent to fracture. Graded I-III: ▪ Grade I: Wound < 1 cm, minimal soft tissue injury/contamination. ▪ Grade II: Wound 1–10 cm, moderate soft tissue injury/contamination. ▪ Grade III: Wound > 10 cm, severe soft tissue injury/contamination.	**Orthopaedic emergency**. Initial management includes limb reduction, splinting, IV antibiotics, tetanus prophylaxis. Urgent (< 6 hours) surgical irrigation and debridement, open reduction, and external fixation. Wound is left open with delayed 1° closure after 3–4 days.

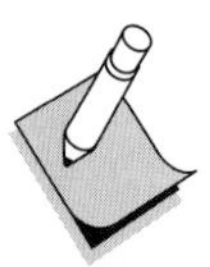

Criteria for ARDS–

- *Hypoxia refractory to O_2 supplementation (Pao_2/Fio_2 ≤ 200 mm Hg)*
- *Presence of bilateral infiltrates (CXR, chest CT)*
- *Absence of left heart failure (PCWP < 18 mm Hg, normal LV function on echo, normal CVP)*

TREATMENT

Use mechanical ventilation with **low tidal volumes (6 mL/kg)** to keep plateau pressures < 30 cm H_2O. **Use PEEP to keep Fio_2 < 60%.** Identify and treat underlying causes. Diurese aggressively.

Sepsis and Systemic Inflammatory Response Syndrome

DEMOGRAPHICS/RISK FACTORS

Though the true incidence of systemic inflammatory response syndrome (SIRS) is not known, mortality is ~7% from SIRS and ~15% from sepsis. SIRS results from an inflammatory response to either infectious or noninfectious insults. Sepsis is SIRS due to an infectious etiology (eg, pneumonia, bacteremia, urinary tract, abdominal source). Noninfectious etiologies include trauma, pancreatitis, and massive transfusion.

SIGNS/SYMPTOMS

Signs and symptoms are dependent upon etiology. Two of four criteria must be met to diagnose SIRS:

1. T > 38°C or < 36°C
2. HR > 90 bpm
3. RR > 20 breaths/min or $Paco_2$ < 32 mm Hg
4. WBC > 12 K/μL or < 4 K/ μL or PMN > 10%.

Sepsis is the combination of SIRS and infection.

APACHE score–

Measure of severity of disease based on age, chronic health problems, and 12 acute physiologic parameters. Score = 0–4 associated with a 4% mortality rate. Score > 34 associated with 85% mortality.

DIAGNOSIS

Confirm criteria listed above to diagnose SIRS. To diagnose sepsis, must also identify etiology: perform exam, CXR, urinalysis, blood cultures, and CT scan.

TREATMENT

Early diagnosis is key. Control source (eg, abscess drainage), give broad-spectrum antibiotics, and provide supportive care with fluid resuscitation and vasopressors. **Patients with high acute physiology and chronic health evaluation (APACHE) scores may benefit from drotrecogin alfa (activated protein C).** Evaluate and treat for adrenal insufficiency, if present (see Chapter 12).

Multisystem Organ Failure

A leading cause of late mortality. Commonly due to shock and severe trauma. Risk factors include age, high injury severity score, transfusions, hypotension, acidosis, and infection. Patients may demonstrate respiratory failure (eg, ARDS), cardiac failure (eg, hypotension requiring vasopressors), renal failure (eg, ↑ creatinine, oliguria, need for dialysis), gastrointestinal ischemia (eg, ileus, pancreatitis, acalculous cholecystitis), hepatic failure (eg, jaundice, ↑ liver function tests, ↑ PT), neurologic dysfunction (eg, delirium, AMS), hematologic abnormalities (eg, thrombocytopenia, leukocytosis, leukopenia, disseminated intravascular coagulation [DIC]), and metabolic derangement (eg, lactic acidosis, hyperglycemia). Management is supportive: mechanical ventilation, fluids, vasopressors, dialysis, blood products, nutrition, and sedation.

Calciphylaxis

Affects up to 4% of patients with **chronic renal failure**. Carries a mortality as high as 80%. Due to **vascular (arteriolar) calcifications and microthrombi → skin and soft tissue necrosis.** Often affects fatty tissues, particularly in the lower extremities. Usually a clinical diagnosis but may see calcification of the vessels and subcutaneous tissues on radiographs. Treat with **Na^+ thiosulfate** (↑ Ca^{2+} solubility) and normalize Ca^{2+} and PO_4^{3-}. Necrotic tissue may require debridement and burn wound care.

Stevens-Johnson Syndrome and Toxic Epidermal Necrolysis Syndrome

Demographics/Risk Factors

Severe cutaneous adverse drug reactions, which cause blisters and epidermal detachment. Differ only in the extent of dermal involvement: **Stevens-Johnson syndrome (SJS) involves < 10% total body surface area (TBSA) and toxic epidermal necrolysis syndrome (TENS) involves > 30% TBSA**. Likely an autoimmune reaction to medications (eg, anticonvulsants, **sulfonamides**, nonsteroidal anti-inflammatory drugs [NSAIDs], allopurinol, steroids) or infections (eg, *Mycoplasma pneumoniae*). Mortality approaches 35% with TEN.

Signs/Symptoms

Fever, cough, malaise, painful skin, burning eyes, and mucosal erosions may occur days before skin lesions. Skin changes progress from erythema → necrosis → bullae → full thickness loss of epidermis (exposed red dermis). Mucosal involvement of the eyes, oropharynx, lungs, and urethra can cause vision loss, dysphagia, ARDS, and dysuria, respectively.

Diagnosis

Clinical diagnosis based on history and characteristic lesions. Exam demonstrates **Nikolsky's sign** (ie, skin separation with horizontal traction). Biopsy shows **keratinocyte necrosis at dermal-epidermal junction.**

Treatment

Control pain and **withdraw inciting medications**. Provide wound care (similar to burn treatment). Early intravenous immunoglobulin (IVIG) may be beneficial in TENS. Consider antibiotics for neutropenia or infection.

Burns: Thermal, Chemical, and Electrical Injuries

Burns can result from thermal (eg, flame, scald, contact), chemical (eg, hydrofluoric acid [HF]), or electrical insults. Diagnosis and management are based on the depth and extent of the burns:

- First-degree: Affects epidermis only. Blanching erythema and pain.
- Second-degree: Involves full thickness of epidermis and partial thickness of dermis. Erythema with or without blanching, blisters, and pain. Intact dermal appendages (ie, hair follicles, glands) allow regrowth of epidermis in 7–14 days. Deeper, second-degree burns appear pale or mottled but may still heal (14–28 days), but with severe scarring.
- Third-degree: Extends through full-thickness dermis and into subcutaneous tissue. Characteristic white leathery eschar is insensate.
- Fourth-degree: Involving deep structures (eg, muscle, bone).

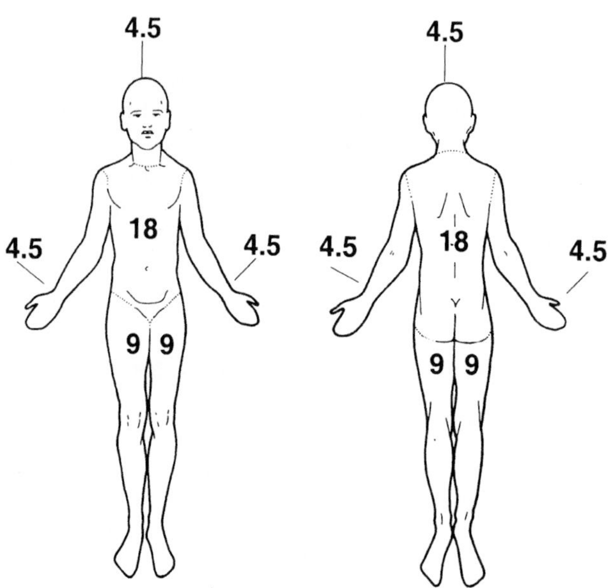

FIGURE 18-4. Determination of TBSA—"Rule of 9s."

(Reproduced, with permission, from Feliciano DV, et al. *Trauma*, 6th ed. New York: McGraw-Hill, 2008:1055.)

The palm of the hand approximates 1% TBSA.

TBSA is determined as a percentage of skin affected with 2° to 3° burns (see Figure 18-4).

Specific types of burns are particularly important.

- Inhalation injury and CO poisoning: Inhalation of hot smoke particles can lead to **thermal injury to the airways and lungs**. May be associated with singed facial hairs and carbonaceous sputum. Obtain a **carboxyhemoglobin level** to evaluate for CO poisoning.
- Electrical burns: Most severe injury occurs at entry and exit sites and can include **extensive soft tissue destruction that is not visible externally.**
- HF burns: HF exposure results in **liquefaction of tissues and Ca^{2+} precipitation.** Patients present with exquisite pain and edema of affected area. Necrosis may be present.

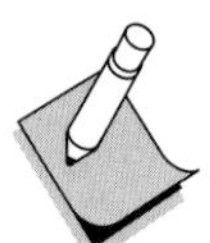

Parkland formula–
Crystalloid requirement for the first 24 hours (mL): 4 × weight (kg) × % TBSA

Rapidly assess the burn patient. Secure airway early (due to risk of oropharyngeal edema), obtain IV access, start fluid resuscitation, and keep patient warm. Initial 24-hour fluid requirements are estimated by the **Parkland formula**.

Topical antibiotics are applied to prevent infection. Options include

- Bacitracin: Painless. Less antibacterial coverage.
- Silver sulfadiazine: Broad-spectrum, painless. Does not penetrate eschar. **Avoid in patients with sulfa allergy**.
- Mafenide acetate: Broad-spectrum coverage (except fungal), penetrates eschar. Painful. Can cause **metabolic acidosis.**
- Silver nitrate: Broad spectrum, painless. Stains skin black. Can cause **methemoglobinemia.**

Diagnose burn wound infection by biopsy (> 10^5 organisms/g tissue or invasion of viable tissue); culture swab is unreliable.

Circumferential burns to chest and extremities with thick eschar can impair chest wall excursion and distal perfusion; if present, perform immediate escharotomy. Deep second- and third-degree burns require excision and split thickness skin graft due to inability to heal spontaneously.

Chemical burns should be copiously irrigated. Treat CO poisoning with **100% O_2**, and consider hyperbaric oxygen in severe exposures to prevent delayed neurologic sequelae. For electrical burns, titrate resuscitation to urine output (1.5 mL/kg/h), treat myoglobinuria, check cardiac enzymes, perform cardiac monitoring, and obtain baseline ophthalmic exam (due to risk of cataracts). For HF burns, apply **Ca^{2+} gluconate** gel to the wound, monitor serum Ca^{2+} levels and QT interval prolongation, and administer IV Ca^{2+} gluconate when necessary.

Do not neutralize chemical burns.

TRAUMA, BURNS, AND CRITICAL CARE

Hypothermia

Decrease in core body temperature to < 35°C. Most commonly caused by environmental exposure. Mild hypothermia results in vague complaints of nausea, dizziness, and shivering; moderate-to-severe hypothermia (< 32.2°C) may result in loss of shivering, rigidity, AMS, and cardiac arrhythmias (ie, tachycardia → bradycardia → VF, asystole). **Hypothermic patients in cardiac arrest** (eg, **drowning after falling through ice) must be aggressively resuscitated because of high tolerance to cerebral ischemia.** Consider external (eg, warming blankets, water baths, forced warm air) or internal (eg, heated humidified O_2, warmed fluids, and heated peritoneal, chest tube, gastric, and bladder lavage) rewarming. In severe cases (eg, cardiac dysrhythmia), consider cardiopulmonary bypass or hemodialysis.

▶ SAMPLE QUESTIONS

A 35-year-old male presents with blood at the urethral meatus after a MVC. What is his injury?	Urethral disruption. There is a high likelihood of associated pelvic fracture.
A 45-year-old female with severe alcoholic pancreatitis develops respiratory distress. CXR shows bilateral infiltrates. What is the diagnosis? What are the three criteria to make this diagnosis?	ARDS: (1) O_2 refractory hypoxia (2) Bilateral infiltrates (3) Absence of left heart failure.
An 18-year-old man presents after a MVC with a lateral skull injury and loss of consciousness. He is now lucid. He develops progressive obtundation, a dilated ipsilateral pupil, and contralateral hemiparesis. What vessel is injured?	Middle meningeal artery is most commonly lacerated after a temporal bone fracture → epidural hematoma. Requires emergent craniotomy and evacuation.
A 17-year-old female is the unrestrained front-seat passenger in a head-on MVC and has contusions of her knee. What associated injury should you look for?	Posterior hip dislocation or posterior acetabular wall fracture (from knee hitting the dashboard while sitting).
A 45-year-old male fell from a three storey deck and landed on both feet. What two injuries should you look for?	Calcaneal fractures, thoracolumbar vertebral compression fractures (axial loading).
A 62-year-old pedestrian is struck and has bilateral tibial shaft fractures. He develops respiratory distress on posttrauma day 2. What is his diagnosis? What other signs should you look for?	Fat embolus syndrome. The triad is petechiae, respiratory distress (ARDS), and mental status changes.
A 72-year-old female in a MVC is hypotensive with a + DPL. She undergoes laparotomy and splenectomy; a large pelvic hematoma is identified. What is the next step in management?	Never open a pelvic hematoma for blunt trauma. Obtain angiogram +/– embolization of the bleeding source. If pelvic fracture is identified → perform external fixation (wrap with sheet if fracture found outside of OR).
A 30-year-old female is obtunded and hypotensive after a rollover MVC. Her DPL is grossly +. What is the next step?	Go directly to the OR. Follow the priority of ABCs → hemorrhage control is the first priority.

A 45-year-old male sustains a severe crush injury to the distal femur and knee with a comminuted femur fracture. There are no distal pulses. Does the vascular or orthopedic procedure take priority?	Stabilize the bone (quickly) before definitive repair of vasculature. However, if this will take > 6 hours of ischemia time, place a temporary vascular shunt first.
A 23-year-old male in a MVC is hypotensive with an unstable pelvis. Where should the DPL be performed?	Perform a supraumbilical DPL when pelvic hematoma is suspected.

▶ BASIC SCIENCE

Anatomy of Fetal Circulation

Shunts reflect pressure gradients of the pulmonary and systemic circulation. Blood enters the fetal circulation via the **single umbilical vein** and bypasses the hepatic circulation as the **ductus venosus** shunts blood from the umbilical vein to the inferior vena cava (IVC). Next, blood is shunted from the right to left heart via the **foramen ovale**. The small volume of blood that does enter the pulmonary circulation is directed to the systemic circulation via the **ductus arteriosus** (left pulmonary artery → descending aorta). A large portion of the cardiac output (CO) exits the fetus via **two umbilical arteries for gas exchange in the placenta** (see Figure 19-1).

Neonatal Physiology

Cardiac System

Normal pediatric vital signs vary with age and are summarized in Table 19-1.

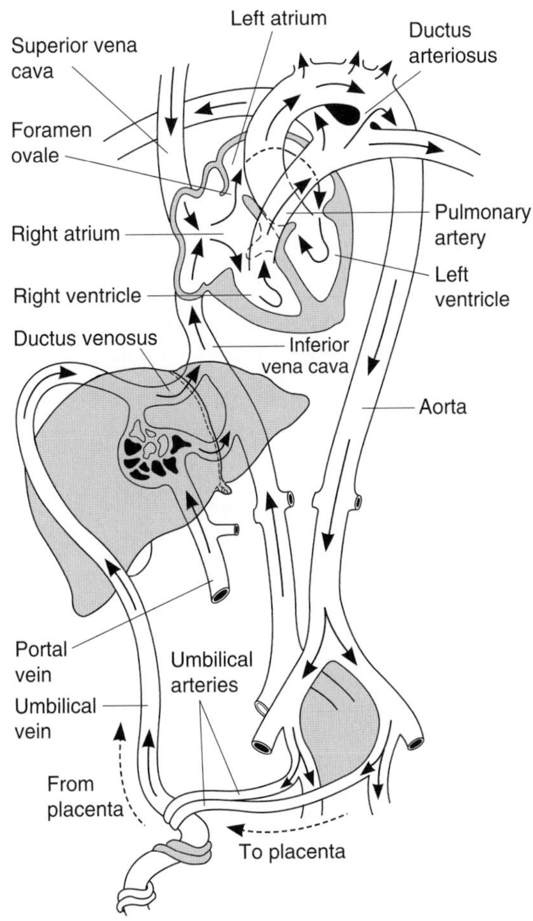

FIGURE 19-1. Fetal circulation.

(Reproduced, with permission, from Ganong WF. *Review of Medical Physiology*. 22nd ed. New York: McGraw-Hill, 2005:628.)

PEDIATRIC SURGERY

TABLE 19-1. Pediatric Vital Signs

AGE	SBP (mm Hg)	HR (bpm)	RR (bpm)
Newborn–1 month	> 60	120–160	40–60
1 month–1 year	70–95	100–140	25–50
1–8 years	80–110	80–100	15–30
8 years-adulthood	90–140	60–100	12–20

PULMONARY SYSTEM

Not fully developed until 8 years of age. Alveoli are identifiable in the fetus at 24 weeks' gestation. Infants are **preferential nasal breathers** between 6 months and 6 years of age. Diaphragm is the 1° muscle for respiration.

Adequate urine output for an infant is 2–3 mL/kg/h.

RENAL SYSTEM

Neonatal kidneys receive only 2–4% of the CO (vs 20–25% in adults). Glomerular filtration rate (GFR) of a full-term newborn is about 2–4 mL/min, which ↑ 5- to 10-fold over the first week of life. Newborn kidneys have a limited ability to concentrate urine (maximum urine osmolality = ~500 mOsm). Adequate urine output for an infant is **2–3 mL/kg/h.**

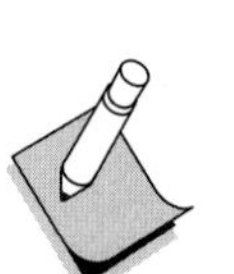

Key immunoglobulins–

IgG = Crosses placenta

IgA = Transferred in breast milk

IMMUNE SYSTEM

Fetus obtains maternally acquired immunity in the form of **immunoglobulin G (IgG)**, which **crosses the placental barrier**. The breast fed infant also receives **immunoglobulin A (IgA)** in the **breast milk**. The infant immune system is slow to produce IgG. Additionally, newborns exhibit ↓ polymorphonuclear neutrophil (PMN) activity, complement fixation, and chemoattraction.

Pediatric Fluid and Nutritional Requirements

FLUID REQUIREMENTS

Newborn fluid maintenance is determined by the **Holliday and Segar formula**.

- 4 mL/kg/hr for the first 10 kg
- 2 mL/kg/hr for the second 10 kg
- 1 mL/kg/hr for each kilogram thereafter

Unique considerations for newborn volume resuscitation include ↑ insensible water losses (compared to adults) and a physiologic diuresis during the first week of life (caused by ↑ GFR).

For schock associated with pediatric trauma, first bolus 20 mL/kg twice; if hemodynamic instability persists, give packed red blood cells (PRBC; 10 mL/kg). Best indicator of shock is **tachycardia** (> 150 bpm in neonate, > 120 bpm if < 1 year, > 100 bpm if > 1 year).

NUTRITIONAL REQUIREMENTS

Caloric and protein requirements are based on age.

- Preterm: 120–130 kcal/kg/d (3–4 g protein/kg/d)
- Full term: 110–120 kcal/kg/d (2–2.5 g protein/kg/d)
- 6 months–3 years: 100 kcal/kg/d (1.2–1.6 g protein/kg/d)
- 7–10 years: 70 kcal/kg/d (1.0–1.5 g protein/kg/d)
- 10–18 years: 50–60 kcal/kg/d (1.0 g protein/kg/d).

▶ CLINICAL SCIENCE

Choanal Atresia

Occlusion of the posterior nares. Slight predilection for twins and unilaterality. Presents with **intermittent respiratory distress** (**retractions**), poor suckling, and a normal cry. Diagnosis is confirmed when a **nasogastric tube (NGT) will not pass the anterior nares**. Treat with surgical resection and postoperative stent to maintain patency.

Thyroglossal Duct Cyst

DEMOGRAPHICS

Most common congenital neck anomaly. Arises from embryonic ectodermal rests after thyroid descent. Often presents < 30 years of age, though up to 50% may not be diagnosed until adulthood.

SIGNS/SYMPTOMS

Palpable, asymptomatic (unless infected), **midline neck mass** below the level of the hyoid bone that **moves with swallowing**. On exam, the mass will move cephalad with tongue protrusion.

DIAGNOSIS

Clinical diagnosis.

TREATMENT

Sistrunk procedure, which involves excision of cyst, tract up to base of tongue, and central portion of the hyoid bone.

Branchial Cleft Anomalies

Anomalies of the **lateral neck** that may include cysts, sinuses, or fistulas. Greater than 90% arise from the **second branchial cleft,** resulting in drainage from small pit in the skin anterior to the lower one-third of the sternocleidomastoid (SCM). Diagnosis is suggested by clear fluid draining from anterior neck. Though imaging is rarely necessary, CT or MRI can confirm a fluid-filled mass in the anterior neck. Treat with complete resection of the cyst and tract. The tract may extend to the pharynx between the major carotid artery branches.

Childhood neck masses–
Lateral: Branchial cleft cysts
Midline: Thyroglossal duct cysts

Cystic Hygroma

Benign lymphatic lesions that can affect any body area, but most commonly involve the **posterior triangle of the neck, supraclavicular area, and axilla**. Exam reveals a soft, painless, **compressible** mass that **transilluminates**. Confirm diagnosis with ultrasound (in utero), CT, or MRI. Imaging is not always necessary but will show the deep extent into the mediastinum or chest. Treat with injection of sclerosing agent or surgical excision. Primary complication is **infection,** which should delay intervention by 3 weeks.

Torticollis

Due to SCM trauma during birth or due to uterine positioning. Infants appear healthy at birth; over days to weeks, infants develop SCM swelling with eventual contracture. Diagnosis is clinical, but plain radiographs can rule out bony abnormality. Treat with physical therapy, though 50–70% will resolve by 8 months of age if left untreated.

A newborn girl, born with normal APGAR scores, demonstrates early feeding intolerance with choking. An NGT is unable to be placed due to hypopharyngeal resistance. What is the most common radiographic presentation of the disease? This child has esophageal atresia (EA) and a tracheoesophageal fistula (TEF). The most common type is proximal EA with a distal fistula. Radiograph may show the NGT coiled in the proximal esophagus and copious gas throughout the abdomen.

Esophageal Atresia and Tracheoesophageal Fistula

Demographics/Risk Factors

VACTERL syndrome:
Vertebral anomalies
Anorectal anomalies
Cardiac anomalies
Tracheo-**E**sophageal fistulas
Renal/**R**adial anomalies
Limb anomalies

Congenital communication between the trachea and esophagus occurring in approximately 0.2% of live births. Ten percent are associated with the **VACTERL syndrome**.

Types

Five major types are shown in Figure 19-2. The most common type consists of **EA with a distal TEF**.

Signs/Symptoms

EA and TEF type determine symptomatology. EA usually presents with **drooling and inability to tolerate feeds**, while proximal TEFs present with **coughing and respiratory distress after eating**. Pure atresia may be suspected prenatally when **maternal polyhydramnios** is severe.

Diagnosis

Confirm with bronchoscopy, esophagoscopy, and **failure to pass NGT** (all except type E fistulas). Contrast radiographic studies are seldom indicated and carry a high risk of aspiration pneumonitis. Evaluate for concurrent VACTERL anomalies.

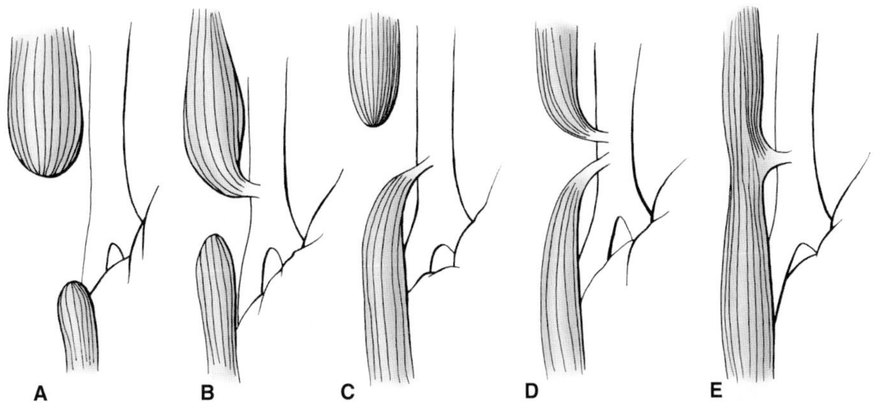

FIGURE 19-2. Types of tracheoesophageal fistulas. Note: Type-E TEF is often referred to as "H type."

(Reproduced, with permission, from Brunicardi FC, et al. *Schwartz's Principles of Surgery*. 8th ed. New York: McGraw-Hill, 2005.)

TREATMENT

Surgical intervention includes an extrapleural thoracotomy (to avoid pleural contamination if a leak occurs), division of fistula, and 1° reanastomosis of esophagus. Leak (15%) and stricture (10%) are the most common complications. Pure atresia or long gap atresia may need a staged repair. Pure TEF (ie, type E fistula) can be repaired via a cervical incision.

Congenital Lobar Emphysema

Bronchial obstruction due to cartilage malformation or external compression (eg, left atrial enlargement). **Progressive air trapping** leads to **hyperexpansion** with eventual mediastinal shift and respiratory failure. Most commonly affects the left upper or right middle lobes. Often asymptomatic at birth, but a hyperinflated lung may lead to compression of other lobes and respiratory distress. Diagnose with CXR or CT. Treatment includes lobectomy of affected area. It is important not to misdiagnose congenital lobar emphysema (CLE) as a pneumothorax and place a chest tube, as this may have disastrous consequences.

Congenital Cystic Adenomatoid Malformation

Proliferation of the lung with intercommunicating cysts at the level of the terminal bronchioles. Develops as a consequence of bronchiolar overgrowth. Cysts can air trap and become infected. These are often seen on prenatal ultrasounds and may regress completely. Clinical presentation ranges from asymptomatic to severe **respiratory distress** at birth. Diagnose with CXR or CT. Given the theoretical risk of malignant degeneration, treatment is resection.

Pulmonary Sequestration

Cystic lung mass composed of primitive lung tissue that **does not communicate with the tracheobronchial tree**. Arterial supply is always systemic, but venous drainage depends on type:

- **Extralobar**: Drains primarily through **systemic (azygous) veins.**
- **Intralobar**: Most common. Drains primarily through **pulmonary veins.**

Extralobar sequestrations tend to affect males and are diagnosed early (due to coexistent anomalies). Most commonly presents as a left lower lobe consolidation; exam may reveal a systolic bruit over affected site. CT angiography (CTA) or MR angiography (MRA) demonstrate systemic blood flow to the involved tissue. Embolization of the functional vascular shunt may be useful for compromised cardiovascular status. Definitive treatment includes excision for extralobar lesions and lobectomy for intralobar lesions. The systemic arteries often traverse the inferior pulmonary ligament and should be carefully identified and ligated to avoid having the vessel retract below the diaphragm and causing uncontrolled bleeding.

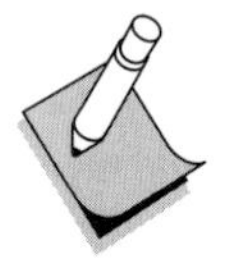

Childhood mediastinal masses–

Most common: Neurogenic tumors

Anterior: Lymphoma, teratoma (or other germ cell tumor), thymoma, thyroid cancer

Middle: Lymphoma, teratoma, bronchogenic cyst, cardiogenic cyst

Posterior: Neuroblastoma, neurofibroma, ganglioneuroma, meningioma

Bronchogenic Cyst

Most common mediastinal cystic mass. Filled with milky fluid and lined with respiratory epithelium. Symptoms are related to location: central cysts cause airway compression and respiratory distress, while peripheral cysts become infected. Diagnose with CXR and localize with CT. Due to risk of hemorrhage, infection, and proposed risk of malignant degeneration, all lesions (even if asymptomatic) **should be excised**. Excision can be accomplished with video-assisted thoracoscopic surgery.

Congenital Diaphragmatic Hernia

Demographics/Risk Factors

Herniation of abdominal viscera into the thoracic cavity with associated **pulmonary hypoplasia**. Affects 1/3000 of live births and may be transmitted with autosomal dominant or recessive inheritance.

Types

Two 1° types are **Bochdalek's** (left posterior; 85% of cases) and **Morgagni's** (anterior). Left-sided hernias allow displacement of small and large bowel; right-sided defects allow herniation of liver and large bowel.

Signs/Symptoms

Most common presenting sign is **respiratory distress and cyanosis within the first hours of life**, though **scaphoid abdomen**, **barrel chest**, and pulmonary HTN may also be present. Auscultation of bowel sounds over the chest wall can occasionally be appreciated.

Diagnosis

Often diagnosed in utero by ultrasound. CXR shows bowel in the chest, often with NGT above the diaphragm. Evaluate all organ systems, as 80% of patients will have additional anomalies.

Treatment

Perform initial stabilization with gentle ventilation and delayed operation until the pulmonary HTN resolves. Surgical repair is via the abdomen or chest and includes 1° or prosthetic repair. Critically ill infants may require **extracorporeal membrane oxygenation** to temporize. Overall survival is reported at 50% but can approach 80% in specialized centers.

In spite of an elemental formula diet, a 6-week-old firstborn male presents to the ED with nonbilious projectile vomiting. Serum K^+ and Cl^- are 2.9 mEq/dL and 89 mEq/dL, respectively. An ultrasound confirms pyloric stenosis. How should this patient be managed? Correct his hypovolemia with aggressive fluid resuscitation. Bolus with 20–40 mL/kg of normal saline followed by D5$^1/_2$NS with 20 meq/L KCl at 1.5 times maintenance. Perform pyloromyotomy when electrolytes are corrected.

Pyloric Stenosis

Demographics/Risk Factors

Affects 1/500 of births with an incidence four times greater in **males**. Other risk factors include a **family history of the disease and firstborn status.**

Signs/Symptoms

Typically presents with feeding intolerance progressing to **nonbilious, projectile emesis** at **3–6 weeks of age**. Exam may reveal the classic **"olive"** in upper abdomen. Labs often reveal **hypochloremic, hypokalemic metabolic alkalosis.**

Diagnosis

Confirm clinical suspicion with ultrasound findings: muscle thickness > 4 mm, diameter > 14 mm, channel length > 17 mm.

Treatment

After correction of hypovolemia and electrolyte disturbances, perform open or laparoscopic pyloromyotomy.

Choledochal Cyst

Demographics

A congenital dilation of the biliary tree with **malignant potential**. Though rare in the United States, it is relatively common in Asian populations. Females are affected four times as frequently as males.

Types

Classification includes (see Figure 19-3):

- Type I: **Most common.** Dilation of long segment(s) of the duct.
- Type II: Single diverticulum of the extrahepatic duct.
- Type III (choledochocele): Cyst arising from the segment of the bile duct that traverses the duodenal wall.

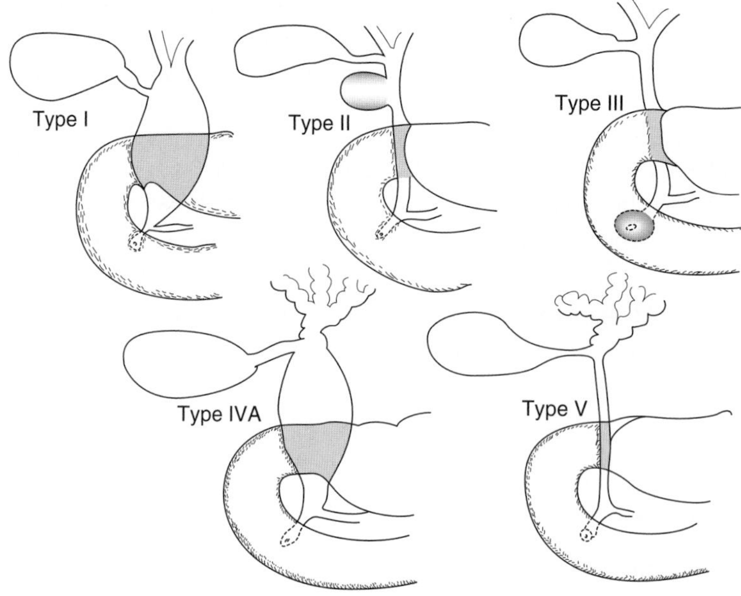

FIGURE 19-3. Classification of choledochal cysts.

- Type IVA: Multiple cysts involving intrahepatic and extrahepatic ducts.
- Type IVB: Multiple cysts involving only extrahepatic ducts.
- Type V (**Caroli's disease**): Multiple cysts involving only intrahepatic ducts.

SIGNS/SYMPTOMS

Classic triad of **pain, jaundice, and palpable mass** is present in less than one-third of patients. Clinically, jaundice is minimal and pain is episodic. May be associated with cholangitis.

DIAGNOSIS

Often diagnosed prenatally by ultrasound. After birth, ultrasound, CT, or magnetic resonance cholangiopancreatography (MRCP) are useful, though CT and MR provide the most information about relationships to adjacent structures.

TREATMENT

Types I, II, and IVB require total cyst excision. Type III cysts are treated with sphinterotomy or transduodenal excision. Types IVA and V cysts require hepatectomy if limited to one lobe of the liver; if both lobes are involved, consider transplant. Complications of unresected cysts include pancreatitis, cholangitis, obstructive jaundice, and **cholangiocarcinoma**.

Biliary Atresia

Disorder of the extrahepatic bile ducts, progressing to hepatic fibrosis. Affects 1/20,000 infants. May be an immune response to a viral infection. Sixty percent of cases are isolated, while the remainder are associated with disorders such as situs inversus, polysplenia, or preduodenal portal vein. Patients present with clay colored stools, jaundice that does not resolve by 2 weeks of life, and failure to thrive. Associated with **conjugated hyperbilirubinemia. Hepatobiliary iminodiacetic acid (HIDA) scan** has high sensitivity (but marginal specificity) and shows brisk radiotracer uptake without excretion to the duodenum. Ultrasound and endoscopic retrograde cholangiopancreatography (ERCP) can rule out other causes of biliary obstruction. Liver biopsy demonstrates an obstructive (rather than hepatocellular) cause of stasis. **Early hepaticoportoenterostomy** (**Kasai procedure**) is associated with less frequent progression to transplant: about one-third of Kasai patients can be considered cured, one-third go on to liver transplant, and one-third die before transplant.

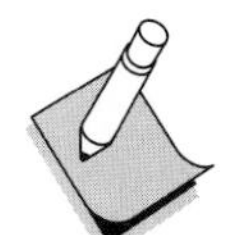

Neonatal jaundice is commonly due to low glucuronyl transferase activity (↑ unconjugated bilirubin) and is benign. ↑ Conjugated bilirubin should prompt search for surgically treatable causes of jaundice: biliary atresia, choledochal cysts, cholestasis.

Annular Pancreas and Pancreatic Divisum

Faulty rotation of the ventral pancreatic bud (annular pancreas) or failure of fusion of the ventral duct with the dorsal duct of Santorini (pancreatic divisum). Annular pancreas causes duodenal obstruction, while pancreatic divisum is a normal variant affecting 10% of the population. Annular pancreas is treated with an intestinal bypass procedure rather than resection of the encircling pancreas. Divisum may cause recurrent pancreatitis because of relative obstruction as the minor duct that inadequately drains the bulk of the exocrine pancreas. Treat with sphinteroplasty of the minor papillae.

Intestinal Stenosis and Atresia

Due to a failure of duodenal recanalization (stenosis) or mesenteric infarcts (atresia) during embryologic development. Twenty percent of patients with duodenal stenosis will also have Down's syndrome. Presents as **inability to tolerate feeds, bilious emesis** (as obstruction is distal to ampulla of Vater) **without distension**. Can diagnose as early as the second trimester by ultrasonographic "**double bubble**" (ie, dilated stomach and duodenum). Similar finding is seen on postnatal abdominal radiograph. Congenital duodenal atresia and stenosis are treated surgically with duodenoduodenostomy or duodenojejunostomy.

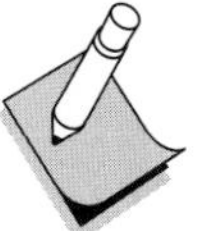

Have a high level of suspicion for intestinal stenosis/atresia in a newborn with bilious emesis.

PEDIATRIC SURGERY

Malrotation of Midgut Volvulus

Demographics

Failure of normal 270° counterclockwise rotation of mingut during sixth week of embryonic development. May affect as many as 1 in 500 births. Up to 90% are symptomatic by 1 year of age.

Signs/Symptoms

Some cases remain clinically silent, but most present with bilious vomiting and failure to thrive. Older children may have vague abdominal pain.

Bilious vomiting in an infant is malrotation until proven otherwise.

Diagnosis

Gold standard for diagnosis is an upper gastrointestinal (GI) series with small bowel follow through (SBFT), which shows proximal small bowel obstruction (SBO) and abnormal duodenal sweep (ie, **does not cross midline**).

Always perform appendectomy during Ladd's procedure for malrotation of midgut volvulus.

TREATMENT

Perform **immediate** operative detorsion of volvulus: evisceration, counterclockwise detorsion with placement of small bowel on right and colon on left, division of Ladd's bands, and appendectomy.

Omphalocele and Gastroschisis

Involve an anterior abdominal wall defect resulting in organ herniation (see Table 19-2).

Meconium Ileus

DEMOGRAPHICS

Mucous secreted by the small intestine (SI) is thickened, eventually leading to SBO. Occurs in > 10% of cystic fibrosis (CF) patients.

SIGNS/SYMPTOMS

Abdominal distension, **bilious emesis,** and failure to pass meconium postnatally. Abdominal radiographs show **ground glass** or **soap bubble** appearance as viscous meconium mixes with air (**Neuhauser's sign**).

DIAGNOSIS

Clinical diagnosis based on history, exam, and radiographic findings.

TREATMENT

Treat initially with rehydration and NGT decompression. This, along with gastrograffin enema, is successful in 80% of cases. If conservative management fails,

TABLE 19-2. Omphalocele Versus Gastroschisis

	OMPHALOCELE	GASTROSCHISIS
Pathogenesis	Failure of umbilical sac to close after developmental intestinal herniation.	Proper sac closure but with 2° paraumbilical (right) hernia.
Hernia contents	Small/Large bowel, stomach, and solid viscera possible.	Small bowel
Associated abnormalities	85%. Most common = cardiovascular. Associated with **Beckwith-Wiedemann syndrome** (macroglossia, macrosomia, omphalocele), cloacal extrophy.	< 5%. Associated with intestinal atresia, Hirschsprung's disease.
Diagnosis	Prenatal ultrasound.	Prenatal ultrasound
Management	Abdominal closure (either 1° or with staged-silo). Must complete evaluation for other anomalies.	Abdominal closure (either 1° or with staged-silo). Urgent repair if child is stable: first step is to cover bowel with moist towel and keep the mesentery from kinking and causing venous obstruction.

perform laparotomy with enterotomy and evacuation. May require irrigation of mucosa with N-acetylcysteine, gastrograffin, or saline. Consider appendectomy due to high risk of appendicitis in children with CF.

Hirschsprung's Disease

Demographics/Risk Factors

Defect in neural crest cell migration → absence of ganglion cells in Auerbch's plexus → absence of peristalsis → distal bowel obstruction. Affects 1 in 5000 of births. Associated with the *RET* proto-oncogene.

Signs/Symptoms

Failure to pass meconium, **bilious emesis,** abdominal distension.

Diagnosis

Confirm with rectal suction biopsy, which demonstrates **absence of ganglion cells.**

Treatment

Either one- or two-staged colectomy with resection of all involved tissue and a pull-through procedure.

Imperforate Anus

Due to faulty division as the cloaca separates into the rectum and urogenital sinus. Males are more commonly affected. Associated with the VACTERL syndrome. **High anomalies** (ie, above levator muscles) usually do not exhibit ectopic perineal opening on exam but may fistulize with urinary system; **low anomalies** (ie, below levators) show perineal opening in boys and a fistulous tract to lower vagina in girls. Ultrasound assists in diagnosis. Treat high lesions with colostomy and later anal reconstruction with posterior sagittal anoplasty. Treat low lesions with posterior sagittal anoplasty and subsequent anal dilation. Sphincter anatomy is usually preserved in low lesions.

Necrotizing Enterocolitis

Demographics/Risk Factors

Necrotizing enterocolitis (NEC) is the most common GI emergency among neonates in the ICU. Associated with prematurity, infections, hypoxia, hypotension, enteral feeding, and use of umbilical catheter.

Signs/Symptoms

May include feeding intolerance, abdominal distension, **bloody stools,** ileus, or in advanced disease, hemodynamic instability, and abdominal wall erythema.

Diagnosis

Clinical diagnosis confirmed with abdominal radiographs demonstrating **pneumatosis intestinalis, portal venous air, or free air.**

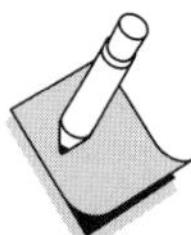

Indications for operation in NEC—

Free air

Persistent acidosis

Abdominal wall erythema

Persistent "fixed loop" of bowel on radiographs

TREATMENT

Uncomplicated NEC is medically managed with bowel rest, decompression, fluid resuscitation, and broad-spectrum antibiotics. **Presence of free air, persistent acidosis, persistent "fixed loop" on abdominal radiographs, or abdominal wall erythema** are indications for surgery. Definitive therapy involves resection of perforated or gangrenous bowel. Consider a second look procedure for bowel of questionable viability. Postoperative complications include recurrence, sepsis, disseminated intravascular coagulation (DIC), and stricture. Overall mortality for those requiring surgery may be as high as 60%. **Prior to ostomy reversal, obtain barium enema** to evaluate for distal stricture.

> A 13-month-old child presents to the ED with a 12-hour history of colicky abdominal pain. A week earlier, he was been seen by his pediatrician for a fever and runny nose. Today, his stool is guaiac + and he has a mass in his left upper quadrant. What is the proper management for this disorder? Perform ultrasound to see characteristic target lesion of intussusception. Air- or water-soluble contrast enema may be used as a diagnostic tool as well as a therapeutic means to reduce the intussuscepted segment. Surgery is indicted if maximal pressures (1-m column height of fluid or 120 mm Hg of air) fail to reduce intussusception.

Intussusception

DEMOGRAPHICS/RISK FACTORS

Telescoping of bowel into a distal segment. Peak incidence **3 months to 2 years of age**. Most cases are idiopathic, though hypothesized lead points include enlarged lymphoid patches, polyps, Meckel's diverticula, duplication cysts, or tumors. Most common site is the **ileocecal (IC) junction.**

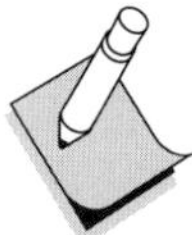

Indications for surgical management of intussusception—

Failure of radiographic reduction

Duration > 12 hours

Recurrent symptoms

Presence of a pathologic lead point

Bowel obstruction or signs of peritonitis

SIGNS/SYMPTOMS

Classic triad of acute abdominal pain, currant jelly stools, and palpable abdominal mass is present in < 50%. Crampy abdominal pain, intermittent vomiting, and recent viral illness are clues to diagnosis.

DIAGNOSIS

Air contrast enema is diagnostic and curative in 80% of cases.

TREATMENT

If nonoperative treatment fails, surgery is required. Via open or laparoscopic technique, milk intussusceptum from distal bowel. Resect any ischemic bowel and evaluate for pathologic lead point. Appendectomy may be required if intussusception at IC junction results in vascular compromise.

Meckel's Diverticulum

DEMOGRAPHICS/RISK FACTORS

Most common congenital abnormality of the SI occurring in 2% of the population. Caused by **persistence of the vitelline (omphalomesenteric) duct**

remnant ~2 ft proximal to the IC valve. Usually diagnosed before age 2; 75% diagnosed before 10 years of age.

Meckel's diverticulum "Rule of 2s"–

2% of population

2 feet from IC valve

2% symptomatic

Presentation by age 2

2 types of mucosa (gastric, pancreatic)

SIGNS/SYMPTOMS

Often asymptomatic, though 2% present with **bleeding**, obstruction, perforation, volvulus, or intussusception. Ectopic gastric or pancreatic mucosa found in 80% of patients.

DIAGNOSIS

^{99m}Tc pertechnetate (Meckel's scan) confirms presence of ectopic gastric mucosa and is the diagnostic modality of choice.

TREATMENT

Surgery is required in the presence of symptoms and may entail resection with end-to-end anastomosis or wedge resection of diverticulum with transverse closure of ileum.

Acute appendicitis is discussed in Chapter 10.

Pectus Excavatum

Concave deformity of the sternum and anterior chest wall associated with ↓ exercise tolerance and ↓ lung volumes. Exam confirms diagnosis. Treatments include sternal osteotomy with cartilage resection (Ravitch procedure) or insertion of sternal bar (Nuss procedure).

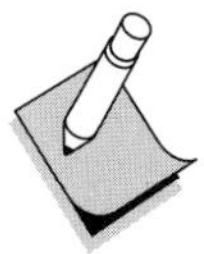

Hernias are discussed in Chapter 8.

Hydrocele

Most common in preterm infants. Typically presents as a nontender fluid collection within the processus vaginalis. Transillumination is not advised to differentiate from hernias, as a newborn's bowel will transilluminate as well. Communicating hydroceles (ie, communicates with peritoneal cavity) change in size as fluid transfers between scrotum and peritoneal cavity. These require surgical intervention as they carry the same risk of incarceration as inguinal hernias. Noncommunicating hydroceles (ie, fluid is confined to the scrotum) are constant in size and generally resolve without intervention.

Testicular Torsion

Painful scrotal swelling and edema due to twisted spermatic cord with subsequent impairment of blood flow. Classically associated with the **"bell clapper" deformity** caused by elevation of testicle within the scrotum. Associated with loss of the ipsilateral cremasteric reflex. Though a clinical diagnosis, Doppler ultrasound confirms impaired blood flow. Treatment is operative detorsion with **bilateral orchidopexy**.

Cryptorchidism

Occurs most commonly in premature, low birth weight, or twin neonates. Diagnosed due to absence of palpable testicle(s) on exam; confirm diagnosis with MRA. As many testes will spontaneously descend, re-examine patient at 6 months. Treatment involves retrieval and fixation of testis in the scrotal pouch. If untreated, one-third of patients progress to testicular involution, resulting in lack of germ cells by 2 years of age. Also associated with **infertility** and **testicular germ cell cancer.**

> A 6 year old girl presents with bilateral periorbital ecchymosis. Her exam reveals a large abdominal mass. Is her prognosis better or worse than a 3 month old with the same disease? The child likely has a neuroblastoma. Outcome is worse in older children (compared to younger children) as the disease usually presents at later stages.

Neuroblastoma

DEMOGRAPHICS

Most common solid extracranial tumor of children < 2 years of age. Often arises from the adrenal gland.

SIGNS/SYMPTOMS

Often asymptomatic though may present with abdominal pain, emesis, weight loss, anorexia, fatigue, bone pain, and chronic diarrhea. Exam may reveal a **palpable abdominal mass, opsoclonus myoclonus, and periorbital ecchymoses**. In a small proportion of infants < 6 months, disease presents with a small 1° tumor and metastatic disease confined to the liver, skin, and bone marrow. These patients have a favorable prognosis.

DIAGNOSIS

Urine catecholamines, vanillylmandelic acid (VMA), homovanillic acid (HMA), and serum neuron specific enolase may all be ↑. Staging workup includes CXR, bone marrow biopsy, and nuclear medicine scans for metastases.

TREATMENT

Complete resection is recommended for stages I and II. If stage III or greater, initiate multiagent chemotherapy with complete resection (after some regression).

STAGING/OUTCOME

Stage and age at diagnosis are the most important prognostic factors. In children < 1 year, tumors often show a lower stage and often spontaneously regress. In children > 1 year, tumors present in advanced stages, and prognosis is poor. Stages are designated after intervention and include:

- Stage I: Localized tumor with complete excision.
- Stage IIA: Localized tumor with incomplete excision.
- Stage IIB: Localized tumor with incomplete excision and + ipsilateral lymph nodes.
- Stage III: Unresectable tumor that crosses the midline or is associated with + contralateral lymph nodes.
- Stage IV: 1° tumor with distant lymph node involvement.
- Stage IVS: Localized tumor with spread to skin, liver, and with minimal bone marrow involvement. **Found only in children < 1 year of age.**

Common solid childhood tumors—

Neuroblastoma: Most common < 2 years

Wilm's tumor: Most common > 2 years

PEDIATRIC SURGERY

Wilms' Tumor

Demographics/Risk Factors

Most common malignant renal tumor of childhood. Most commonly diagnosed at 2–3 years of age. Ten percent are bilateral. Associated with deletions on chromosome 11 and a number of syndromes: WAGR (Wilm's tumor, aniridia, genitourinary malformations, mental retardation), Beckwith-Wiedemann (omphalocele, visceromegaly, macroglossia, gigantism), Denys-Drash (Wilm's tumor, intersex disorders, nephropathy), sporadic aniridia, and isolated hemihypertrophy.

Staging for Wilm's tumor–
Stage I: Limited to kidney, completely excised
Stage II: Beyond kidney, completely excised
Stage III: Residual, nonhematogenous metastases
Stage IV: Hematogenous metastases
Stage V: Bilateral renal involvement

Signs/Symptoms

Usually presents with a large asymptomatic abdominal mass noticed by parents during dressing or bathing. Other signs include **HTN**, **left-sided varicocele, hematuria, and abdominal or flank pain**.

Diagnosis

Abdominal and chest CT are used to confirm diagnosis, evaluate contralateral kidney, and to rule out metastases. Abdominal ultrasound can evaluate the renal vein and IVC for tumor extension.

Treatment

Treatment is surgical resection (ie, nephrectomy) with examination of contralateral kidney and neoadjuvant chemotherapy (eg, actinomycin, vincristine, doxorubicin). Partial nephrectomy is commonly used for bilateral disease. Radiation may be used for stage III disease. Prognosis is based on grade; anaplastic or sarcomatous types carry a worse prognosis.

Hepatoblastoma

An embryonal tumor occurring in children < 3 years of age. Most commonly affects males and is found in association with Beckwith-Wiedemann syndrome and familial adenomatous polyposis. Typically presents late as an asymptomatic ↑ in abdominal girth. Can have precocious puberty due to production of human chorionic gonadotropin (hCG). Ninety percent have ↑ α-fetoprotein. Confirm diagnosis with MRI and biopsy. Treat with resection and neoadjuvant or adjuvant chemotherapy (eg, doxorubicin, cisplatin) to limit metastatic disease. Approximately 75% of cases are curable, particularly with prefetal histology.

Staging for hepatoblastoma–
Stage I: Completely excised
Stage II: Microscopic residual tumor
Stage III: Partially resected, unresected specimen confined to liver, or tumor spill during surgery
Stage IV: Distant metastases

▶ SAMPLE QUESTIONS

What mutation is associated with most cases of familial Hirschsprung's disease? What is the diagnostic procedure of choice?	*RET* proto-oncogene. Rectal suction biopsy to look for hypertrophic nerve endings and an absence of ganglion cells.
What is the proper treatment of pediatric inguinal hernias?	Herniorrhaphy with high ligation of the sac and possibly contralateral exploration.
What is the proper timing of a Kasai procedure?	Prior to 2 months of age.
What is the origin of the blood supply to most cases of pulmonary sequestration?	Systemic, off the aorta.
What is the classic radiographic sign of duodenal atresia?	"Double bubble" → dilated stomach and duodenum, decompressed SI.
What are the indications for surgical intervention in NEC?	Free air, persistent acidosis, persistent "fixed loop" of bowel on radiographs, abdominal wall erythema.
Of gastroschisis or omphalocele, which is more likely to be accompanied by other congenital anomalies?	Omphalocele.
Where is the fistula likely to be in a case of high imperforate anus?	Males: rectovesicular. Females: rectovaginal, rectovesicular.
A 3-week-old infant presents to the ED with bilious emesis. What needs to be done immediately?	Upper GI with SBFT to rule out malrotation.
What is the most common site of congenital diaphragmatic hernia?	Left posterior.
What is the proper maintenance fluid for a 1 month old infant?	D5 $^1/_4$ NS with 20 mEq/L KCL, according to the Holliday and Segar formula.
What distinguishes a stage III from stage II Wilm's tumor?	The ability to obtain a complete excision with stage II tumors.
A 10-year-old presents with a painless swelling along her lateral neck. Ultrasound reveals a fluid-filled cyst. What is the most common origin of this anomaly?	The second branchial arch.
What are causes of posterior mediastinal cystic masses in children?	Bronchogenic cysts, esophageal duplication, necrotic lymph nodes, meningoceles.

CHAPTER 20

Transplantation

Timothy M. Millington, MD
Reviewed by Dicken S.C. Ko, MD, FRCSC

Antibody Review

HLA Types

HLA type refers to the human form of the major histocompatibility complex (MHC).

- **MHC I**: Three major genes (ie, HLA-A, HLA-B, HLA-C) encode proteins that combine to form receptors present on almost all **nucleated cells** and platelets. These present antigens produced inside the cell to **CD8 T lymphocytes** and allow virally infected or cancerous cells to be targeted for apoptosis.
- **MHC II**: Three major genes (ie, HLA-DP, HLA-DQ, HLA-DR) encode proteins that combine to form a receptor expressed on **antigen presenting cells** (eg, macrophages). After phagocytosis of a potential pathogen, foreign antigens are presented in association with MHC to **CD4 T lymphocytes,** leading to activation of the immune response.

Important criteria in donor-recipient matching–
ABO, HLA, lymphocytoxic crossmatch, donor-recipient organ size match

Donor-Recipient Crossmatching

Crossmatching (cytotoxicity assay) is the process of combining donor lymphocytes and recipient serum to determine if there are preformed antibodies against the potential graft (see Hyperacute Rejection). The routine screening of recipients for **panel reactive antibodies** (PRA) uses a standard panel of cells and determines the percentage of preformed antidonor antibodies. PRAs may be ↑ by sensitizing conditions, such as prior history of organ or cellular transplant, multiple pregnancies, and blood transfusions.

Organ Rejection

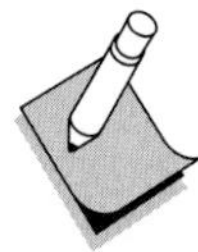

Timing of rejection–
Hyperacute: Minutes to hours
Accelerated: < 1 week
Acute: 1 week to anytime
Chronic: Years

Hyperacute Rejection

Occurs immediately after transplantation (minutes to hours) due to preformed recipient antibodies that are present against the donor organ. This can occur after transplantation from an **ABO incompatible donor or to a crossmatch + recipient**. Humoral-mediated immune response results in thrombosis of vessels in the donor organ. The variety of pretransplant studies (ie, multiple ABO studies, HLA compatibility test) makes such rejections rare. Treatment is **graft removal** because the allograft is a thrombosed organ, has no viability, and is a source of further complications.

Accelerated Rejection

Occurs within the first week of transplant as a result of **recipient T cells that are sensitized to donor antigens**. This also may occur in the setting of crossing the ABO incompatible barrier or transplantation in the setting of a crossmatch + recipient. These circumstances are more prevalent today as many centers have ABO incompatible and desensitization protocols designed to allow selected recipients an opportunity for transplantation. Treatment of humoral-mediated rejection includes plasmapheresis, antilymphocyte antibodies (eg, monoclonal antibodies, thymoglobulin), anti-CD20 (B cell) antibodies, calcineurin inhibitors (eg, tacrolimus), and antimetabolites (eg, mycophenolate mofetil). Intravenous immunoglobulin (IVIG) may be used as an adjunct to therapy in these patients.

ACUTE REJECTION

Can occur **anytime after transplantation**. May be divided into cellular or humoral rejection. Cellular rejection is treated with steroid pulses; if resistant, administer antilymphocyte therapy. Humoral rejection is treated with plasmapheresis, IVIG, antilymphocyte therapy, calcineurin inhibitors, and antimetabolites.

Humoral immunity: B cell-mediated
Cellular immunity: T cell-mediated

CHRONIC REJECTION

Occurs usually **months to years after transplantation**. Although thought to result from the combination of humoral and cellular responses over time, the actual mechanism is not well elucidated. Confirm diagnosis with biopsy.

Antirejection Medications

Tacrolimus and CsA are metabolized by the P-450 system. Levels are affected by other drugs metabolized by this system.

The immune response is a complex biological response to foreign antigens that occurs through numerous pathways (both known and unknown). Targeted immunosuppression is preferred over broad-spectrum immunosuppression. Multimodality therapy allows for tailoring of immunosuppression and minimization of individual drug side effects (see Table 20-1). Sites of action are summarized in Figure 20-1.

▶ **CLINICAL SCIENCE**

A 62-year-old woman with diabetic nephropathy undergoes a cadaveric kidney transplant. Her initial urine output is 150 mL/hr but abruptly ceases 6 hours postoperatively. What are the next appropriate steps in diagnosis and management? Ensure BP and HR are appropriate, irrigate urinary catheter to rule out catheter obstruction, and obtain urgent graft Doppler ultrasound to rule out vascular thrombosis and hydronephrosis.

A 57-year-old man undergoes kidney transplantation, and his renal function normalizes. Five years later, he develops increasing HTN with a creatinine = 3.3 mg/dL. His immunosuppressive drugs are at appropriate therapeutic levels. What are the next appropriate diagnostic steps? Renal ultrasound to initially evaluate possible vascular stenosis or hydronephrosis. Ultrasound-guided percutaneous renal biopsy is indicated to determine etiology of dysfunction.

Kidney Transplantation

INDICATIONS

Preferred treatment for dialysis-dependent end-stage renal disease (ESRD). Compared to dialysis, transplantation **is more cost-effective and offers a better quality of life and longer survival**.

Preoperative evaluation and contraindications include:

- **Medical**: Underlying **cardiac disease is the most common cause of post-transplant mortality**. Patients with risk factors (eg, age, DM, prior

TABLE 20-1. Antirejection Medications

Medication	Mechanism	Role	Side Effects	Notes
AZA	Inhibits purine synthesis, T-cell production.	Maintenance immunosuppression.	**Bone marrow suppression**, hepatotoxic.	Converted to active form in **liver.**
Steroids (prednisone, methylprednisolone)	Inhibit DNA/RNA synthesis via many pathways. Mechanism of action is related to nuclear factor of activated T cells → ↓ T-cell count, inhibits inflammatory cytokine (eg, IL-1, IL-2) production.	Pulses during acute rejection episodes; low dose for long-term maintenance.	Cushing's syndrome DM, abnormal fat deposition, osteoporosis), gastric ulcers, poor wound healing.	Taper as possible to eventual goal of steroid-free or steroid-reduced therapy.
Mycophenolate mofetil	Similar to AZA but targets alternative pathway of purine synthesis that affects T cells more specifically.	Maintenance immunosuppression.	Bone marrow suppression, diarrhea.	More T cell–specific than AZA.
CsA	Binds cyclophilin and forms complex that binds to **calcineurin**. Prevents T-cell activation, IL-2 transcription.	Maintenance immunosuppression.	**Nephrotoxic**, hepatotoxic, ↑ **K^+**, ↑ glucose, **hirsutism**, neurotoxicity. Does not target proliferating cells so **no bone marrow suppression**.	Target trough 200–300 g/mL. Metabolized by **P-450 system**. However, long-term trough levels can be very low and and maintain efficacy.
Tacrolimus (FK506)	Same as CsA but binds FK binding protein rather than cyclophilin. Inhibits T-cell activation, maturation.	Maintenance immunosuppression.	Similar to CsA. Diarrhea. Main difference is more DM, less hirsutism, perhaps more neurotoxicity.	Target trough 5-15 ng/mL depending on protocol. **More potent than CsA.** Metabolized by **P-450 system**.
Sirolimus	Binds to target of rapamycin but does not interfere with calcineurin. Inhibits B and T-cell activation and proliferation, blocks IL-2 receptor signal transduction.	Maintenance immunosuppression.	More side effects than CsA or FK506 but **less nephrotoxic**. Pulmonary complications, oral ulcers, delayed wound healing, intolerability, significant DVTs.	Has been used off-label in patients with a history of tumors (eg, skin) that developed after transplantation.

TABLE 20-1. Antirejection Medications (*Continued*)

MEDICATION	MECHANISM	ROLE	SIDE EFFECTS	NOTES
Antithymocyte globulin	Polyclonal antisera against T-cell antigens. Derived by injecting lymphocytes into various species (antithymocyte globulin [ATGAM] = horse; thymoglobulin = rabbit).	Acute rejection, induction therapy.	Fever, rigors, **serum sickness**, anemia, viral infection, **PTLD,** thrombocytopenia.	Can develop immune response to antibody over time.
Monoclonal antibodies (OKT3)	Monoclonal antibody against CD3. Prevents T-cell receptor complex formation, T-cell opsonization/ function.	Acute rejection	Flulike symptoms (fevers, chills, nausea, diarrhea, rash, headache, ↓ BP) related to cytokine release. Also pulmonary edema, bronchospasm.	Less well-tolerated but more specific than polyclonal antibodies. Can develop sensitization to antibodies, which ↓ effect.

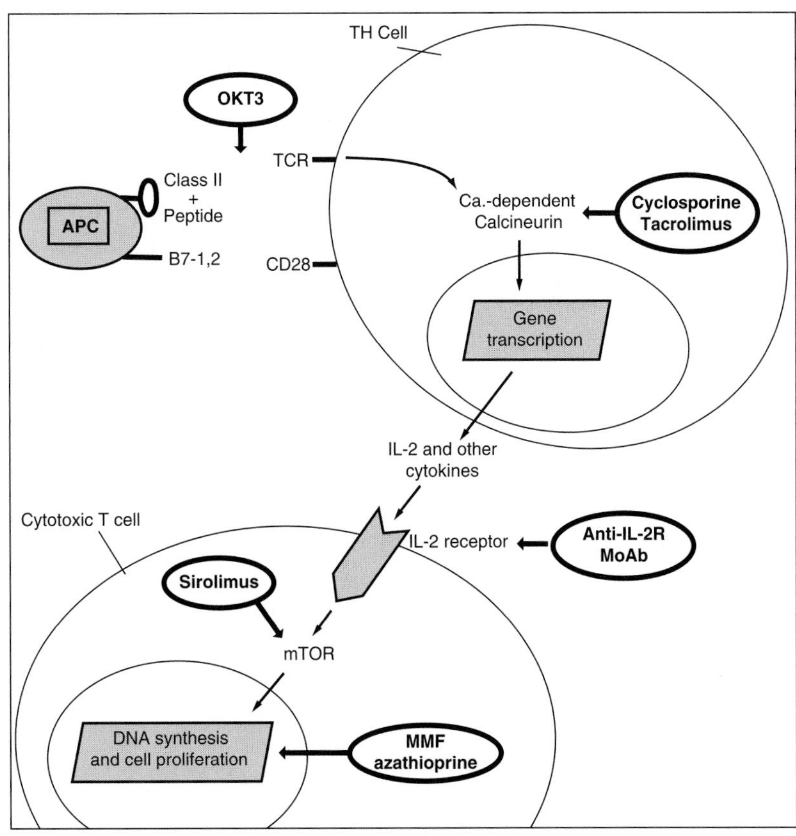

FIGURE 20-1. Sites of immunosuppressive drug actions.

(Reproduced, with permission, from Brunicardi FC, et al. *Schwartz's Principles of Surgery*. 8th ed. New York: McGraw-Hill, 2004:301.)

myocardial infarction [MI]) require preoperative evaluation and treatment, if necessary. Cancer and chronic infection must be adequately treated before immunosuppression can be administered. An interval of 2 years after curative treatment of malignancy is recommended before kidney transplantation. However, the absolute necessity for such duration is under debate for many malignancies (eg, prostate cancer that is treated). Sometimes the mortality rate for staying on chronic dialysis is much worse than tumor recurrence. There are a paucity of studies that clearly define the absolute causality of immunosuppression to specific tumors. **Hepatitis B virus (HBV) or hepatitis C virus (HCV) with cirrhosis or acute hepatitis are relative contraindications to kidney transplant, but patients may be considered for combined liver and kidney transplant, if candidacy for both is determined to be medically suitable.**

- **Surgical**: Severe arterial occlusive disease may make a transplant technically impossible and should be evaluated and treated prior to transplant. Consultation with the vascular surgeon is also indicated to determine any future plans. Chronic infection, bleeding, or mass effect (eg, polycystic kidney disease) of the native kidney may necessitate a native nephrectomy at the time of transplant.
- **Immunologic**: Includes ABO compatibility, HLA tissue typing, and screening for preformed anti-HLA antibodies.
- **Psychosocial**: Ability to adhere to a posttransplant medical regimen should be addressed preoperatively. More importantly, under the current medical system, the ability to obtain insurance and medical coverage for expensive immunosuppression has an impact on compliance in the long-term. **In the adolescent population, the most common cause of long term allograft loss is noncompliance.** Therefore, psychosocial support and stability must be achieved in the best possible manner to impact long-term success.

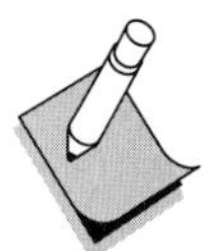

Transplant vocabulary–
Autograft = Organ from the same individual
Allograft = Organ from the same species but not genetically identical
Xenograft = Organ from different species
Orthotopic = Organ transplanted into its usual anatomic site (heart, lung, liver)
Heterotopic = Organ transplanted into a foreign site (kidney, pancreas)

OPERATIVE DETAILS

Preferred transplant site is in the **extraperitoneal iliac fossa** because of the ease of vascular access, shorter donor ureter, better blood supply, and simplicity of percutaneous biopsy. Arterial inflow can be provided by the common, external, or internal iliac (rare) arteries (see Figure 20-2). Venous drainage can be via the external or common iliac (end-to-side) veins. The urinary reconstruction is usually via an extravesical reimplantation technique that forms a ureteric tunnel in an attempt to prevent reflux into the allograft.

POSTPROCEDURE CARE

Requires attention to hemodynamic stability and electrolyte balance to protect graft function. **Graft function is most readily monitored with urine output, blood urea nitrogen (BUN), and creatinine.** Immediate function is associated with a brisk diuresis and rapid clearance of creatinine. Slow graft function demonstrates a slower improvement and may require posttransplant dialysis.

COMPLICATIONS

Early complications include

- **Bleeding**: Rare but are becoming more problematic in the light of the ↑ use of clopidogrel or anticoagulation (eg, patients with coronary stents

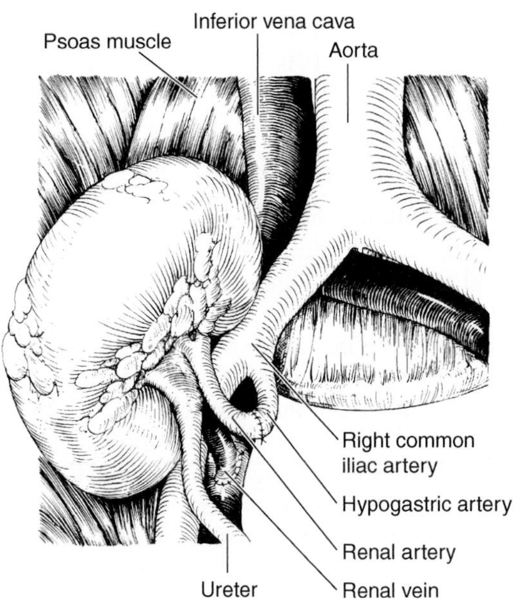

FIGURE 20-2. Anatomy of kidney transplantation.

(Reproduced, with permission, from Doherty GM, Way LW. *Current Surgical Diagnosis and Treatment*, 12th ed. New York: McGraw-Hill, 2006:1359.)

who are now undergoing renal transplantation). In addition, the presence of hypercoagulable states, such as antiphospholipid syndrome or factor V Leiden, will require initiation of anticoagulation intraoperatively. Although bleeding usually tamponades, re-exploration is indicated for evacuation of compressive hematoma.

- **Thrombosis**: Arterial thrombosis is usually caused by a technical problem (eg, intimal dissection, torsion). Diagnose with Doppler ultrasound. Requires **urgent thrombectomy**. Venous thrombosis is less common and **may be due to the extension of a native DVT.** Diagnosis and treatment are similar. Both arterial and venous thromboses usually result in **graft loss** as the thrombotic event extends well into the peripheral vessels. Treatment of the main vessel does not have any impact on the rest of the organ's perfusion.
- **Urinary leak and obstruction:** Leak usually occurs at anastomosis due to anastomotic **tension or ischemia**. Small leaks may potentially be treated by cystoscopy and ureteric stenting; large leaks require exploration and re-implantation. Obstruction may be the result of blood clots, hematoma, torsion, or postoperative edema. Because the ureter is re-implanted in a nonanatomic position, cystoscopic insertion of a stent is difficult, and the manipulation of a stent through a new suture line can further disrupt the anastomosis. Often, the best option is to simply take the recipient back to the OR for open exploration to definitively address the underlying problem. The surgical length of stay and future complications will likely be reduced.
- **Lymphocele**: Occurs in up to 5–10% of patients and can cause compression of adjacent graft structures. Diagnose with ultrasound in most settings. Can usually be percutaneously aspirated if hematoma, urinoma, or abscess are suspected. Treatment includes creation of a peritoneal window to allow drainage and reabsorption of the collection. This can be accomplished by

open or laparoscopic techniques. Although it is an off-label use, fibrin sealant has also been used to inject the lymphocele with good results and without the need for further surgical procedures.

- **Acute rejection**: Discussed earlier.

Late complications include:

- **Chronic rejection**: Often referred to as **chronic allograft nephropathy (CAN)** and is actually a multifactorial decline in kidney function with immunologic and nonimmunologic causes. Results from a combination of chronic rejection, nephrotoxic side effects of some immunosuppressant drugs, and donor-related factors. The usual course of CAN is progressive renal dysfunction that leads to ESRD and subsequent chronic dialysis. At that time, patients are re-evaluated to determine medical suitability of a retransplant.
- **Arterial stenosis**: Results in HTN and graft dysfunction. Angiography and stenting is preferred treatment. Surgery is reserved for nonresponders.
- **Ureteral stenosis:** Due to scarring from chronic anastomotic ischemia. Ultrasound demonstrates hydronephrosis. Treat with stenting or surgical re-implantation.
- **Opportunistic infections**:
  - **Bacterial:** Usually occur early in common postsurgical locations (eg, surgical wound, lungs, urinary tract, bloodstream). Preoperative immunizations for *Haemophilus influenzae*, *Streptococcus pneumoniae*, and *Neisseria meningitis* are recommended.
  - **Viral:** Cytomegalovirus (CMV) can cause flu-like symptoms or severe tissue-invasive disease (eg, pneumonitis, hepatitis). Treatment includes **ganciclovir** or **valganciclovir**.
  - **Fungal:** Most commonly involves *Candida* and *Aspergillus*. Usually treated with amphotericin B. *Pneumocystic carinii* (PCP) can cause pneumonia. Prophylaxis against PCP includes **trimethoprim-sulfamethoxazole**.
- **Malignancy**: If cancer develops, considering discontinuing immunosuppression and initiating dialysis.
  - **Skin cancers: Most common malignancies in recipients.** Compared to normals, ↑ incidence of 1° (3- to 7-fold) and metastatic disease. **Unopposed human papilloma virus** may play a role. Minimize sun exposure and reduce antimetabolite immunosuppression.
  - **Lymphoma: Most common noncutaneous malignancies in recipients.** More than 95% of these are **B cell lymphomas** associated with **Epstein-Barr virus (EBV**; ie, **PTLD)**. Treatment includes ↓ immunosuppression, ganciclovir, chemotherapy, and specific monoclonal antibodies targeting CD20.
  - **Kaposi's sarcoma**

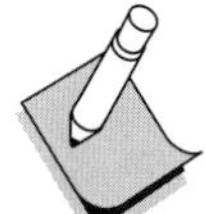

The most common cause of late kidney graft loss is recipient death from cardiovascular causes.

OUTCOMES

Outcomes are better if organ is from a living donor rather than cadaveric donor (see Table 20-2).

A 58-year-old man with end-stage alcoholic cirrhosis undergoes a cadaveric liver transplant. His sensorium initially clears, and output from his biliary T-tube is brisk. On postoperative day 2, he is confused, and his bilirubin increases. What studies are appropriate? Determine trend of his transminases, obtain Doppler ultrasound of his hepatic vasculature, T-tube cholangiogram, and CT scan of his head.

TABLE 20-2. Graft and Patient Survival After Renal Transplantation

DONOR TYPE (YEARS)	GRAFT SURVIVAL (%)	PATIENT SURVIVAL (%)
Cadaveric		
1	88	94
5	63	77
10	36	56
Living		
1	94	98
5	80	90
10	59	79

Liver Transplantation

INDICATIONS

Treatment of choice for acute (fulminant hepatic failure) and chronic (end-stage liver disease [ESLD]) liver failure. About 15,000 patients are awaiting liver transplants in the United States; about 4500 transplants are performed annually.

Common causes of acute, **fulminant hepatic failure** requiring liver transplant include acetaminophen toxicity, acute HBV infection, and Wilson's disease.

Common forms of ESLD necessitating transplant include:

- **Chronic hepatitis**: **Alcohol-induced cirrhosis**, viral hepatitis (HCV, [**most common cause of ESLD in the United States**], HBV), autoimmune hepatitis.
- **Metabolic causes**: Hemochromatosis, α_1-antitrypsin deficiency, Wilson's disease.
- **Cholestatic disorders**: Biliary atresia is the **most common cholestatic disorder leading to liver transplantation in children. Primary biliary cirrhosis** involves destruction of the interlobular biliary tree, leading to cirrhosis. Commonly found in **middle-aged women. Primary sclerosing cholangitis** involves injury to bile duct. Commonly found in **young men** and in **association with inflammatory bowel disease** (70% of cases).
- **Malignancy**: Transplant may be considered when curative resection of hepatic malignancy is not possible. Best outcomes are demonstrated in recipients with a single lesion < 5 cm or < 3 lesions that are each < 2 cm. Contraindications include metastatic disease and vascular invasion.
- **Budd-Chiari syndrome**: Obstructing thrombus of the hepatic vein results in ESLD.
- **Polycystic liver disease**.

ESLD patients may progress to decompensated cirrhosis. Manifestations include ascites, encephalopathy, spontaneous bacterial peritonitis, hepatorenal syndrome, and portal hypertensive bleeding.

Contraindications to liver transplant are similar to those for kidney transplant. Severe cirrhosis can cause hypoxic pulmonary HTN (**hepatopulmonary syndrome**), which may render a patient unable to tolerate a transplant. **The most frequent contraindication to liver transplantation is continuing substance abuse.**

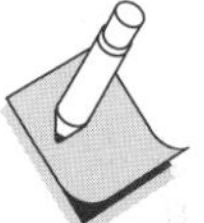

Hepatitis is discussed in Chapter 20.

HCV cirrhosis is most common cause of ESLD in the US.

Wilson's disease is an autosomal dominant disorder of copper excretion. Treatment includes penicillamine, but liver transplant might be necessary.

Most common contraindication to liver transplant–
Continuing substance abuse

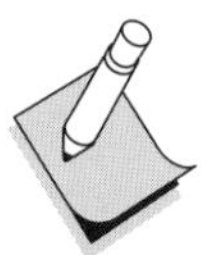

Safe cold ischemic times vary among different organs–

Kidney: Up to 36–40 hours

Pancreas: Up to 24 hours

Liver: Up to 16 hours

Heart/Lung: Up to 6 hours

Choice of donor hepatectomy depends on liver size required by recipient–

Pediatric recipients: Left lateral segment (25%), left lobe (40%)

Adult recipients: Right lobe (60%)

OPERATIVE DETAILS

During the **preanhepatic phase,** the native liver is mobilized, and its blood supply and venous drainage are isolated. Portal HTN and coagulopathy may lead to large amounts of blood loss during the pre-anhepatic phase. The **anhepatic phase** begins when the portal vein, hepatic artery, and hepatic veins are divided, and the native liver is removed. The suprahepatic and infrahepatic venae cavae and portal vein are anastomosed to the donor liver. Historically, **venovenous bypass** may be used to return blood from the lower body and gastrointestinal (GI) tract via cannulas in the femoral and portal veins. Currently the more popular method is the "piggy-back" caval anastomosis in which the recipient vena cava is not resected but longitudinally opened to anastomose to the widely spatulated donor vena cava. The liver is reperfused via the portal and caval anastomoses. The hepatic artery may be anastomosed before or after reperfusion. The biliary anastomosis is performed during the **postanhepatic** phase. **Severe coagulopathy** and **electrolyte disturbances** leading to cardiac arrhythmias may occur during this phase as the donor liver is reperfused. Prophylactic treatments include ε-aminocaproic acid and aprotinin.

Living donor liver transplantation allows for ↓ waiting time so that transplant can be performed before decompensated hepatic failure occurs. The major disadvantages of this procedure are donor and recipient complications (occurring in 10–15%) including **bile leaks** and donor death (< 0.5%). Additionally, issues related to graft size relative to recipient might negatively impact survival.

POSTPROCEDURE CARE

Goals of **early postprocedure care** are hemodynamic stability, graft function monitoring, and complication detection. Indications of a functioning graft include: rapid awakening from anesthesia, clear postoperative mental status, normalization of the coagulation panel, resolution of any preoperative hypoglycemia, ↓ serum lactic acid and bilirubin levels, normalization of transaminases, color of biliary tube output, and normalizing renal function.

COMPLICATIONS

Abnormal graft function can be caused by **early** complications.

- **Primary graft nonfunction (PNF)**: Occurs in 1–2% of patients and has an **80–100% mortality if retransplantation is not performed**. Risk factors relate primarily to the donor and include ↑ age, hepatic steatosis, prolonged cold ischemia, and prolonged hospitalization. Though treatment includes IV prostaglandin E_1, a clearly established diagnosis of PNF requires urgent **retransplantation**.
- **Hemorrhage: Common postoperative complication**. Monitor abdominal drains closely. Re-exploration is usually necessary.
- **Hepatic artery thrombosis**: Occurs in 3–5% of liver transplants. Symptoms vary from asymptomatic ischemia to biliary complications to liver abscesses. Diagnose with Doppler ultrasound; confirmation with angiography or magnetic resonance angiography (MRA) might be necessary. Treatment includes **re-exploration and thrombectomy**.
- **Portal vein thrombosis**: Leads to **portal HTN** with variceal bleeding and ascites. Diagnose with Doppler ultrasound. Early cases may be treated with thrombectomy.

- **Bile leaks**: Occur in up to 5–15% of patients. May present with rising liver function tests, fever, and abdominal pain. Treatment includes endoscopic retrograde cholangiopancreatography (ERCP) and stenting; re-exploration is much less common.
- **Medical complications**: Includes pulmonary (eg, edema, pneumonia, effusion, acute respiratory distress syndrome), renal (eg, acute tubular necrosis, drug toxicity), and infectious complications.

Late complications include

- **Primary disease recurrence**: **Most common late complication**, especially with hepatitis. HCV recurrence is **almost universal**, and recurrent cirrhosis is becoming more common.
- **Rejection**: Can be monitored with serial serum bilirubin and transaminases and with percutaneous liver biopsy. Treat with high-dose steroids or antilymphocyte antibodies (although this is becoming increasingly less common with today's use of immunosuppression). Treating patients with steroids in the setting of hepatitis can result in rapid recurrence and complications.
- **Biliary stricture:** Can result in cholangitis or cholestasis. Treat with ERCP stenting or surgical revision (Roux-en-Y).
- **Arterial stenosis or pseudoaneurysm**: Caused by deterioration of the vascular anastomosis.
- **Late portal venous thrombosis**: Results in portal HTN (collateral blood flow may be sufficient to preserve graft function).
- **Infection**
- **Malignancy**

1-year graft and patient survival is influenced by early postoperative complications and patient's overall health.

OUTCOMES

Living donor organ outcome benefit is not as significant as that with kidney transplantation (see Table 20-3).

Pancreas and Small Intestine Transplantation

PANCREATIC TRANSPLANTATION

Commonly performed in combination with kidney transplants in diabetic patients with renal failure.

TABLE 20-3. Graft and Patient Survival After Liver Transplantation

DONOR TYPE (YEARS)	GRAFT SURVIVAL (%)	PATIENT SURVIVAL (%)
Cadaveric		
1	86	86
5	64	72
10	45	59
Living		
1	76	85
5	73	85
10	43	85

Cardiac transplant is discussed in Chapter 15. Lung transplant is discussed in Chapter 16.

SMALL INTESTINE TRANSPLANTATION

Least frequently transplanted organ. May be transplanted as part of a multiple-organ transplant (eg, liver transplant in short bowel syndrome [SBS]). Indications include SBS, long-term total parenteral nutrition (TPN) dependence, and life-threatening complications caused by underlying pathology. **Highest rejection rate and lowest graft survival.** Currently there is no simple test to monitor for rejection other than repeated endoscopy and random biopsies of the intestine.

▶ SAMPLE QUESTIONS

What is the mechanism of hyperacute rejection after kidney transplantation? Treatment?	Preformed recipient antibodies bind to transplanted organ, causing complement activation and thrombosis. Requires transplant nephrectomy when kidney is nonviable.
What is the mechanism of acute rejection? Treatment?	T cell–mediated destruction of graft. Treatment can include steroid pulses, ↑ immunosuppression, antilymphocyte antibodies.
What is the mechanism of chronic rejection after kidney transplantation? Treatment?	Multifactorial (drug side effects, chronic allograft nephropathy). Treat by titrating immunosuppression (lowering calcineurin inhibitor dose). May institute therapy for chronic humoral rejection. If patient's disease progresses to ESRD, consider possible retransplant.
A 56-year-old man presents with ESRD due to diabetic nephropathy. He also has peripheral vascular disease, stable angina, melanoma, and HCV. What preoperative workup and treatment is necessary to list him for kidney transplant?	Cardiac clearance (stress test and catheterization), vascular evaluation (ensure adequate blood supply for potential graft), melanoma treatment with 2- to 5-year period without recurrence, hepatic evaluation (rule out cirrhosis or active hepatitis).
What factors ↑ the risk of 1° graft failure after liver transplantation?	Problems with the donor: advanced age, hepatosteatosis, prolonged hospitalization, excessive ischemia time.
What is the correct sequence of anastomoses in a liver transplant?	Venous (caval then portal), arterial, biliary.
What is the cause of PTLD?	B cell lymphoma, most likely due to EBV.
What is the first appropriate test in a kidney transplant recipient who develops an early postoperative rise in creatinine?	Doppler ultrasound (look for venous and arterial thrombosis, hydronephrosis, extraluminal fluid collection).
What is the differential diagnosis for an extraluminal fluid collection immediately after a kidney transplant?	Urinoma (anastomotic leak), hematoma, lymphocele, seroma. Abscess is not likely this early.
Which of the following drugs has a mechanism of action most different from the other three: tacrolimus, sirolimus, AZA, CsA?	AZA inhibits de novo purine synthesis. The others inhibit T cell activation and maturation.

Describe the hepatic carcinoma (by tumor size and number of tumors) most likely to benefit from liver transplantation.	Single lesion < 5 cm or < 3 lesions all < 2 cm. Vascular invasion or metastatic disease must not be present.
What is the best initial treatment for a urine leak after kidney transplant?	Cytoscopy with stent, drainage of urinoma. Will most likely require open exploration and re-implantation.
What unusual infections must be considered in a transplant recipient presenting with pneumonia?	CMV, PCP, fungi (*Aspergillus*, *Candida*).
What is the most common cause of death in kidney transplant recipients?	Coronary artery disease.

CHAPTER 21

Surgical Subspecialties

Mark M. Melendez, MD, MBA
Reviewed by Alexander B. Dagum, MD, FRCSC, FACS

▶ OTOLARYNGOLOGY

Basic Science

TRIANGLES OF THE NECK

Anterior and posterior triangles are depicted in Figure 21-1. Specific contents of each triangle are summarized in Table 21-1. The **sternocleidomastoid (SCM)** divides the neck into the anterior and posterior triangles.

Clinical Science

APPROACH TO THE NECK MASS

Evaluation of a patient with a neck mass includes a **thorough history** (eg, duration and extent of symptoms, risk factor exposure), exam (including lymph nodes), and special investigations (eg, **CT**, **MRI**, **panendoscopy**, **biopsy**; see Figure 21-2). Fine needle aspiration (FNA) is always preferred.

Causes of neck masses–

Child: Congenital

Adult: Infectious or neoplastic

A 45-year-old woman with a history of tobacco use presents with a painless mass near the left ear. On exam, a mass measuring 4 cm is palpable anterior to the left tragus. FNA of the mass shows a pleomorphic adenoma. What is the next step in the management of this patient? Treat benign tumors with superficial parotidectomy.

Clues to the diagnosis of a neck mass: "Rules of 7s"–

Symptoms for 7 days: Infectious.

Symptoms for 7 weeks/months: Neoplastic.

Symptoms for 7 years: Congenital.

SALIVARY GLAND TUMORS

Majority of salivary gland tumors originate in the parotid gland (80%) and are benign (80%). Tumors of **smaller glands are more likely to be malignant (80% malignant)**. Risk factors include advanced age, tobacco use, and previous

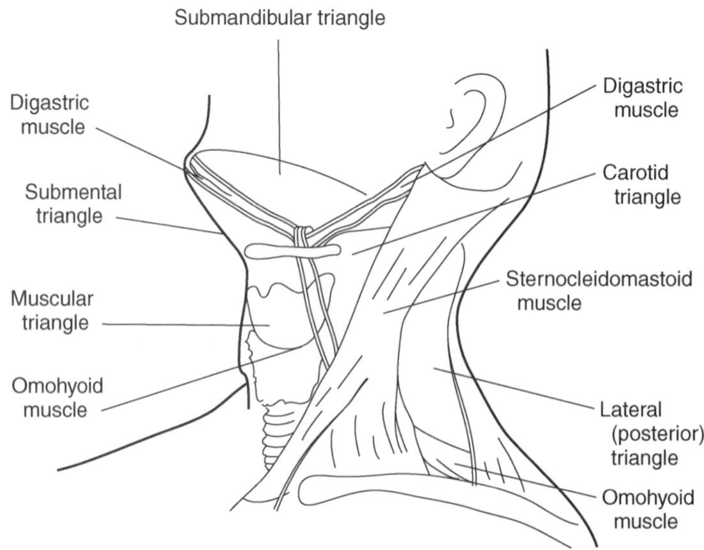

FIGURE 21-1. Anterior and posterior triangles of the neck.

(Reproduced, with permission, from Lalwani AK. *Current Diagnosis & Treatment in Otolaryngology—Head & Neck Surgery*, 2nd ed. New York: McGraw-Hill, 2008:426.)

TABLE 21-1. **Contents of Triangles of the Neck**

STRUCTURES	ANTERIOR TRIANGLE	POSTERIOR TRIANGLE
Nerves	Glossopharyngeal (lingual branches; CN IX), vagus (CN X), hypoglossal (CN XII), nerve to the mylohyoid.	Accessory (CN XI).
Arteries	Facial, internal/external carotid.	Subclavian artery.
Veins	Facial, interior/anterior jugular.	External jugular, subclavian vein.
Lymph nodes	Submental, submandibular.	Cervical.
Glands	Submandibular, parotid, thyroid.	
Muscles	SCM, digastric, suprahyoid, infrahyoid.	SCM, trapezius, splenius capitis, levator scapulae, scalenus medius, scalenus posterior.

Salivary gland "Most Commons"–

#1 Benign tumor: Pleomorphic adenoma

#2 Benign tumor: Warthin's tumor

#1 Malignant tumor: Mucoepidermoid

#2 Malignant tumor: Adenoid cystic (#1 in minor glands)

#1 Childhood tumor: Hemangioma

radiation exposure. The most common benign tumors are **pleomorphic adenomas,** followed by **Warthin's tumors**. Warthin's tumors tend to affect males and occur bilaterally. **Mucoepidermoid cancers**, followed by **adenoid cystic cancers**, are the **most common malignant tumors**, though adenoid cystic cancers are the most common in the minor glands. Tumors usually present as **painless masses**, but **pain** and **facial paralysis** are associated with **neural invasion** and should ↑ suspicion for malignancy. **History and exam** are often the **most useful diagnostic** tools for differentiating benign from malignant disease. **FNA** for tissue diagnosis may be performed on the mass itself or on a suspicious cervical lymph node. CT is best for demonstrating surrounding tissues and lymph nodes; MRI is optimal for showing the mass in greatest detail. **Size** determines stage (T1 < 2 cm, T2 2–4 cm, T3 > 4 cm). Treat **benign tumors** with **superficial parotidectomy**. Treatment of **malignant tumors** includes **resection of the gland** of origin (including facial nerve for parotid lesions), modified radical neck dissection (MRND), and when indicated, **postoperative radiation** (eg, + margins, recurrent disease, T3 or T4 parotid disease, high-grade lesion, invasion in adjacent structures). Low-grade malignant

Major risk factors for malignant parotid tumors–

Age (55–65 years)

Prior radiation exposure

Tobacco use

Remote history of incomplete resection of benign tumor.

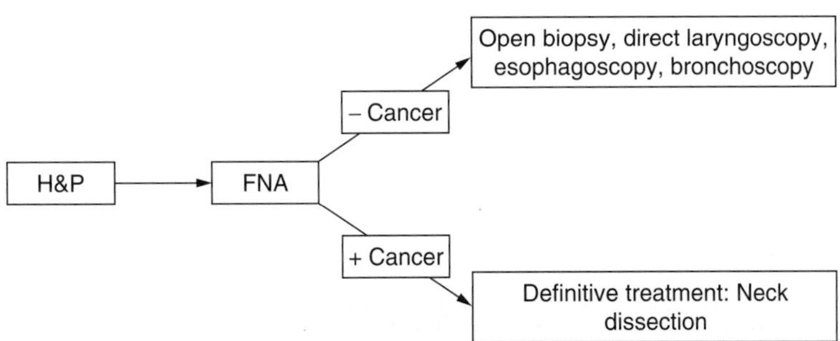

FIGURE 21-2. **Clinical approach to the neck mass.**

Recent parotid surgery plus sweating while eating—
Think Frey's syndrome and damage to the auricotemporal nerve. Results from abnormal re-innervation of the parasympathetic fibers from CN IX to the sympathetic fibers of the skin.

tumors < 4 cm in diameter, which are confined to the superficial lobe, may be amenable to superficial parotidectomy. Common postoperative complications include injuries to CN VII (mandibular branch), CN XII, lingual nerve, greater auricular nerve (may be sacrificed intentionally), and auricotemporal nerve. Damage to the latter results in **Frey's syndrome** with characteristic **gustatory sweating**.

ORAL CAVITY TUMORS

About 90% are **squamous cell carcinomas (SCC)**, most commonly affecting the **tongue** of men. May be preceded by premalignant lesions such as **leukoplakia** (ie, white patch) or **erythroplakia** (ie, red patch). Risk factors include alcohol and tobacco use. Typically present as a **painless mass** or ulcer. May be associated with pain, bleeding, **otalgia**, and change of speech. Labs may be unremarkable. **CT** and **MRI** confirm lesion and determine size and relation to adjacent structures. Biopsy during direct laryngoscopy confirms diagnosis. Local control of T1 or T2 lesions includes wide local excision (WLE) or radiation; if possible, treat T3 and T4 lesions with WLE and radiation. Neck dissection is used therapeutically (for clinically + nodes) or prophylactically for those at high risk for occult metastases (eg, T2 or higher). Chemotherapy is reserved for select cases (eg, large tumors prior to salvage surgery).

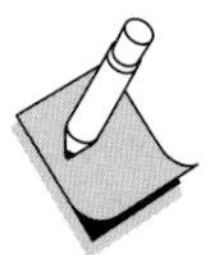

Always look for other head and neck cancers—
Risk of second 1° tumor = 14%

Tumor, node status, and metastasis (TNM) staging includes

- T: T1 (tumor < 2 cm), T2 (tumor > 2 cm and < 4 cm), T3 (tumor > 4 cm), T4 (tumor invades adjacent structures; a→resectable, b→unresectable)
- N: N0 (– regional lymph nodes), N1 (+ ipsilateral lymph node ≤ 3 cm), N2a (+ ipsilateral lymph node > 3 cm and < 6 cm), N2b (multiple + ipsilateral lymph nodes all < 6 cm), N2c (+ bilateral or contralateral lymph nodes all < 6 cm), N3 (+ lymph nodes > 6 cm)
- M: M0 (metastatic disease absent), M1 (metastatic disease present).

Staging includes

- Stage I: T1N0M0
- Stage II: T2N0M0
- Stage III: T3N0M0 *or* T1-3N1M0
- Stage IVa: T4aN0-1M0 *or* T1-4aN2M0
- Stage IVb: Any T, N3M0 *or* T4b, any N, M0
- Stage IVc: Any T, any N, M1

Modified radical neck dissection preserves—
- *Internal jugular vein*
- *CN XI*
- *SCM*

Five-year survival varies from 80% with T1 disease to 20% with T4 disease.

LARYNGEAL TUMORS

Similar to oral cavity cancer, laryngeal cancer is most commonly **SCC** of the glottic, supraglottic, or subglottic regions. Tends to affect men in the fifth to seventh decades. **Risk factors** include **tobacco** and **alcohol** use. Typically presents with hoarseness, dysphagia, otalgia, odynophagia, or airway obstruction. Workup and diagnostic tests are similar to oral cavity cancer. Treatment varies by tumor location and effect on vocal cord function: T1-2 glottic and supraglottic lesions respond to **radiation**; T3-4 lesions require **neoadjuvant chemoradiation and surgery** (eg, partial or total laryngectomy) if possible. **MRND is indicated for lymph node involvement**. Tracheostomy is necessary in most cases to secure airway. Five-year survival varies from up to 95% with stage I disease to as low as 20% with stage IV disease.

Peritonsillar Abscess

Polymicrobial infection commonly caused by extension of acute tonsillitis. Most commonly affects young adults. Presenting symptoms include trismus, odynophagia, dysphagia, dehydration, voice change (**"hot potato" voice**), **uvular deviation toward the contralateral side**, and **bulging of the anterior tonsillar pillar**. Though exam will usually confirm diagnosis, **needle aspiration** can be both diagnostic and therapeutic. If aspiration fails, consider tonsillar incision and drainage. Empiric coverage of ***Streptococcus*** is indicated.

A 12-year-old male presents to the ED with fever, dyspnea, and drooling. Exam reveals bulging of the posterior pharyngeal wall. What is the main complication of this disease? This is a retropharyngeal abscess, which can cause severe laryngeal edema, airway obstruction, and abscess rupture (with subsequent aspiration pneumonia or asphyxia).

Retropharyngeal Abscess

Infection of the retropharyngeal space from aerobic (eg, ***Staphylococcus***, β-hemolytic ***Streptococcus***), anaerobic (eg, ***Peptostreptococcus***), or Gram - (eg, ***Haemophilus parainfluenzae***) organisms. May occur in children and adults. Symptoms can include fever, irritability, **drooling**, nuchal rigidity, dyspnea, dysphagia, and **airway obstruction (Ludwig's angina)**. Patient may hold neck rigidly towards the unaffected side. Exam will reveal a **posterior pharyngeal wall bulge**. Diagnosis should be clinically suspected, and treatment should begin immediately. Labs will reveal leukocytosis. Lateral cervical spine radiograph will demonstrate **retropharyngeal widening. First priority is securing the airway,** followed by exploration, drainage, and IV antibiotics. Complications include **mediastinitis** (**50% mortality**), airway loss, aspiration pneumonia, empyema, and death.

▶ OBSTETRICS AND GYNECOLOGY

Basic Science

Anatomy of Female Reproductive System

Summarized in Figure 21-3. Pertinent structures include

- Median umbilical ligament: Obliterated urachus
- Medial umbilical ligament: Obliterated umbilical artery
- Ovarian artery and uterine artery (ovarian branch): Arterial supply to the ovary

*Ureter travels **UNDER** the uterine vessels.*

The cervix consists of a stratified squamous epithelium separated from the columnar epithelium by the **squamocolumnar junction**. This is the **most common site of cervical neoplasia.**

The ovary is composed of epithelial and stromal cells. Additionally, oocyte-containing follicles are embedded in the stroma.

Physiology of the Female Reproductive System

The menstrual cycle is typically 28 days, divided among follicular, ovulatory, and luteal phases.

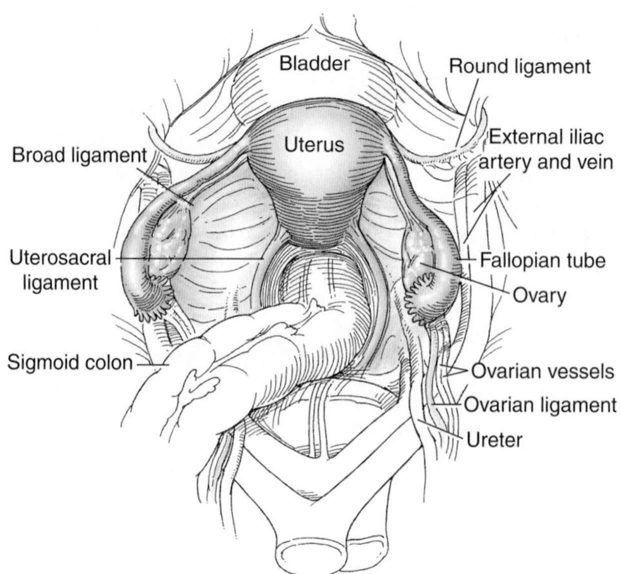

FIGURE 21-3. Female reproductive system.

(Reproduced, with permission, from Brunicardi FC, et al. *Schwartz's Principles of Surgery*, 8th ed. New York: McGraw-Hill, 2005:1562.)

- Follicular: Follicle stimulating hormone (FSH) and luteinizing hormone (LH) are released from the pituitary to stimulate estrogen release as well as growth and maturation of the oocyte. Increasing estrogen levels inhibit FSH. A dominant follicle persists and continues to produce estrogen.
- Ovulatory: Begins ~14 days into the menstrual cycle. Increasing estrogen → ↑ LH → release of dominant follicle egg from the ovary. Egg released during ovulation enters the fallopian tube. Increased mucous amount and thickness prepare cervix for sperm.
- Luteal: Empty dominant follicle regresses to corpus luteum, which secretes estrogen and progesterone. Fertilization may occur.

Clinical Science

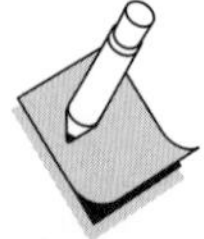

Gynecologic causes of acute abdomen–
Pelvic inflammatory disease
Ovarian torsion
Ectopic pregnancy (particularly ruptured).

ENDOMETRIOSIS

Affects about **20% of reproductive aged women** and may result in infertility. Etiology is unknown but may be caused by **retrograde menstruation**. Functional endometrial tissue is **most commonly found in extrauterine sites** (eg, ovaries, uterosacral ligaments, cul-de-sac). May present with infertility, menorrhagia, chronic pelvic pain, and spotting; exam can reveal pelvic mass or **tender nodularity of the uterosacral ligament.** Diagnosis is suspected with ultrasound or MRI and confirmed with laparoscopy. Lesions are typically blue-black lesions resembling "**gunpowder burns**" or "**chocolate cysts.**" Treatment is supportive: pain control (nonsteroidal anti-inflammatory drugs [NSAIDs]), oral contraceptive pills (OCPs), danazol, and GnRH agonists. Surgery is reserved to restore fertility and normal anatomy.

ENDOMETRIAL CANCER

Most common malignancy of the female reproductive tract, affecting ~39,000 women annually, with a peak incidence at 60 years of age. **Most commonly**

adenocarcinoma; endometrial sarcoma is rare. Associated with unopposed estrogen, HTN, diabetes mellitus (DM), tamoxifen use, obesity, polycystic ovarian syndrome, early menarche or late menopause, nulliparity, and presence of atypical complex endometrial hyperplasia. Most commonly presents with **postmenopausal vaginal bleeding**. Confirm diagnosis with endometrial biopsy, curettage, or vaginal ultrasound. Total abdominal hysterectomy and bilateral salpingo-oophorectomy (TAH BSO) with peritoneal washings and lymph node sampling may be curative. Adjuvant radiotherapy may be required in select patients (eg, high grade lesion, deep myometrial involvement, + lymph nodes).

FIGO staging for endometrial cancer–
Stage 0: Carcinoma in situ
Stage I: Tumor limited to corpus uteri
Stage II: Tumor invades cervix; does not extend beyond uterus
Stage III: Local and/or regional spread of disease
Stage IV: Bowel or bladder invasion or distant metastases

A 55-year-old woman presents with a 3-month history of lower abdominal pain and increasing abdominal girth. Exam reveals a pelvic mass. CA 125 is markedly elevated; ultrasound demonstrates a solid right ovarian mass. What is the next best step in the evaluation of this patient? Patient likely has ovarian cancer with ascites. Perform TAH BSO, pelvic and para-aortic lymph node dissection, and total omentectomy.

Ovarian Cysts and Ovarian Cancer

May be divided into benign or malignant lesions. While benign lesions (eg, ovarian cysts including follicular, corpus luteal, thecal luteal, endometriomas) do not progress to cancer, neoplastic lesions (see Table 21-2) result in the greatest number of gynecologic cancer deaths. All ovarian masses should be evaluated with respect to the mass consistency (ie, solid or cystic) as well as patient age and menopausal status. **Age > 50 years is associated with a higher risk of malignant ovarian growth.** Most women with ovarian cancer present with vague symptoms such as lower abdominal pressure, bloating, and early satiety; exam may reveal a pelvic mass and ↑ abdominal girth. A **solid, irregular, fixed pelvic mass, particularly one in a peri- or postmenopausal woman** that is enlarging or that is found in conjunction with an upper abdominal mass or ascites, is highly suggestive of an ovarian malignancy. **Krukenberg tumors are metastatic lesions to the ovaries** that can arise from a number of different 1° lesions and are commonly found bilaterally.

Meig's syndrome–
Hydrothorax
Ascites
Ovarian tumor

Pseudomyxoma peritonei–
Extension of mucinous tumors (ovarian, appendiceal) to the peritoneal surfaces, filling abdomen with mucin.

CA-125 is helpful in differentiating benign or malignant processes, though it may be - in half of early stage ovarian cancers. Although transvaginal ultrasound and abdominal-pelvic CT are useful in identifying masses, it is often impossible to determine the nature of an ovarian tumor without laparotomy and histopathological analysis.

Treatment varies by type of lesion:

- Ovarian cyst in prepubertal female: Observe or cystectomy.
- Ovarian cyst in premenopausal female: Observe, repeat ultrasound. If persistent, cystectomy.
- Ovarian cyst in postmenopausal female: TAH BSO, peritoneal washings, omental biopsy.
- Ovarian cancer: TAH BSO, pelvic and para-aortic lymph node biopsy, total omentectomy, peritoneal washings.

Chemotherapy is very effective in ovarian cancer as adjuvant therapy and in achieving clinical remission. **Dysgerminoma** in is particularly **sensitive to chemoradiation.**

FIGO staging of ovarian cancer—
Stage I: Tumor limited to ovaries.
Stage II: Tumor extending beyond ovaries into pelvis.
Stage III: Tumor extending beyond pelvis and/or retroperitoneum or inguinal lymph nodes. Involvement of small intestine, omentum, superficial liver.
Stage IV: Metastases outside peritoneum.

TABLE 21-2. Malignant Ovarian Tumors

Type of Tumor	Key Facts
Dysgerminoma	**Most common malignant germ cell ovarian tumor.** Presents in second to third decade. ↑ **LDH,** ↑ **CA 125.** Radiation- and chemotherapy-sensitive.
Immature teratoma	Typically present in young females. ↑ **AFP.** Mature forms are generally benign and contain tissue resembling adult (eg, hair, teeth) rather than embryonic features.
Choriocarcinoma	Malignant trophoblastic proliferation, most commonly following **hydatiform molar pregnancy** (gestational trophoblastic disease). ↑ **hCG.** Treat with chemotherapy or TAH, if necessary.
Granulosa-thecal tumor	Sex cord stromal tumor. Results in **precocious puberty** and transformation of estrogen-responsive tissues.
Sertoli-Leydig tumor	Sex cord stromal tumor. Produces **excess testosterone → virilization.**
Serous cystadenoma	**Serous, fluid-filled lesion** with tubal-like, tall columnar, ciliated epithelium. May be bilateral.
Mucinous cystadenoma	Tall, columnar epithelium with **mucin production**; similar to intestinal or endocervical epithelium.

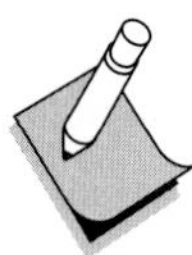

Cervical cancer—
Most commonly SCC at the transformation zone.

CERVICAL CANCER

Second most common cancer of the female reproductive system, most commonly seen in women aged 45-55 years. Risk factors include **human papilloma virus** (HPV; types 16, 18, 31), early sexual activity, multiple partners, multiparity, tobacco use, and chronic cervical inflammation. Classic symptom is **painless, postcoital vaginal bleeding.** As Pap smear is only ~50% sensitive, colposcopic biopsy is required for suspicious areas. Loop electrical excision procedure (LEEP) with conization should be done when cytologic examination reveals moderate or severe dysplasia, particularly in the setting of - or discrepant colposcopic results. Treatment varies by stage:

- Carcinoma in situ or stage IA1: Removal of transformation zone (eg, cauterization, cryotherapy, laser vaporization, cone biopsy, LEEP). TAH if fertility is not desired.
- Stages IA2, IB, II: Radical hysterectomy, bilateral pelvic lymph node dissection.
- All others: Internal or external radiation.

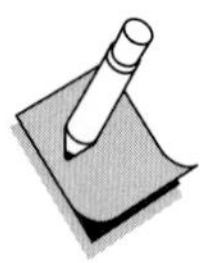

FIGO staging for cervical cancer—
Stage I: Limited to the cervix.
Stage II: Spread to the upper two-thirds of the vagina with or without parametrium.
Stage III: Spread to the lower one-third of the vagina or to pelvic wall.
Stage IV: Invades bladder, rectum, areas beyond true pelvis, + distant metastases.

VULVAR AND VAGINAL CANCER

Most commonly **SCC** associated with HPV infection. ↑ Risk of **vaginal clear cell adenocarcinoma** with in utero **diethylstilbestrol** (DES) exposure. Signs and symptoms include abnormal **vaginal bleeding**, discharge, and pruritus. For vulvar cancer with microinvasion, WLE is acceptable; other lesions require WLE or radical vulvectomy with lymph node dissection. Vaginal cancer may be treated with vaginectomy, with or without radiation.

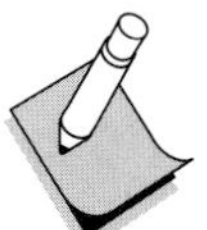

HPV vaccine is now available for prevention of cervical cancer caused by certain types of HPV.

▶ UROLOGY

Basic Science

ANATOMY OF THE GENITOURINARY SYSTEM

Kidneys are retroperitoneal solid organs enveloped in Gerota's fascia. Arterial supply is via the right and left (shorter) renal arteries. Venous drainage is via the right (shorter) and left renal veins. On the **right**, the gonadal and adrenal veins drain into the **inferior vena cava (IVC)**; on the **left**, they drain into the **left renal vein**.

In both men and women, the bladder stores and expels urine. Unlike women, though, male urinary continence and ejaculation is mediated by the presence of both internal and external sphincters.

The male reproductive system includes the prostate, seminal vesicles, and testes. With the seminal vesicles, the prostate produces seminal fluid. The **Sertoli cells** of the testes are involved in **spermatogenesis.** Sperm travels from the testes, through the vas deferens (see Figure 21-4) to the ejaculatory duct, which is formed by the vas deferens and the seminal vesicles. Testicular **Leydig cells** are involved in **testosterone production**.

FIGO staging of vulvar cancer–

Stage I: Involving vulva +/– perineum, – lymph nodes; ≤ 2 cm

Stage II: Involving vulva +/– perineum, – lymph nodes; > 2 cm

Stage III: Involving lower urethra, vagina, anus + ipsilateral regional lymph nodes

Stage IV: Involving upper urethra, bladder, rectum, + bilateral regional lymph nodes, + pelvic lymph nodes, or + distant metastases

PHYSIOLOGY OF THE GENITOURINARY SYSTEM

Renal functions are described in see Table 21-3.

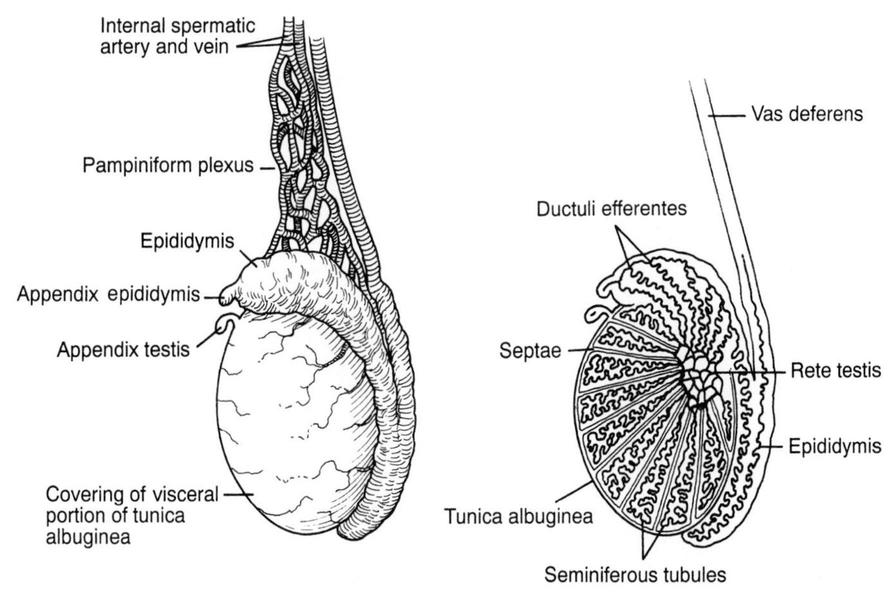

FIGURE 21-4. Anatomy of the male reproductive system.

(Reproduced, with permission, from Brunicardi FC, et al. *Schwartz's Principles of Surgery*, 8th ed. New York: McGraw-Hill, 2005:521.)

FIGO staging of vaginal cancer–

Stage I: Involving vaginal wall

Stage II: Involving subvaginal tissue but not pelvic wall

Stage III: Involving pelvic wall

Stage IV: Involving bladder, rectum, or structures beyond true pelvis

Renal vein lies anterior to the artery, which lies anterior to the ureter.

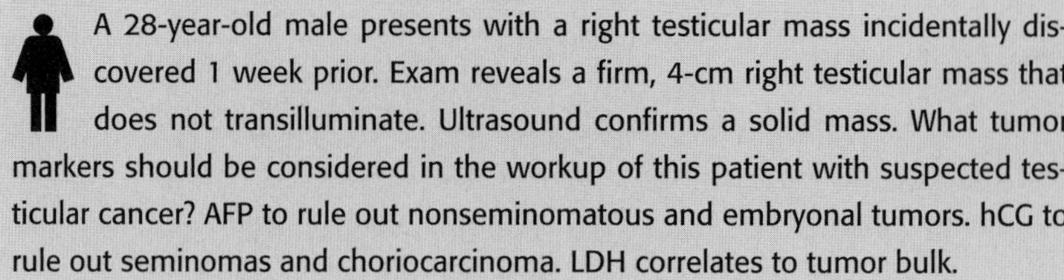

A 28-year-old male presents with a right testicular mass incidentally discovered 1 week prior. Exam reveals a firm, 4-cm right testicular mass that does not transilluminate. Ultrasound confirms a solid mass. What tumor markers should be considered in the workup of this patient with suspected testicular cancer? AFP to rule out nonseminomatous and embryonal tumors. hCG to rule out seminomas and choriocarcinoma. LDH correlates to tumor bulk.

Clinical Science

Testicular Tumors

Most common cancer in men aged 20–35 years. Risk factors include cryptorchidism (↑ risk for both testicles). Exam will reveal a **solid, firm testicular mass that may be painless.** Confirm diagnosis with testicular ultrasound; rule out metastatic disease with abdominal-pelvic CT and CXR. Definitive diagnosis and treatment includes **radical orchiectomy (inguinal approach)**. **Seminomas** are also **radiosensitive**.

Left gonadal vein drains into the left renal vein. Right gonadal vein drains into the IVC. For this reason, rule out abdominal pathology in the setting of an isolated right sided varicocele.

Nephrolithiasis

Most commonly affects males aged 20–50 years. Stone types are summarized in Table 21-4. Classic symptoms of an obstructing kidney stone include **colicky flank pain and hematuria**. Approximately 90% of stones are **radio-opaque** and can be **visualized on a kidney, ureter, and bladder (KUB)** radiograph; however, **noncontrast abdominal CT** is the preferred diagnostic study. May demonstrate a stone at the **ureteropelvic junction,** pelvic brim, or uterovesicular junction. Conservative management entails hydration and pain

Renin-angiotensin-aldosterone system–

↓ Osmolarity

↓

↑ Renin

↓

Cleavage of angiotensinogen → angiotensin I (AT-I)

↓

AT-I → AT-II (via ACE in lungs)

↓

↑ A ldosterone

TABLE 21-3. Renal Functions

Function	Description
Regulation of red blood cell (RBC) production	Erythropoietin → ↑ RBC production.
Regulation of vitamin D production	Vitamin D is converted to its **active form** (calcitriol; 1,25-dihydroxycholecalciferol) in the kidneys.
Excretion of waste and bioactive substances	Excretes drug metabolites, hormones, and breakdown products of protein (urea), creatine (creatinine), and hemoglobin.
Regulation of H_2O and electrolyte balance	Involved in reabsorption of substances including Na^+, K^+, glucose, and H_2O. H_2O regulation at the collecting ducts is regulated by **antidiuretic hormone (ADH; vasopressin).** Na^+ reabsorption is controlled by **aldosterone**.
Regulation of BP	Juxtaglomerular apparatus responds to renal blood flow **(pressure and osmolarity).** ↓ Perfusion pressure, osmolarity → renin release → ↑ aldosterone → Na^+ reabsorption.

A solid mass of the testicle is cancer until proven otherwise.

TABLE 21-4. Characterization of Nephrolithiasis

TYPE	ETIOLOGIES	DIAGNOSIS/MANAGEMENT
Calcium oxalate/phosphate	**Most common type**. Associated with 1° hyperparathyroidism, hypercalciuria, hyperuricosuria, dietary/enteric hyperoxaluria.	Radio-opaque. Treat with hydration.
Struvite ($MgNH_4PO_4$)	Caused by urease-producing bacteria (eg, ***Proteus mirabilis***).	Radio-opaque, **staghorn calculi**. Treat with hydration, antibiotics for UTI.
Cystine	Caused by defect in transport of cystine.	Radio-opaque. Treat with hydration, urine alkalinization.
Uric acid	Found with **high purine turnover** (Lesch-Nyhan), dehydration, high uric acid states (gout).	**Radiolucent**. Treat with hydration and **urine alkalinization**.

control (stones < 5 mm will usually pass spontaneously). Other options include extracorporeal shock wave lithotripsy for nonobstructing stone < 3 cm or **percutaneous nephrolithotomy** for larger stones.

RENAL CELL CARCINOMA

Comprises about 95% of renal neoplasms. Found most commonly in men during the sixth decade of life. Risk factors include tobacco use and family history of renal cancer or associated syndromes (ie, von Hippel-Lindau [vHL] disease). Typically presents with triad of **flank pain, palpable mass, and hematuria** (micro- or macroscopic). Also associated with **paraneoplastic syndromes** (eg, polycythemia, hypercalcemia, HTN, Cushing's syndrome) or signs of distant disease (eg, bone pain). Confirm diagnosis with renal ultrasound or abdominal CT, which demonstrate a solid, hypervascular mass. CXR and bone scan can help assess for metastatic disease. Must determine whether lesion is metastatic from a **distant 1° (eg, lung, breast, stomach, contralateral kidney).** Treatment includes a combination of modalities including **nephrectomy** (generally radical), chemotherapy, radiotherapy, immunotherapy, and hormonal therapy. Five-year survival for stage I disease is ~94%, but survival dramatically ↓ with stage IV disease (< 20%).

Staging of renal cell carcinoma–
Stage I: ≤ 7 cm, limited to kidney, – lymph nodes
Stage II: > 7 cm, limited to kidney, – lymph nodes
Stage III: Any sized tumor limited to kidney with 1 + regional lymph node or *any sized tumor that invades the major veins, adrenal gland, or perinephric tissue (not beyond Gerota's fascia) with or without 1 + regional lymph node*
Stage IV: Any tumor that invades beyond Gerota's fascia, > 1 + regional lymph node, or *+ distant metastases*

PROSTATE CANCER

Most common cancer of men; second leading cause of cancer death in men. Most commonly an **adenocarcinoma** that affects men during their eighth decade of life. Risk factors include ↑ **age**, family history of cancer, high dietary fat, and African American race. May present as an asymptomatic, incidentally discovered mass during digital rectal exam. If metastatic, might present with bone pain, lower-extremity edema, or urinary abnormalities. Prostate specific antigen (**PSA**) will be ↑. As PSA is also ↑ in prostatitis and benign prostatic hypertrophy (BPH), confirm diagnosis with **transrectal ultrasound-guided biopsy**. CXR and bone scan are necessary to rule out metastatic disease, which is typically **osteoblastic and radio-opaque**. Treatment options include watchful waiting, radical prostatectomy (with pelvic lymph node dissection), radiation (external beam or brachytherapy), androgen deprivation (eg, flutamide), or a combination of modalities. Antiandrogen therapy is recommended for metastatic disease. Complications of prostatectomy include **incontinence and impotence**. Five-year survival for stage I disease is nearly 100%; the rate ↓ to ~30% with stage IV disease.

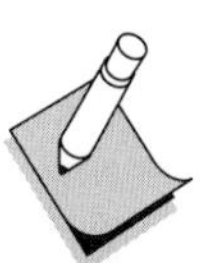

Staging for prostate cancer–
Stage I: Incidentally discovered tumors, – regional lymph nodes.
Stage II: Palpable disease confined to prostate, – regional lymph nodes.
Stage III: Disease extends beyond prostatic capsule with or without invasion into seminal vesicles, – regional lymph nodes.
Stage IV: Disease extends into adjacent structures (other than seminal vesicles), lymph nodes, or distant locations.

URINARY INCONTINENCE

Disorder affecting ~13 million patients in the United States, particularly women with ↑ age. Risk factors include childbirth, UTI, drug effect, BPH, birth defect, spinal cord abnormality or other nerve disorder (eg, neuropathy), bladder or pelvic floor weakness, and prolapse. Types include:

- **Stress: Involuntary incontinence** when intra-abdominal pressure exceeds that of the urethral sphincter (eg, coughing).
- **Urge: Detrusor muscle overactivity**. Associated with feeling the need void with the inability to prevent incontinence.
- **Overflow: Continuous inability to fully empty bladder**, resulting in continuous dribbling of urine. Associated with urethral obstruction (eg, BPH) or spinal cord abnormalities (eg, spina bifida, meningocele, multiple sclerosis, trauma).
- **Mixed type**: Combination of different types.

Diagnosis is clinical. Urodynamic studies may elucidate the type of incontinence. Conservative management can include Kegel exercises, timed voiding, lifestyle changes (eg, tobacco cessation, diuretic avoidance, antihistamines), and various medications (eg, anticholinergic [oxybutynin] for urge incontinence; α_1-antagonists [doxazosin], tamsulosin, or transurethral resection of prostate [TURP] for BPH-induced overflow incontinence). Stress incontinence may be amenable to pessary placement or retropubic urethropexy and suburethral sling procedures. Urge incontinence may be treated with bladder augmentation.

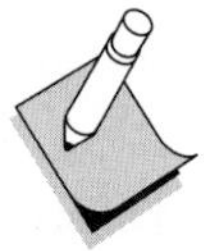

Staging for bladder cancer–
Stage I: Carcinoma in situ
Stage II: Invades the urothelium but does not extend to muscular layer
Stage III: Invades beyond muscle to fatty layer around bladder or invades the prostate, uterus, or vagina
Stage IV: Invades pelvic side wall, abdominal wall, + regional lymph nodes, or + metastatic disease

BLADDER CANCER

Usually **transitional cell carcinoma** affecting men in the seventh decade of life. Risk factors include **tobacco use**, ↑ age, chronic inflammation, or chemical exposure (eg, **aniline**, benzidine, polyaromatic hydrocarbons, cyclophosphamide, phenacetin). **Schistosomiasis** infection is associated with **SCC**. Most common symptoms include micro- or macro-scopic **hematuria** and bladder irritability. Confirm diagnosis with cystoscopy with biopsy; urine cytology may be +. Superficial tumors may be treated with **transurethral resection of bladder tumor** and intravesical chemotherapy (eg, doxorubicin, thiotepa, mitomycin C, **bacillus Calmette-Guérin vaccine**). For invasive but localized cancers, treat with **radical cystectomy** with urinary diversion or partial cystectomy with chemotherapy. Treat advanced bladder cancer with chemotherapy (eg, cisplatin-based regimen).

▶ NEUROSURGERY

Basic Science

ANATOMY OF THE CENTRAL NERVOUS SYSTEM

Brain is divided into right and left hemispheres. Key functional cortical areas are summarized in Figure 21-5.

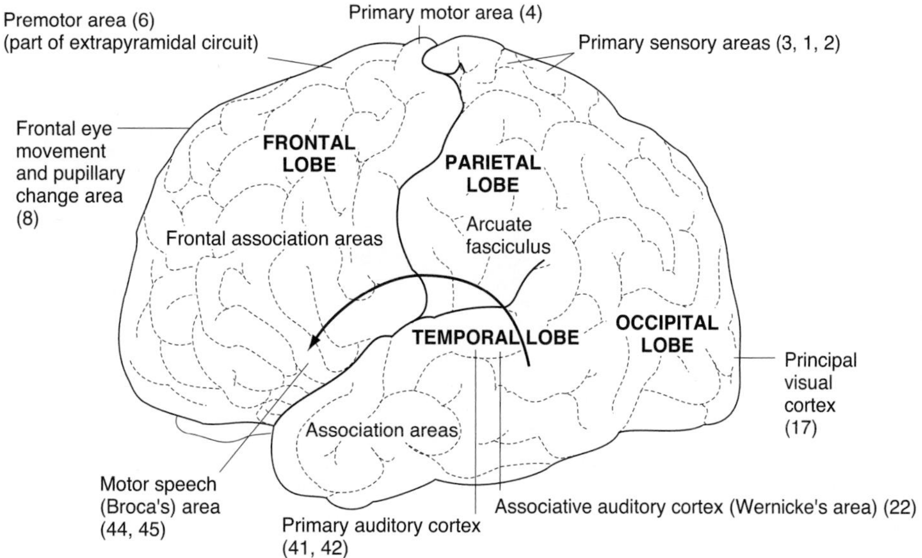

FIGURE 21-5. Cerebral cortex and its functions.

(Reproduced, with permission, from Le T, et al. *First Aid for the USMLE Step 2*, 4th ed. New York: McGraw-Hill, 2003:279.)

Blood supply from the brain derives from the internal carotid (ICA; supplies hemispheres) and the vertebral arteries (supplies hemispheres, cerebellum, brain stem). The ICA gives off the anterior and middle cerebral arteries; the vertebrals give off the basilar artery and ultimately, the posterior cerebral artery. The two sources anastomosies at the Circle of Willis. The **artery of Adamkiewicz**, found in the T10-L2 region, supplies the lower thoracic cord and conus medullaris.

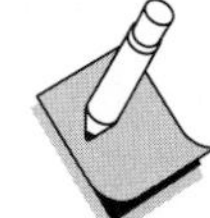

Prognosis for patients with bladder cancer is dependent on depth of invasion and presence of + lymph nodes and metastatic disease.

Spinal cord anatomy with relevant sensory pathways are depicted in Figure 21-6. Pathologies specific to these pathways include:

- **Brown-Sequard syndrome**: Unilateral hemisection. Ipsilateral loss of motor function, deep touch, vibration, and proprioception. Contralateral loss of light touch, temperature, and pain.
- **Central cord syndrome**: Caused by hyperextension injury or damage to central cord (eg, hemorrhage, infarct). Results in weakness of the upper extremities (relative to lower extremities) with variable sensory loss below the affected level.
- **Anterior cord syndrome**: Loss of blood supply to anterior spinal cord. Results in bilateral loss of motor function as well as pain and temperature sensation. Proprioception, vibration, and deep touch sensation are intact.

Clinical Science

ARTERIOVENOUS MALFORMATIONS

Congenital vascular malformations. Most commonly acutely symptomatic at 20–40 years of age. Hallmark sign is **hemorrhage**. Additionally, may present with sudden **headache** of intense proportion (1° symptom of subarachnoid hemorrhage). May also be associated with loss of consciousness, seizures, neck stiffness (meningismus), and focal neurologic defects. A **noncontrast brain CT** will confirm hemorrhage; cerebral angiogram defines vascular anatomy in preparation for surgical intervention. Initial treatment includes control of

Cerebral hemorrhage is discussed in Chapter 18.

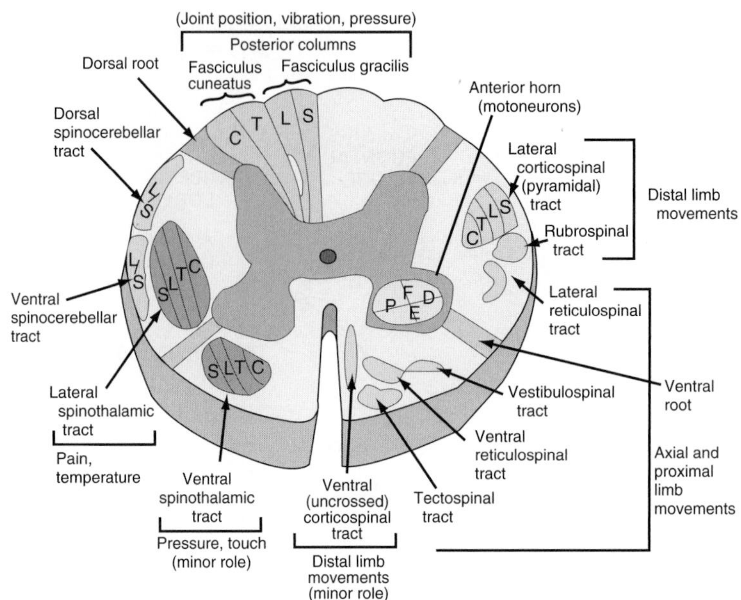

FIGURE 21-6. Spinal cord anatomy with pertinent sensory pathways.

(Reproduced, with permission, from Kasper DL, et al. *Harrison's Principles of Internal Medicine*, 16th ed. New York: McGraw-Hill, 2005:2440.)

HTN, seizure prophylaxis, and Ca^{2+} channel blockers to **prevent vasospasm**. Surgical therapy includes **embolization** or **radiosurgery**.

BRAIN TUMORS

Tumor types are summarized in Table 21-5. CT and MRI are usually diagnostic for all lesions.

▶ ORTHOPAEDIC SURGERY

Basic Science

ANATOMY OF THE PERIPHERAL NERVOUS SYSTEM

Upper extremity innervation is provided by way of the brachial plexus (see Figure 21-7). At the level of the hand, sensation is provided by the median, radial, and ulnar nerves (see Figure 21-8).

Hand musculature with respective innervation and functions are summarized in Table 21-6.

PHYSIOLOGY OF THE MUSCULOSKELETAL SYSTEM

Bone is composed of collagen (primarily **type I**), H_2O, and hydroxyapatite crystals. According to Wolff's Law, bone is laid along lines of stress. Can be characterized by both its microscopic and macroscopic structures:

- **Macroscopic**: Trabecular, cancellous (ie, spongy architecture, much less dense than cortical) versus cortical (ie, contains osteons with Haversian canals).
- **Microscopic**: Woven (randomly distributed collagen; abundant in newborns) versus lamellar (mature bone with organized collagen matrix).

TABLE 21-5. Brain Tumors

Tumor	Description	Management
Astrocytoma	Presents similarly to glioblastoma multiforme (GBM) but over longer time period. **Low-grade → young age. High-grade → older age.**	Resection, if possible (usually for cerebellar lesions). Radiation, chemotherapy. Most eventually degenerate to GBM.
GBM (astrocytoma grade 4)	**~25% of 1° brain tumors.** Hemorrhage, ↑ intracranial pressure (ICP), focal neurologic deficits.	Resection, if possible. Radiation, chemotherapy, and dexamethasone to control edema. **Poor prognosis. Average survival = 11 months.**
Oligodendroglioma	**Slow-growing** tumor of young/middle aged patients. More common in children. Affects cerebral hemispheres. Presents with long history of **seizures. + Calcifications.**	Resection. Chemoradiation for malignancy.
Meningioma	Arise from the meninges. ~20% of brain tumors. **Middle-aged women**. Presents with **unilateral, painless proptosis, anosmia**. **+ Calcifications**.	Resection. Prognosis excellent if fully resectable, otherwise recurrence is the norm.
Ependymoma	**Most commonly involves fourth ventricle/central canal. Childhood → posterior fossa; adult → supratentorial.** Presents with ↑ ICP, childhood hydrocephalus.	Resection +/– radiation.
Medulloblastoma (primitive neuroectodermal tumor; PNET)	Most commonly affects **children**, fourth ventricle. Presents with ↑ ICP, **cerebellar dysfunction.** Can involve cerebrospinal fluid (CSF).	Resection, radiation, chemotherapy.
Acoustic neuroma	Schwannoma of **CN VIII**. Associated with **neurofibromatosis**. Presents with **unilateral hearing loss, tinnitus, vertigo**, facial numbness, hydrocephalus.	Resection.
Pituitary adenoma	Lesion of pituitary **stalk/optic chiasm**. Presents with amenorrhea, **galactorrhea, acromegaly,** visual disturbances (loss of peripheral vision).	**Trans-sphenoidal resection, bromocriptine.**

(Adapted, with permission, from McPhee SJ, et al. *Current Medical Diagnosis & Treatment* 2008, 47th ed. New York: McGraw-Hill, 2008:861.)

Major cell types include **osteoblasts** (create bone) and **osteoclasts** (resorb bone). Balance between bone formation and resorption is governed by the interactions between Ca^{2+}, vitamin D, and parathyroid hormone (see Chapter 12). Bone formation occurs via intramembranous (bone deposited by mesenchyme) or endochondral (cartilaginous framework is replaced by bone) ossification. Bone healing occurs via induction and hematoma formation, inflammation, soft callus formation, hard callus formation, and bone remodeling.

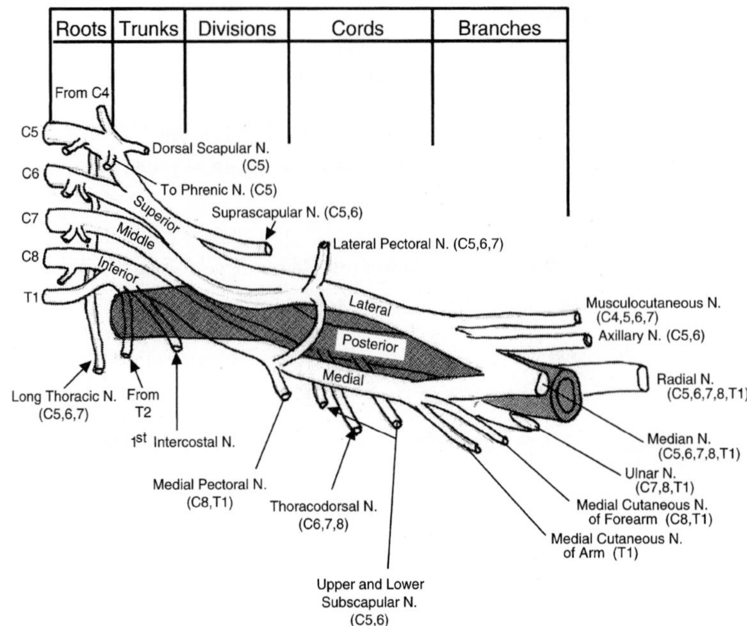

FIGURE 21-7. Anatomy of the brachial plexus.

(Reproduced, with permission, from Brunicardi FC, et al. *Schwartz's Principles of Surgery*, 8th ed. New York: McGraw-Hill, 2005:1725.)

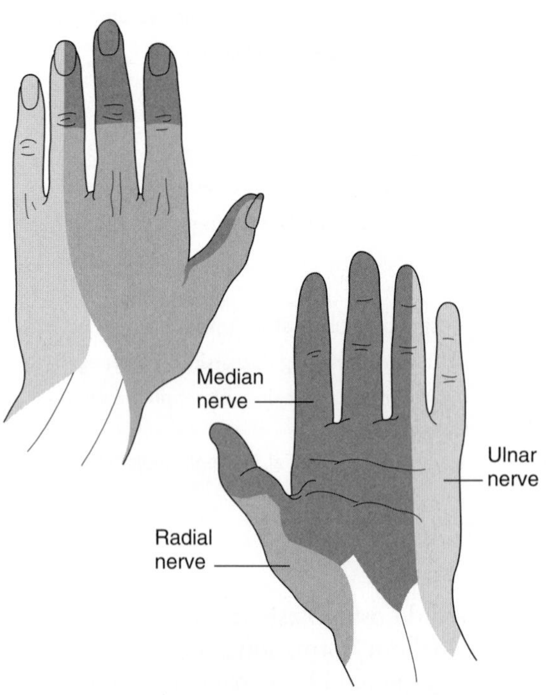

FIGURE 21-8. Sensory distribution of the hand.

(Reproduced, with permission, from Doherty GM, Way LW. *Current Surgical Diagnosis and Treatment*, 12th ed. New York: McGraw-Hill, 2006:1253.)

TABLE 21-6. Muscles of the Hand

MUSCLE	NERVE	FUNCTION
Adductor pollicis	Ulnar	Adducts thumb toward middle digit.
Abductor pollicis brevis	Median	Abducts thumb.
Flexor pollicis brevis	Median, ulnar	Flexes thumb.
Opponens pollicis	Median	Opposes thumb.
Adductor digiti minimi	Ulnar	Abducts little finger.
Flexor digiti minimi brevis	Ulnar	Flexes proximal phalanx of little finger.
Opponens digiti minimi	Ulnar	Opposes little finger.
Lumbricals	Median (2 radial lumbricals), ulnar (2 ulnar lumbricals)	Flexes proximal phalanx, extends interphalangeal (IP) joint.
Dorsal interossei	Ulnar	Adducts digits, extends IP joint (with lumbricals), flexes metacarpophalangeal (MCP) joint.
Palmar interossei	Ulnar	Moves index, ring, little fingers toward middle finger.

Clinical Science

PATHOLOGIC CONDITIONS OF THE PERIPHERAL NERVOUS SYSTEM

Pathologies associated with the peripheral nervous system are summarized in Table 21-7. Majority of neuropathies improve without surgical intervention. Surgery is reserved for those with progressive worsening of deficits or pain.

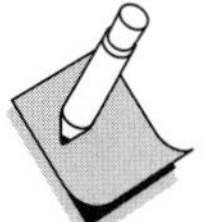

L5-S1 and L4-L5 *–Most common site for lumbar disc herniation.*

COMMON ORTHOPAEDIC INJURIES

Refer to Table 18-14.

COMMON ORTHOPAEDIC NEOPLASMS

Refer to Table 13-4.

TABLE 21-7. Pathologic Conditions of the Peripheral Nervous System

Nerve(s)	Signs/Symptoms
Upper Extremity	
C5 root	**Shoulder weakness,** supraspinatus/deltoid weakness.
C6 root	Weakness of bicep strength, ↓ thumb/index finger sensation and **biceps reflex**.
C7 root	Weakness of triceps strength, middle finger sensation, **triceps reflex**.
C5-C6 trunk	**Erb's palsy** = waiter tip position (shoulder adducted, internally rotated elbow extended with wrist flexed).
C8-T1 trunk	**Klumpke's palsy** = claw hand (affects intrinsic hand muscles).
Long thoracic nerve (C5-C7)	**Winged scapula** = serratus anterior weakness because of long thoracic nerve injury or trapeziurs weakness. CN XI injury will cause an even more severe winging of the scapula.
Axillary nerve (C5-C6)	**Weakness of deltoid** (weak arm abduction); ↓ sensation of lateral upper arm.
Median nerve (C5-T1)	**Weakness of thenar muscles**, wrist flexion, pronation; ↓ sensation of radial aspect of palm, radial $3^1/_2$ fingers.
Musculocutaneous nerve (C5-C7)	**Weakness in elbow flexion and supination**; ↓ sensation of lateral forearm.
Radial nerve (C5-T1)	**Saturday night palsy** = wrist drop (inability to extend wrist and fingers and thumb at MCP joint); ↓ sensation of dorsum of hand, posterolateral forearm.
Ulnar nerve (C8-T1)	**Weakness in thumb adduction**, MCP joint abduction/adduction, **clawing** of the ring and little fingers (eg, MCP extension, PIP/DIP flexion); ↓ sensation in little and ulnar half of ring fingers as well as medial palm.
Lower Extremity	
L4 root	Weakness of **patellar reflex**, knee/foot dorsiflexion; ↓ sensation to medial leg.
L5 root	Weakness of **great toe and other toes, ankle dorsiflexion**; ↓ sensation to top the first webspace.
S1 root	Weakness of **Achilles reflex**, ankle plantar flexion; ↓ sensation to lateral foot/heel.

▶ SAMPLE QUESTIONS

What are the nerves of the anterior triangle?	Glossopharyngeal, vagus, hypoglossal, nerve to mylohyoid.
A FNA of a neck mass in a 62-year-old male is for malignant cells. What is the next step in management?	Open biopsy, direct laryngoscopy, esophagoscopy, bronchoscopy.
What are the most common benign salivary tumors?	#1: Pleomorphic adenomas. #2: Warthin's tumors.
A patient with leukoplakia is at risk for what type of cancer?	SCC.
What is the treatment for a patient with early stage laryngeal cancer?	T1-2 glottic and supraglottic lesions respond to radiation. T3-4 lesions require neoadjuvant chemoradiation and surgery (partial or total laryngectomy), if possible. Perform a MRND for + lymph nodes.
What is the management for a patient with trismus, odynophagia, dysphagia, muffled voice, and uvular deviation?	Likely diagnosis is peritonsillar abscess. Treat with needle drainage. Perform incision and drainage if pus not evacuated.
A 40-year-old woman presents with a history of severe pelvic pain, dyspareunia, and tenesmus. Exam reveals a pelvic mass and tender nodularity of the uterosacral ligament. What is the likely diagnosis? Treatment?	Endometriosis. Pain control (NSAIDs), OCPs, danazol, GnRH agonists. Reserve surgery to restore fertility and normal anatomy.
What is the treatment for a patient who presents with flank pain, palpable mass, and hematuria?	After confirmation of renal cell carcinoma, treatment includes nephrectomy, chemotherapy, radiotherapy, immunotherapy, and hormonal therapy.
The most common site for lumbar disc herniation?	L5-S1 or L4-L5.
A 35-year-old male presents with the inability to extend his wrist after his girlfriend fell asleep on his arm (Saturday night palsy). What is the most likely nerve injured?	Radial nerve.
A 24-year-old female in a motor vehicle collision (MVC) has a flexed, adducted, internally rotated leg. What is the	Posterior hip dislocation or femoral neck fracture.

diagnosis?	
A 26-year-old male sustains a supracondylar fracture of his left arm. The arm feels tense, and exam reveals pain with passive movement and paresthesias. What is the next best step in the management?	The likely diagnosis is Volkmann's contracture. Treat with fasciotomy. May also need exploration of brachial artery.

INDEX

D

E

H

I

J

K

L

M

N

O

P

R

T

U

V

THE RESIDENT-TO-RESIDENT INSIDER'S GUIDE TO ABSITE SUCCESS

- Complete coverage of all the must-know basic science AND clinical surgery topics in one study package
- Up-to-date coverage reflects the reorganized ABSITE
- High-yield information, illustrations, mnemonics, and clinical images great for initial review or last-minute cramming
- From authors who know exactly what it takes to pass the ABSITE with flying colors

A RESIDENT-TO-RESIDENT GUIDE

LOOK FOR THESE OTHER GREAT SURGERY REVIEWS FROM McGRAW-HILL:

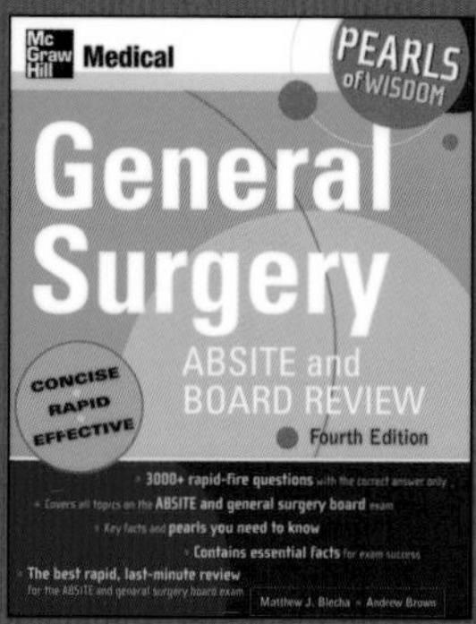

BLECHA:
General Surgery ABSITE and Board Review, 3e
ISBN: 978-0-07-146431-4

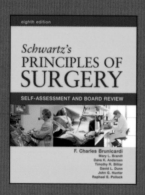

BRUNICARDI:
Schwartz's Principles of Surgery: Self-Assessment and Board Review, 8e
ISBN: 978-0-07-144687-7

ABOUT THE AUTHORS:

Jennifer LaFemina, MD, graduated from UCLA School of Medicine in 2003 and is a surgical resident at Massachusetts General Hospital.

Robert Todd Lancaster, MD, MPH, graduated from Emory University School of Medicine in 2003 and is a surgical resident at Massachusetts General Hospital.

Tao Le (Series Editor), MD, MHS, is Assistant Clinical Professor of Pediatrics in the Division of Allergy and Immunology at the University of Louisville. He is also the author of *First Aid for the USMLE Step 1* and many other *First Aid* series books.

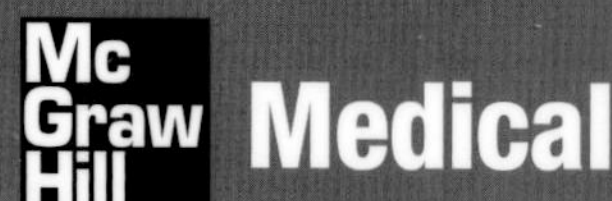

mcgraw-hillmedical.com

ISBN 978-0-07-154547-1
MHID 0-07-154547-6